THE BIOLOGY
OF NICOTINE
DEPENDENCE

The Ciba Foundation is an international scientific and educational charity. It was established in 1947 by the Swiss chemical and pharmaceutical company of CIBA Limited—now CIBA-GEIGY Limited. The Foundation operates independently in London under English trust law.

The Ciba Foundation exists to promote international cooperation in biological, medical and chemical research. It organizes about eight international multidisciplinary symposia each year on topics that seem ready for discussion by a small group of research workers. The papers and discussions are published in the Ciba Foundation symposium series. The Foundation also holds many shorter meetings (not published), organized by the Foundation itself or by outside scientific organizations. The staff always welcome suggestions for future meetings.

The Foundation's house at 41 Portland Place, London W1N 4BN, provides facilities for meetings of all kinds. Its Media Resource Service supplies information to journalists on all scientific and technological topics. The library, open five days a week to any graduate in science or medicine, also provides information on scientific meetings throughout the world and answers general enquiries on biomedical and chemical subjects. Scientists from any part of the world may stay in the house during working visits to London.

Ciba Foundation Symposium 152

THE BIOLOGY OF NICOTINE DEPENDENCE

A Wiley-Interscience Publication

1990

JOHN WILEY & SONS

Chichester · New York · Brisbane · Toronto · Singapore

©Ciba Foundation 1990

Published in 1990 by John Wiley & Sons L[
Baffins Lane, Chichester
West Sussex PO19 1UD, England

Other Wiley Editorial Offices

John Wiley & Sons, Inc., 605 Third Avenue,
New York, NY 10158-0012, USA

Jacaranda Wiley Ltd, G.P.O. Box 859, Brisbane,
Queensland 4001, Australia

John Wiley & Sons (Canada) Ltd, 22 Worcester Road,
Rexdale, Ontario M9W 1L1, Canada

John Wiley & Sons (SEA) Pte Ltd, 37 Jalan Pemimpin 05-04,
Block B, Union Industrial Building, Singapore 2057

Suggested series entry for library catalogues:
Ciba Foundation Symposia

Ciba Foundation Symposium 152
264 pages, 41 figures, 19 tables

Library of Congress Cataloging-in-Publication Data
The Biology of nicotine dependence.
     p. cm.—(Ciba Foundation symposium; 152)
    Editors: Greg Bock and Joan Marsh.
    Proceedings of a symposium held at the Ciba Foundation, London,
7–9 November 1989.
    'A Wiley–Interscience publication.'
    Includes bibliographical references.
    ISBN 0 471 92688 4
    1. Nicotine—Physiological effect—Congresses. 2. Nicotinic
receptors—Congresses. 3. Tobacco habit—Physiological aspects—
Congresses. I. Bock, Gregory.   II. Marsh, Joan.   III. Series.
    [DNLM: 1. Nicotine—pharmacology—congresses. 2. Substance
Dependence—congresses.   W3 C161F v. 152/QV 137 B615 1989]
QP801.N48B56   1990
616.865—dc20
DNLM/DLC
for Library of Congress   90-12213
                                            CIP

British Library Cataloguing in Publication Data
The biology of nicotine dependence.
   1. Man. Effects of nicotine
   I. Bock, Greg   II. Marsh, Joan, *1960–*   III. Series
   615.78
   ISBN 0 471 92688 4

Phototypeset by Dobbie Typesetting Limited, Devon.
Printed and bound in Great Britain by Biddles Ltd., Guildford.

Contents

Participants

M. Awad Department of Pharmacology, Faculty of Medicine, Technion—Israel Institute of Technology, POB 9697, Haifa 31096, Israel

D. J. K. Balfour Department of Pharmacology & Clinical Pharmacology, University of Dundee Medical School, Ninewells Hospital, Dundee DD1 9SY, UK

N. L. Benowitz Division of Clinical Pharmacology & Experimental Therapeutics, Building 30, 5th Floor, San Francisco General Hospital Medical Center, 1001 Potero Avenue, San Francisco, California 94110, USA

J.-P. Changeux Unit of Molecular Neurobiology, Department of Biotechnology, Institut Pasteur, 28 rue de Dr Roux, F-75724 Paris, cedex 15, France

P. B. S. Clarke Department of Pharmacology & Therapeutics, McGill University, Suite 1325, McIntyre Medical Sciences Building, 3655 Drummond Street, Montreal, Quebec, Canada H3G 1Y6

A. C. Collins Institute for Behavioral Genetics, University of Colorado, Campus Box 447, Boulder, Colorado 80309-0447, USA

D. Colquhoun Department of Pharmacology, University College London, Gower Street, London WC1E 6BT, UK

K. Fuxe Department of Histology, Karolinska Institute, Box 60400, S-104 01 Stockholm 60, Sweden

J. A. Gray Department of Psychology, Institute of Psychiatry, De Crespigny Park, Denmark Hill, London SE5 8AF, UK

N. E. Grunberg Department of Medical Psychology, Uniformed Services University of the Health Sciences, 4301 Jones Bridge Road, Bethesda, Maryland 20814-4799, USA

S. Heinemann   Molecular Neurobiology Laboratory, The Salk Institute, PO Box 85800, San Diego, California 92138-9216, USA

J. E. Henningfield   NIDA Addiction Research Center, PO Box 5180, Baltimore, Maryland 21224, USA

H. Howald   K-125.12.20, CIBA-GEIGY Ltd, CH-4002 Basle, Switzerland

L. L. Iversen   Neuroscience Research Centre, Merck, Sharp & Dohme Research Laboratories, Terlings Park, Eastwick Road, Harlow, Essex CM20 2QR, UK

K. J. Kellar   Department of Pharmacology, Georgetown University Medical Center, 3900 Reservoir Road, Washington DC 20007, USA

J. Lindstrom   Receptor Biology Laboratory, The Salk Institute for Biological Studies, PO Box 85800, San Diego, California 92138-9216, USA

P. Lippiello   RJ Reynolds Tobacco Co, Winston-Salem, North Carolina 27102, USA

E. D. London   Neuropharmacology Laboratory, NIDA Addiction Research Center, POB 5180, Baltimore, Maryland 21224, USA

G. G. Lunt   Biochemistry Department, University of Bath, Claverton Down, Bath BA2 7AY, UK

O. F. Pomerleau   Department of Psychiatry, Behavioral Medical Program, University of Michigan, Riverview Building, 900 Wall Street, Ann Arbor, Michigan 48105, USA

J. E. Rose   Nicotine Research Laboratory, VA Medical Center—Research (151), 508 Fulton Street, Durham, North Carolina 27705, USA

M. A. H. Russell   Health Behaviour Unit, Institute of Psychiatry, De Crespigny Park, 101 Denmark Hill, London SE5 8AF, UK

R. D. Schwartz   Department of Pharmacology, Box 3813, Duke University Medical Center, Durham, North Carolina 27710, USA

J. H. Steinbach   Department of Anesthesiology, Washington University School of Medicine, 660 South Euclid Avenue, St Louis, Missouri 63110, USA

I. P. Stolerman   Department of Psychiatry, Institute of Psychiatry, De Crespigny Park, 101 Denmark Hill, London SE5 8AF, UK

T. H. Svensson   Department of Pharmacology, Karolinska Institute, Box 60400, S-104 01 Stockholm, Sweden

R. J. West   Department of Psychology, Royal Holloway & Bedford New College, Egham Hill, Egham, Surrey TW20 0EX, UK

S. Wonnacott   Biochemistry Department, University of Bath, Claverton Down, Bath BA2 7AY, UK

Introduction

Leslie Iversen

Neuroscience Research Centre, Merck, Sharp & Dohme Research Laboratories, Terlings Park, Eastwick Road, Harlow, Essex CM20 2QR, UK

The title of this symposium does not include the word 'addiction'. Scientists in general avoid the word because of the confusion between its popular and scientific meanings. The term 'drug dependence' is more precise.

Drug dependence includes several different components. Usually, but not always, continued administration of drugs of dependence leads to tolerance, i.e. larger doses are needed to elicit the same effect after chronic usage. Physical dependence is also a common but not invariable attribute of drugs of dependence; physical dependence means that one can elicit a withdrawal syndrome by removing the drug. In animal models, a more dramatic withdrawal syndrome can sometimes be precipitated by the administration of an antagonist drug that acts at the same receptor as the drug of dependence. In the case of opiates, for example, there is a much better understanding of the withdrawal syndrome in animal models since the advent of opiate antagonists such as naloxone and naltrexone. In some cases it may be quite hard to see a consistent withdrawal syndrome in animals unless an antagonist is used. It is only in the last few years that reliable animal models have been available to study physical dependence and withdrawal after chronic treatment with benzodiazepene tranquilizers. The advent of such drugs as flumazenil (Ro 15-1788) as benzodiazapine receptor antagonists proved to be very valuable in such studies. One of the research tools we would like to have in studying each example of drug dependence is antagonist drugs to probe the level of physical dependence that may develop. A third facet of drug dependence is a very important one in leading to compulsive drug abuse, namely the phenomenon of psychic craving—hard to define scientifically and virtually impossible to understand in terms of brain mechanisms.

This trio of factors describes the overall phenomenon of drug dependence quite well. Some drugs may show only two of the three; some drugs may show predominantly one feature and not the other two. Cannabis users, for example, demonstrate psychic craving and abuse, but there is little evidence for physical dependence or tolerance. Smokers develop some degree of tolerance and a clear psychic craving for nicotine.

When we discuss the neurobiology of nicotine dependence, many of the features are more generally applicable to the large group of psychoactive compounds that have been used and abused throughout the whole of human history. It is important to realize that physical dependence, tolerance and psychic craving can occur to differing degrees. The most intense for all all three is probably elicited by opiate drugs. But milder levels of dependence develop in habitual users of benzodiazepine tranquilizers, nicotine and caffeine and they may find it very difficult to wean themselves off the habit.

One issue which will be important in our discussions is how to help people who are dependent on a drug to wean themselves off that drug. We don't really know how to do that very effectively. There have been a number of attempts, particularly in the opiate field, with rather limited success. An important pharmacological concept is that one agonist compound in a group of related drugs can substitute quite readily for the primary drug. That sometimes proves advantageous, for example in the substitution of methadone for heroin, where replacement by a weaker agonist with different pharmokinetics, that does not give the same peak concentration in blood, can help the addict to recover from drug dependency.

One of the most fascinating aspects of this field is how little we understand the neural mechanisms that underlie the development of drug dependence. Dependence does not arise overnight, it is a slow process, an adaptive plastic change in the nervous system that may take days, weeks or months to develop to its full extent. In the case of morphine and related opiates in experimental animals, the development of physical dependency depends on ongoing protein synthesis. Nevertheless, despite the great upsurge of interest and activity in the area of opiate research during the last 10–15 years, there has been no break-through in understanding the mechanisms underlying opiate dependence.

One of the challenges to neurobiology in the next decade is to try to understand the processes in the brain which underlie the behavioural changes in the organism during the development of drug dependence. That is a fundamentally important challenge, because until we have such an understanding of the basic neuro-biology, we will not be in a position to plan any rational therapy.

Behavioural pharmacology of nicotine: implications for multiple brain nicotinic receptors

I. P. Stolerman

Department of Psychiatry, Institute of Psychiatry, De Crespigny Park, 101 Denmark Hill, London SE5 8AF, UK

Abstract. Behavioural studies can contribute to the characterization of receptors for psychoactive drugs, and attempts have been made to link behavioural effects of nicotinic agonists with the high affinity binding site for [³H]nicotine. Cueing (discriminative stimulus) effects of drugs enable trained humans or animals to recognize when a specific drug is administered. There was a correlation between the potencies of some compounds in the binding procedure and their ability to produce the nicotine discriminative stimulus in rats, supporting the view that the high affinity binding site was a functional receptor. Nicotine also produced complex changes in locomotor activity of rats, characterized acutely by transient depression and chronically by persistent stimulation. The abilities of nicotinic compounds to produce these locomotor effects were not always consistent with the studies on binding and the nicotine discriminative stimulus. Some compounds were relatively more potent in producing locomotor depression or stimulation than the discriminative effect. Some compounds also failed to produce chronic locomotor activation at doses that produced discriminative and acute depressant effects. These findings may be interpreted as preliminary evidence that different behavioural effects of nicotine may be mediated through different mechanisms, possibly involving multiple subtypes of nicotinic receptors.

1990 The biology of nicotine dependence. Wiley, Chichester (Ciba Foundation Symposium 152) p 3–22

Nicotine has a very wide range of behavioural effects. Some of these effects are potentially useful, notably improvements in cognitive functions such as aspects of learning and memory, whereas others generate massive problems, such as the positive reinforcing effect that is a basis for addiction. Understanding the receptor mechanisms upon which nicotine acts in the brain to produce behavioural changes may aid attempts to utilize the former and to minimize the latter type of effect. This paper describes some recent attempts to use nicotinic agonists to correlate behavioural effects with the high affinity binding site for [³H]nicotine. It focuses on the controversial question of multiple nicotinic receptors and outlines a behavioural approach to this question. With rare exceptions, such as Collins et al (1986), behavioural studies with nicotine have not been interpreted in terms of multiple nicotinic receptors.

The behavioural effects of nicotine include changes in the rates of conditioned and unconditioned behaviours, a variety of stimulus properties, and possible influences on cognitive functions. These effects are listed in Table 1, together with notes on their practical significance (reviews by Clarke 1987, Stolerman 1987). The changes in rates of behaviour show a complex pattern, including both decreases and increases in rate depending on (1) the dose and time after administration of nicotine, (2) the amount of previous exposure to nicotine, and (3) the schedule of reinforcement that may be used to maintain the behavioural baseline. Nicotine can also decrease food consumption, particularly of sweet substances of high calorific value, and there is evidence for rebound increases in intake during withdrawal. The stimulus properties of nicotine include

TABLE 1   Summary of major behavioural effects of nicotine

Effect of nicotine	*Notes*
Increases in rates of conditioned behaviour such as working for reward or to avoid aversive stimuli	Less marked than effects of amphetamine
Decreases in rates of conditioned behaviour	Subject to tolerance
Increases in rates of unconditioned behaviour, notably locomotor activity	Increase with repeated exposure to nicotine
Decreases in rates of unconditioned behaviour such as locomotor activity, eating and drinking	Rapid persistent tolerance. Probably a motor deficit rather than a sedative/hypnotic effect
Serves as positive reinforcer in self-administration and, controversially, in place preference procedures	Believed to be a main factor in addiction
Serves as discriminative stimulus (cue)	May contribute to addiction by enabling experienced organisms to identify nicotine
Serves as aversive stimulus in negative reinforcement, punishment, place and taste avoidance conditioning	May oppose or weaken addictive tendency
Improves speed and accuracy of maze learning, memory consolidation, and accuracy in tasks requiring sustained attention	May contribute to addiction by increasing positive reinforcing efficacy
Nausea and vomiting	Partly peripheral origin

This information was taken from reviews by Clarke (1987) and Stolerman (1987).

the ability (1) to maintain self-administration behaviour by serving as a positive reinforcer (reward), (2) to generate distinctive discriminative stimuli that can be used by trained organisms to identify the drug, and (3) to produce aversive effects that may encourage organisms to lessen their exposure to the drug. Nicotine also seems to improve the performance of certain tasks involving learning in ways that cannot be explained by changes in rates of behaviour. These improvements may involve changes in arousal or selective attention, and facilitation of associative processes such as the consolidation of recently acquired information from short-term to longer-term storage.

There is very little evidence that different types of nicotinic receptors mediate these diverse effects. The ganglion-blocking drug mecamylamine seems to block virtually all effects upon which it has been tested, although Collins et al (1986) have reported that unusually small doses of mecamylamine blocked the effect of nicotine on startle responses. Molecular approaches to the question of nicotinic receptor heterogeneity are presented elsewhere in this volume (see paper by Lindstrom et al) and they will not be summarized here.

The first series of experiments used drug discrimination procedures to provide a behavioural assay for sensitivity of the central nervous system (CNS) to nicotine. The discriminative stimulus effect of a drug relates to an ability of the individual to recognize its pharmacological actions in the body, and it may therefore play a significant role in the addiction process. This technique was selected also because of its sensitivity and pharmacological specificity. It was possible for rats to develop a discrimination based upon subcutaneous doses of nicotine as low as 0.1 mg/kg and the resulting dose–response curves typically showed ED_{50} values around 0.04 mg/kg (Stolerman et al 1984). This ED_{50} was associated with plasma nicotine concentrations around 15 ng/ml, which were typical for human cigarette smokers who inhaled. Using rats trained to discriminate nicotine from saline, comparative dose–response studies were carried out with several nicotinic agonists and with many non-nicotinic drugs. The ability of the same series of agonists to inhibit the binding of [^{3}H] nicotine to rat brain membranes in $vitro$ was also determined.

The second, more recent, series of experiments has employed changes in locomotor activity of rats to obtain comparable data for the same series of nicotinic agonists. These behavioural procedures were chosen because there was evidence for possible differences in the relevant CNS mechanisms, and because locomotor activity was readily quantifiable and sensitive to nicotine. Two sets of data were obtained, one for an acute locomotor depressant effect in non-tolerant rats, and one for increases in locomotion in rats chronically exposed to nicotine. The relationship of these effects to addiction is uncertain, although Stolerman et al (1973) have suggested that the acute locomotor depressant effect of nicotine may be a model for the initial aversive effects of the drug in novice smokers. Tolerance develops rapidly to both the locomotor depression in rats and the initial aversive effects in humans.

Experiments on the nicotine discriminative stimulus

Methods

Rats were trained to press bars to obtain food rewards; two bars were present in the test apparatus and it was the presence or absence of nicotine that told the rat which bar to press to obtain food. Thus, an animal could solve the task by identifying whether or not it had received nicotine. For some animals, it was the left bar that always produced food when it was drugged and the right bar that produced food in the absence of drug. After exposure to such conditions, imposed in random order in daily training sessions, the rats started pressing the left bar every time they received nicotine and, in contrast, they started pressing the right bar every time they received saline. In each experiment, the drug–bar pairings were counterbalanced. The rats were trained to identify a 0.1 mg/kg dose of nicotine administered subcutaneously 15 minutes before 15-minute training sessions, and all data were obtained from rats that detected this small dose of nicotine with an accuracy of at least 80%.

Trained rats were used in experiments where responses to different doses of nicotine, and to different agonists and antagonists, were assessed in twice-weekly test sessions. Tests took place in random order, with training continued on intervening days to maintain the baseline of discrimination performance. No food was given during tests to ensure that only the drugs, and not any other cues, determined which bar was pressed. Rosecrans and his colleagues carried out many of the difficult early experiments pioneering the application of this methodology to nicotine (Rosecrans & Chance 1977). Full descriptions of the present procedure have been published (Pratt et al 1983, Stolerman et al 1984).

Results and discussion

A typical dose–response curve for $(-)$nicotine is shown in Fig. 1 (upper left section). The working range of doses under the conditions used rose from a threshold a little above 0.01 mg/kg to 0.1 mg/kg. The ED_{50} value, defined as the dose of drug that produced 50% of the responses on the nicotine-appropriate bar, varied over an approximately twofold range between different groups of rats. Several nicotinic agonists were tested in rats trained in this way. Typically, these compounds increased the percentage of drug-appropriate responses in a dose-related manner, to about the same maximum value as nicotine itself (Fig. 1). Such results were obtained with $(+)$nicotine, $(-)$anabasine, cytisine, $(-)$- and $(+)$nornicotine, N-(3-pyridylmethyl)-pyrrolidine (PMP) and isoarecolone (Stolerman et al 1984, Goldberg et al 1989, Reavill et al 1987, C. Reavill, I. P. Stolerman and J. A. Waters, unpublished data). These results confirmed and extended reports from other laboratories (Chance et al 1978, Romano et al 1981), and were broadly similar to recent findings in squirrel monkeys (Takada et al 1989).

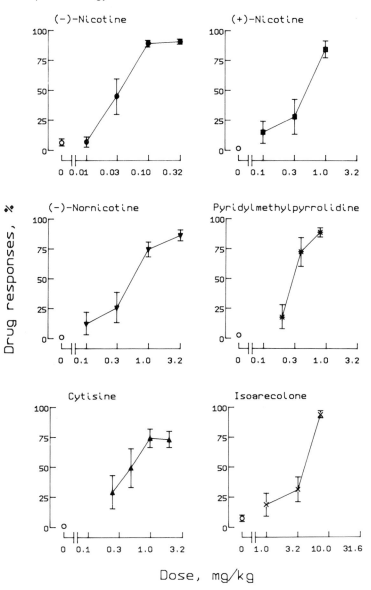

FIG. 1. Dose–response curves for nicotine and related compounds in rats trained to discriminate (−)nicotine (0.1 mg/kg s.c.) from saline. Ordinates, responses on the drug-appropriate bar expressed as a percentage of total responses. Vertical bars in this and subsequent figures represent ± SEM; bars smaller than diameters of symbols are omitted. $n = 8$. All data were obtained in five minute extinction tests. It can be seen that all of the compounds produced nicotine-like discriminative stimulus effects.

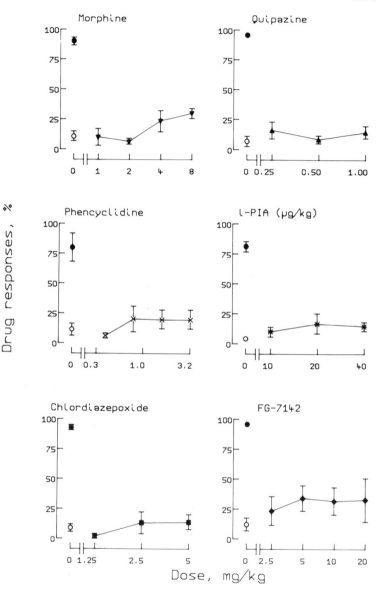

FIG. 2. Dose–response curves for some non-nicotinic compounds in rats trained to discriminate (−)nicotine (0.1 mg/kg s.c.) from saline. Ordinates, responses on the drug-appropriate bar as a percentage of total. Compounds were selected to represent particular pharmacological classes, such as chlordiazepoxide for the benzodiazepines and FG-7142 for the benzodiazepine inverse agonists. None of the compounds produced nicotine-like discriminative stimulus effects. l-PIA, l-phenylisopropyladenosine. $n = 6$–8.

Thus, nicotinic agonists that potently inhibited the binding of [^{3}H]nicotine *in vitro* produced nicotine-like discriminative stimulus effects. These drugs typically increased drug-appropriate responses to 80–90% of total responses. Furthermore, the potency of the agonists as inhibitors of binding was correlated (r = 0.87) with their potency in producing the discriminative effect (Reavill et al 1988, Goldberg et al 1989). These results were interpreted as evidence for mediation of the nicotine cue through the high affinity binding site for [^{3}H]nicotine.

The results with nicotinic agonists were compared with those for non-nicotinic compounds from a wide range of pharmacological classes; only if such drugs failed to produce the nicotine cue could the procedure be considered as specific for nicotinic activity. Considerable numbers of compounds were tested and they rarely increased the rate of drug-appropriate responses above 20–30%. Fig. 2 shows results for some representative non-nicotinic compounds. Similar negative results were obtained with muscarinic agonists, with muscarinic and nicotinic antagonists, and with agonists and antagonists acting at receptors for adenosine, adrenaline, dopamine, opioids and serotonin (review by Stolerman 1987, and unpublished data). The only exception to the negative outcome was with certain agents that shared activity as dopaminergic agonists, which supported other evidence that there was a dopaminergic component in the nicotine cue (Reavill & Stolerman 1987). These results generally suggested that the nicotine cue had a very high degree of pharmacological specificity.

The dose of nicotine used for training influenced characteristics of the nicotine cue (Stolerman et al 1984) in a way that was reminiscent of findings with drugs acting on multiple opioid receptors. Discriminative stimulus methods were therefore used to seek evidence for multiple nicotine receptors, but the results were largely negative. For example, studies of locomotor activity in rats had shown that nicotine has biphasic effects; behavioural depression 5–20 minutes after subcutaneous injections is followed by behavioural facilitation for about 60 minutes. Rats were therefore trained to discriminate nicotine from saline using three different pre-session intervals (5, 20 and 35 minutes before 10-minute training sessions). Then, cross-tests were carried out to determine whether rats trained to recognize nicotine at one pre-session interval also recognized it when tested at other intervals (Stolerman & Garcha 1989). Fig. 3 shows that recognition was complete at all combinations of pre-session intervals. Thus, nicotine produced qualitatively similar discriminative effects at all pre-session intervals used. The pre-session interval influenced the quantitative characteristics of the nicotine cues markedly, but these effects on ED$_{50}$ values were predictable from the interaction of pharmacokinetic factors with known characteristics of drug-produced cues; there was no evidence for multiple nicotinic receptors.

Cytisine was much less potent in the behavioural experiments than was expected from the binding data, which was explained by reference to evidence that it penetrated poorly into the brain (Romano et al 1981). However, in recent

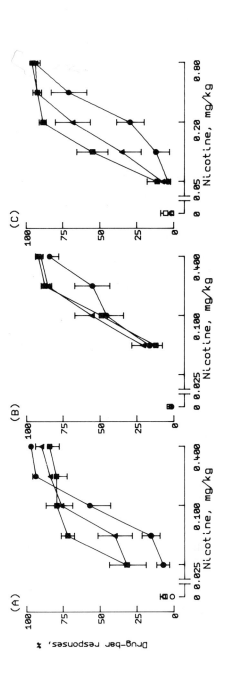

FIG. 3.   Dose–response curves for nicotine in three groups of rats trained to discriminate nicotine (0.4 mg/kg s.c.) from saline with pre-session intervals of five minutes (○, $n = 12$), 20 minutes (▲, $n = 12$) and 35 minutes (■, $n = 8$). Each section of the figure shows results from the three groups of rats when the pre-session intervals during testing were held constant at five minutes (A), 20 minutes (B) and 35 minutes (C). Results after administering saline are also shown (○, △, □). Ordinates, responses on the drug-appropriate bar as a percentage of total. (From Stolerman & Garcha 1989, with permission from Oxford University Press.)

studies carried out in collaboration with Dr B. Testa and Dr B. Walther (University of Lausanne), plasma and brain concentrations of drugs were determined in rats of the same sex, strain and age as those used in behavioural work. For doses of cytisine and nicotine that were approximately equally effective in producing the nicotine cue, the brain concentrations of cytisine were at least three times larger than those of nicotine (Table 2). Since cytisine was several times more potent than (−)nicotine in ligand-binding studies (Reavill et al 1988), its low potency in the discrimination procedure was not explained by poor penetration into the brain. Furthermore, lobeline failed to produce nicotinic agonist or antagonist effects in discrimination experiments (Romano et al 1981, C. Reavill & I. P. Stolerman, unpublished results), but it was a potent inhibitor of nicotine binding *in vitro*. The lack of behavioural effect was not attributable to pharmacokinetic factors because measurements of plasma and brain concentrations of lobeline in Dr Testa's laboratory showed that it penetrated readily into the brain (Table 2). Thus, although the high affinity binding site for [^{3}H]nicotine seems to contribute to the nicotine cue, other mechanisms need to be involved to explain the findings with cytisine and lobeline. Sloan et al (1988) have also maintained that these drugs act through different mechanisms.

Experiments with nicotine on locomotor activity

Methods

Interruptions of parallel beams of infra-red light at opposite ends of activity cages were recorded. Interruptions of either beam that followed interruptions of the other beam were recorded as 'cage crosses' (modified from Clarke & Kumar 1983). To assess the locomotor depressant effect of acutely administered nicotine, rats were placed in activity cages immediately after injection and activity was recorded for the period 5–20 minutes after injection. Each rat was used to test only a single dose of a drug, to prevent tolerance influencing the results. To assess the locomotor stimulant effect of nicotine, rats received daily injections of nicotine (0.4 mg/kg s.c.) and were placed in activity cages for one hour daily.

TABLE 2 Pharmacokinetic measurements of drug concentrations in the plasma and brain of treated rats

Drug s.c.	Dose mg/kg	Plasma ng/ml	Brain ng/ml
Nicotine	0.1	62 ± 5	41 ± 6
Cytisine	1.0	516 ± 27	145 ± 43
Lobeline	4.0	74 + 8	237 + 42

The concentrations of each drug were determined by HPLC 15 minutes after subcutaneous injections at the doses shown (means ± SD, $n = 4$).

This procedure was continued for at least two weeks, to produce tolerance to locomotor depressant effects of nicotine. Then, in rats in which nicotine increased cage crosses by at least 20%, tests of drugs on locomotor activity took place twice weekly. Different doses of drugs were tested in random order, and activity was recorded for 60 minutes beginning immediately after injections. On intervening days the rats continued to receive injections of nicotine.

Results and discussion

Nicotine reliably decreased locomotor activity when administered acutely; Fig. 4 (upper left section) shows results from a typical experiment. All nicotinic agonists tested also reduced locomotor activity in a dose-related manner, and potency

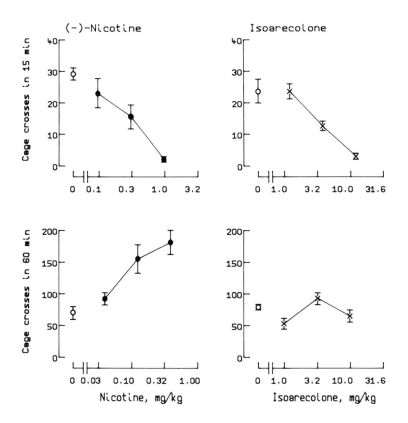

FIG. 4.   Dose–response curves for nicotine and isoarecolone in non-tolerant rats (upper sections) and nicotine-tolerant rats (lower sections). Ordinates, numbers of movements from one side of the activity cage to another. Nicotine and isoarecolone reduced locomotion in non-tolerant rats (H. S. Garcha, C. Reavill, I. P. Stolerman, unpublished data). *n* = 6.

was estimated by a DD_{50} value, defined as the dose of drug decreasing the number of cage crosses to 50% of control values. Table 3 shows that the DD_{50} for the locomotor depressant effect of nicotine was much larger than the ED_{50} for the nicotine cue. Table 3 also shows DD_{50} values for different nicotinic agonists relative to the DD_{50} for nicotine. Whereas the relative doses of PMP were similar in the discriminative and locomotor depression procedures, smaller doses of several other agents were sufficient to decrease locomotor activity. On this basis, cytisine was twice as potent, and isoarecolone was ten times as potent, in locomotor depression as in discrimination. Fig. 4 (upper right section) shows the results for isoarecolone.

Nicotine reliably increased locomotor activity when administered chronically; Fig. 4 (lower left section) shows results from a typical experiment. Some of the other nicotinic agonists tested also increased locomotor activity in a dose-related manner under these conditions, and potency was estimated by a SD_{50} value, defined as the dose of drug stimulating the number of cage crosses to 50% above control values. Table 3 shows that the SD_{50} for (−)nicotine was slightly larger than the ED_{50} for the nicotine cue. By comparing the SD_{50} values for the

TABLE 3   **Concentration of (−)nicotine needed to inhibit nicotine binding _in vitro_ and doses needed to produce three different behavioural effects after subcutaneous injection**

Compound	Binding IC_{50}[a]	Cue CD_{50}[b]	Locomotor activity	
			DD_{50}[c]	SD_{50}[d]
(−)Nicotine (absolute)	9.7 nM	0.04 mg/kg	0.44 mg/kg	0.15 mg/kg
(−)Nicotine (relative)	1.0	1.0	1.0	1.0
Cytisine	0.12	10.6	5.2	—
Lobeline	4.7	—	N.T.	N.T.
Pyridylmethylpyrrolidine	5.3	7.1	7.1	2.1
(+)Nornicotine	12.1	9.7	3.8	2.0
(+)Nicotine	12.9	12.0	4.2	15
(−)Nornicotine	17.4	15.0	N.T.	N.T.
Isoarecolone	46.9	98.0	9.7	—
Anabasine	51.4	57.5	N.T.	N.T.

The table shows the concentrations or doses of various nicotinic agonists that are effective in the different procedures, relative to (−)nicotine which is given a value of 1.0 in each case. A dash indicates that a drug failed to produce the behavioural effect at any dose tested; N.T. indicates drugs not tested in certain procedures.

[a]IC_{50}: Concentration of drug needed to inhibit binding of $[^3H]$(−)nicotine to rat brain membranes by 50% _in vitro_. (IC, inhibitory concentration.)

[b]CD_{50}: Dose of drug needed to increase drug-appropriate responses to 50% in rats trained to discriminate nicotine (0.1 mg/kg) from saline. (CD, cue dose.)

[c]DD_{50}: Dose of drug needed to decrease locomotor activity to 50% of control levels in non-tolerant rats. (DD, depressant dose.)

[d]SD_{50}: Dose of drug needed to stimulate activity to 50% above control levels in rats made tolerant to the locomotor depressant effect of nicotine. (SD, stimulant dose.)

different drugs relative to nicotine (Table 3), it can be seen that the effective doses of (+)nicotine were similar in the discriminative and locomotor stimulation procedures, but differed markedly for other drugs. On the one hand, (+)nornicotine and PMP were relatively more potent as locomotor stimulants; on the other hand, cytisine (up to 2 mg/kg) and isoarecolone (up to 10 mg/kg) lacked stimulant activity entirely. Doses of cytisine and isoarecolone that produced the nicotine cue and the locomotor depressant effect failed to increase locomotor activity. Fig. 4 (lower right section) illustrates the findings with isoarecolone. These experiments are still in progress, hence the incomplete data for certain drugs in Table 3, but the results indicate clearly that the locomotor effects of nicotinic agonists are not correlated with their discriminative stimulus effects, and it is therefore becoming increasingly difficult to interpret the findings in terms of a single nicotinic mechanism.

Conclusions

The major issue is whether the wide range of behavioural effects of nicotine can be explained by action at a single type of receptor. In the drug discrimination procedure, the effects of several nicotine analogues were correlated with their effects at a single, high affinity binding site for [^{3}H]nicotine. This suggests that the binding site may play a key role in the generation of the nicotine stimulus. However, the nicotinic agonist cytisine produced the nicotine cue only at very large doses compared with those expected from binding data, even when pharmacokinetic factors were taken into consideration. This could indicate that a component of the nicotine cue is produced by an action of cytisine at another receptor. The results with both lobeline and cytisine are compatible with an assumption that an effect at the high affinity binding site is necessary, but not sufficient, to produce the nicotine cue. It is therefore possible that an additional nicotinic site is significant for behavioural effects. One strategy for the future will be the use of compounds other than nicotine for training discriminations; this has only recently appeared to be worthwhile, in the light of our rapidly growing knowledge of behavioural effects of different nicotinic agonists.

The results on the locomotor depressant effect of nicotinic compounds in non-tolerant rats were not fully predictable from those obtained with the nicotine cue. Several nicotinic agonists were relatively potent in this procedure, as compared with the cue. Small differences in potency are difficult to interpret, but the tenfold difference in potency of isoarecolone is especially notable. This difference could be explained by an action of isoarecolone at a different receptor; it will require experiments with antagonists to establish whether this is indeed a nicotinic site. Unlike the nicotine cue that is highly specific for nicotine-like activity, locomotor depression can be produced by actions of drugs through a wide range of non-nicotinic mechanisms.

The studies of increases in locomotor activity in tolerant rats reveal further evidence for multiple mechanisms. The potency of the nicotinic compounds in this procedure bore only a weak relationship to their potency in the drug discrimination and locomotor depression procedures. In particular, cytisine and isoarecolone failed to increase locomotor activity at doses that produced nicotine-like discriminative effects and that reduced locomotor activity. In contrast, PMP and (+)nornicotine were relatively potent as stimulants of locomotor activity, compared with their potency in the ligand-binding and discriminative stimulus procedures. These differences could be explained in terms of different subtypes of nicotinic receptor (Sloan et al 1988). There are alternative explanations; for example, different degrees of cross-tolerance may have developed to the different drugs in the studies on locomotor stimulation (where the rats were first made tolerant to the locomotor depressant action of nicotine). Different degrees of cross-tolerance to agonists imply differences in mechanisms, but not necessarily at the level of receptors.

The present results show the feasibility of a behavioural approach to the further characterization of nicotinic receptors. The behavioural effects of nicotine are fairly well defined (Table 1) and it is clear that different nicotinic agonists have different behavioural profiles, although more extensive studies are needed to support interpretations in terms of multiple nicotinic receptors. The immediate path for developing this approach is clear; only partial data are available for just three of the nine behavioural effects (Table 1), and studies with antagonists are essential. However, in the longer term, success will depend upon the availability of a wider range of nicotinic agonists, including some with more selective effects, and upon studies linking the behavioural findings to the results of molecular, neurophysiological and biochemical experiments.

Acknowledgements

I thank the Medical Research Council for financial support, and many present and former colleagues, especially R Kumar, JA Pratt, C Reavill and HS Garcha, for their important contributions to the work summarized here.

References

Chance WT, Kallman MD, Rosecrans JA, Spencer RM 1978 A comparison of nicotine and structurally related compounds as discriminative stimuli. Br J Pharmacol 63:609–616

Clarke PBS 1987 Nicotine and smoking: a perspective from animal studies. Psychopharmacology 92:135–143

Clarke PBS, Kumar R 1983 The effects of nicotine on locomotor activity in non-tolerant and tolerant rats. Br J Pharmacol 78:329–337

Collins AC, Evans CB, Miner LL, Marks MJ 1986 Mecamylamine blockade of nicotine responses: evidence for two brain nicotinic receptors. Pharmacol Biochem Behav 24:1767–1773

Goldberg SR, Risner ME, Stolerman IP, Reavill C, Garcha HS 1989 Nicotine and some related compounds: effects on schedule-controlled behaviour and discriminative properties in rats. Psychopharmacology 97:295–302

Lindstrom J, Schoepfer R, Conroy WG, Whiting P 1990 Structural and functional heterogeneity of nicotinic receptors. In: The biology of nicotine dependence. Wiley, Chichester (Ciba Found Symp 152) p 23–52

Pratt JA, Stolerman IP, Garcha HS, Giardini V, Feyerabend C 1983 Discriminative stimulus properties of nicotine: further evidence for mediation at a cholinergic receptor. Psychopharmacology 81:54–60

Reavill C, Stolerman IP 1987 Interaction of nicotine with dopaminergic mechanisms assessed through drug discrimination and rotational behaviour in rats. J Psychopharmacol 1:264–273

Reavill C, Spivak CE, Stolerman IP, Waters JA 1987 Isoarecolone can inhibit nicotine binding and produce nicotine-like discriminative stimulus effects in rats. Neuropharmacology 26:789–792

Reavill C, Jenner P, Kumar R, Stolerman IP 1988 High-affinity binding of $[^3H](-)$-nicotine to rat brain membranes and its inhibition by analogues of nicotine. Neuropharmacology 27:235–241

Romano C, Goldstein A, Jewell NP 1981 Characterization of the receptor mediating the nicotine discriminative stimulus. Psychopharmacology 74:310–315

Rosecrans JA, Chance WT 1977 Cholinergic and non-cholinergic aspects of the discriminative stimulus properties of nicotine. In: Lal H (ed) Discriminative stimulus properties of drugs. Plenum, New York, p 155–185

Sloan JW, Martin WR, Bostwick M, Hook R, Wala E 1988 The comparative binding characteristics of nicotinic ligands and their pharmacology. Pharmacol Biochem Behav 30:255–267

Stolerman IP 1987 Psychopharmacology of nicotine: stimulus effects and receptor mechanisms. In: Iversen LL et al (eds) Handbook of psychopharmacology. Plenum, New York, vol 19:421–465

Stolerman IP, Garcha HS 1989 Temporal factors in drug discrimination: experiments with nicotine. J Psychopharmacol 3:88–97

Stolerman IP, Fink R, Jarvik ME 1973 Acute and chronic tolerance to nicotine measured by activity in rats. Psychopharmacologia 30:329–342

Stolerman IP, Garcha HS, Pratt JA, Kumar R 1984 Role of training dose in discrimination of nicotine and related compounds by rats. Psychopharmacology 84:413–419

Takada K, Swedberg MDB, Goldberg SR, Katz JL 1989 Discriminative stimulus effects of intravenous *l*-nicotine and nicotine analogs or metabolites in squirrel monkeys. Psychopharmacology 99:208–212

DISCUSSION

Grunberg: It is important to be careful with semantics and nomenclature. You used the terms acute and chronic, but your 'chronic administration' is actually a repetitive acute versus another type of chronic, which is a continuous administration. You are using the behavioural assay to understand the underlying neurobiological mechanisms. When we move into a model of dependence, we are dealing with a different kind of self-administration. Dr Benowitz will talk in more detail about the human smoker and what kind of levels are maintained in the body. In our hands, using acute administration repetitively versus continuous administration by an osmotic minipump, we get different effects on physical activity as well as on other stimuli. I know you are aware of this, but I think it offers another important tool. We can get a lot of information by comparing different paradigms.

Gray: One also has to take into account the possibility of adaptation in systems other than the nicotinic receptors one is looking at, or desensitization in neurophysiological terms. For example, with acute administration of nicotine we've seen increased synthesis of both dopamine in the nucleus accumbens and noradrenaline in the hippocampus. If we repeat the injections over similar periods to the injection regimes used in Ian Stolerman's experiments, we see an increase in the hippocampal response but no change in the accumbens response (Mitchell et al 1989). So one might see different effects later because of the different systems that then get involved.

Stolerman: The points made are all very pertinent, although I think it is reasonable to refer to a regimen of daily nicotine injections over several months as 'chronic'. When comparing an acute with a chronic model, one doesn't know whether it's the different response itself or the acute versus the chronic effect that is of greatest importance. We chose this approach initially because one can see much clearer stimulant effects of nicotine in that way on locomotor activity. We found it more difficult to get clear dose-related increases in activity acutely. The hippocampal effect is probably not a key factor here, because microinjections of nicotine into the dorsal hippocampal area don't produce the motor activity increase in the chronic situation, whereas the mesolimbic dopamine system is implicated (Reavill & Stolerman 1990).

Grunberg: Concerning the brain levels of nicotine and the other drugs, you didn't specify brain loci.

Stolerman: Those are concentrations in whole brain.

Grunberg: The dynamic distribution of these drugs within the brain is important.

Stolerman: I agree, but in some cases we are talking about a difference of nearly 100:1 between the behaviour and the binding. I don't think one is likely to get a 100-fold difference in the concentrations of a drug in different brain areas.

Awad: Dr Stolerman, it is possible that in very low concentrations cytisine produces an increase in locomotor activity.

Stolerman: Yes, it may be that we haven't looked at a wide enough range of concentrations. These results were obtained only recently, but we did include some quite small doses, down to 0.1 mg/kg.

Clarke: I am a little confused with the cytisine locomotor data: we, and you more thoroughly, have shown that if you inject cytisine into certain areas of brain, you do get locomotor activity.

Stolerman: Yes, it is possible to get locomotion; we have shown that by injecting cytisine into the ventral tegmental area it is possible to produce an increase in activity rather like that produced by nicotine (Reavill & Stolerman 1990). This is an unresolved puzzle, and contrasts with the observations made after systemic injections.

Clarke: Is anything known about the metabolism of these nicotinic compounds, cytisine and isoarecolone, and whether any metabolites could be active at nicotinic receptors?

Stolerman: I don't know of any studies on their metabolism. Anabasine, cytisine and lobeline, in our hands, have not been active as antagonists of nicotine.

Balfour: You suggested that the cue is probably mediated in part by the effect of nicotine on dopamine secretion. Most of us would think that the locomotor stimulant action is also mediated by dopamine, but you appear to be indicating that the two responses may be mediated by different systems. Can you comment on that?

Stolerman: Dopamine clearly does play a role in the locomotor activation as well as in the cue. Dr Clarke has shown that lesions of the mesolimbic dopamine system with 6-hydroxydopamine attenuate the locomotor activating effect of nicotine. Nicotine is more potent in releasing dopamine from the mesolimbic system than from the nigrostriatal system. Injections of nicotine into certain areas of the mesolimbic dopamine system produce increases in locomotor activity. So several different lines point to the activity effect being mediated through dopamine. There is some evidence also for the discriminative effect being mediated by dopamine. The recognition site for nicotine may be slightly different but dopamine may be involved in both cases.

Heinemann: Since nicotine has an effect on muscle tone, could all these effects be due to an effect on the motor system? Is there a behavioural test that you can use to be sure that you are looking at an effect on the CNS?

Stolerman: We are fairly sure that these are CNS effects for several reasons. One is that the nicotine blocking drug, chlorisondamine, when injected into the cerebral ventricular system of a rat in doses of 2–5 µg, can block all three effects that I described. Those doses of cholorisondamine given systemically are well below doses that produce blocking effects (Clarke 1984, Kumar et al 1987).

Heinemann: Are you sure that these concentrations of drugs do not affect muscle tone?

Clarke: We have looked at muscle tone in spinal preparations and in anaesthetized rats. The doses Dr Stolerman is using don't affect muscle tone directly, although there is a spinal effect, probably on motoneurons, which probably underlies the depressant effect.

Stolerman: The locomotor depression almost certainly reflects a motor deficit and I do not interpret it as evidence for a sedative-hypnotic action of nicotine. A depressant effect can be obtained by injection of nicotine into the IVth ventricle. It is possibly mediated by adjacent structures such as the cerebellum

(Maiti et al 1986). The activating effect apparently comes from a quite different area of the brain, as discussed earlier. In the discrimination procedure, the motor stimulant and depressant effects of drugs have been completely dissociated from their ability to produce nicotine-like or nicotine-antagonist discriminative effects. Apart from this evidence, it must not be overlooked that discriminative effects are expressed in measures of response choice rather than of response rate. For several classes of drug, discriminative stimulus effects cannot be predicted from motor effects.

Henningfield: I should like to comment on locomotor activity as an assay to characterize drug action. It is a deceptively complex response—for example, amphetamine can increase locomotor activity at some doses, but can also reduce locomotor activity by increasing stereotypy.

Stolerman: Responses that seem simple to measure are actually behaviourally far more complex because there is a range of different behaviours which interact. In this particular case, the decreases in locomotor activity are not explained by stereotyped behaviour produced by nicotine, because such behaviour is not observed, whereas there is a fair indication of a motor deficit of central origin in these animals.

Benowitz: I would like to raise another issue related to pharmacokinetics; a factor that should be considered is the rapidity with which the drug gets into the brain. In humans, the faster the drug gets into the brain, the greater the effect (Porchet et al 1987). If the drug enters the brain slowly, there is time for tolerance or adaptation to develop and the response may be smaller. Drugs that are polar usually enter the brain at a slower rate than do non-polar drugs. Therefore, there could be a pharmacokinetic mechanism for differences in pharmacological response that would not be detected simply by measuring peak concentrations of the drugs in the brain.

Stolerman: That's an interesting possibility, that a drug which enters the brain more slowly may produce a different change at the receptor, a different degree of desensitization for example, that might contribute to the different effects. That needs to be addressed in the future.

Colquhoun: This point about desensitization is interesting. It is one of several reasons why I think it is rash to interpret results of this sort in terms of different receptor subtypes. Differences in response may depend as much, or more, on differences in the extent of desensitization, e.g. as a result of differences in the rate of access, as they do on differences in receptor subtype. There are certainly multiple types of receptor, but it seems unlikely that this sort of experiment will tell us how many. For the muscle nicotinic receptor, components of desensitization have been reported on a 50 msec time scale, a one second time scale and the slowest over a minute or more. All of these times are quite short compared with the time course that you are talking about. The degree of desensitization is usually very intense at equilibrium, with only about 1% of the response left.

Stolerman: I believe we have a strategy to look at behavioural correlates of multiple nicotinic receptors, but there are other interpretations that should be considered. I agree that desensitization is a key problem. We behavioural pharmacologists would like to know what concentrations of nicotine applied for what period of time will produce desensitization in mammalian neurons in the central nervous system. How does this vary with different populations of cells in different areas that might be related to different types of behaviour? How does it vary with different agonists? Neurophysiological studies on this issue would be very valuable.

Colquhoun: As far as I know this hasn't been studied quantitatively with ACh, never mind nicotine, in a central neuron.

Stolerman: When Martin and Gilbert first proposed multiple opiate receptors, primarily on the basis of *in vivo* data which included behavioural measures, there were many other possible interpretations. Now there is good behavioural evidence for subtypes of opioid, dopamine and serotonin receptors, and I expect the same to be true for nicotine in five to ten years.

Heinemann: We've looked at desensitization of some of the receptor subtypes expressed in *Xenopus* oocytes. It is an artificial system but the nicotinic receptor subtypes that we have studied show a slow desensitization that takes seconds in response to micromolar concentrations of nicotine.

Changeux: Using the patch clamp technique, Christopher Mulle in our laboratory has been able to show with isolated neurons from the medial habenula that the response to nicotine desensitizes over a time scale which is not far from that observed with *Xenopus* oocytes. There is an agreement with the results of Heinemann and his collaborators. In addition there is a slow regulation which is called 'wash out'. This is a slow decay of the receptor efficacy which occurs with a much longer time scale, 10 minutes or half an hour. It looks irreversible and we don't know whether it's an artifact.

Heinemann: We see the same thing in oocyte patches. When we go to a different patch on the same cell we recover receptor activity, so it's something happening in the patch.

Kellar: That irreversible desensitization or inactivation of receptor response has been seen in adrenal medullary PC12 cells in culture.

Changeux: It may be due to turnover.

Steinbach: We see a 'wash out' of channel activity in excised patches from PC12 cells or mammalian muscle cells. Channel activity decreases greatly between five and ten minutes after excision. We have only studied it in muscle receptors (Covarrubias & Steinbach 1990). Wash out does not seem to depend on the state of ligation of the receptor or on the degree of desensitization of the receptor. It doesn't depend strongly on temperature or membrane potential. Our guess is that it might result from dissociation of a cytoskeletal protein from the excised patch. I think 'wash out' is a separate phenomenon; it really seems to be different from both desensitization and inactivation.

Stolerman: Do these desensitizing effects occur in these systems at nanomolar concentrations, which is what we are talking about in the behavioural studies? If not, are they relevant to the problem of dependence?

Colquhoun: It's quite difficult to tell. The Feltz & Trautmann study (1982) on muscle was very interesting because they showed intense desensitization with far lower concentrations than people had previously supposed—concentrations which will give apparently quite a good plateau response if applied rather slowly to the preparations.

Steinbach: The concentration dependence would also depend on the muscle receptor. In the case of muscle nicotinic receptors, *Torpedo*-type receptors probably would desensitize at 10 nM because that is the K_d for desensitization, whereas in mammalian skeletal muscle receptors the K_d is 100 or 200 nM.

Schwartz: In binding assays we pick up the phenomenon of a K_d or binding characteristics at nM concentrations. People looking at the membrane and the lipid bilayer in relation to the receptor have calculated the actual concentration of drug molecules per area of lipid membrane at the interface with the receptor protein. If they then re-calculate the K_ds, these are in the μM range, sometimes a 1000-fold higher than the nM concentrations in conventional binding assays. That might be one way of explaining why we are looking at high affinity nM concentrations for characteristics of binding, yet μM concentrations when we look at physiological or biochemical responses.

Stolerman: But the ED_{50} for the nicotine discrimination is at a plasma concentration of 50–100 nM (Stolerman & Reavill 1989). This is not as low as required for the high affinity site but it's not in the μM range. It is a very low concentration that is achieved in the plasma of cigarette smokers who inhale.

Schwartz: But nicotine is probably very good at concentrating in the membrane. The concentration at the receptor site may be very different from the aqueous (extracellular) concentration.

Colquhoun: The conventional view is that in the receptor the agonist binding site is quite a long way from the membrane.

Schwartz: Leo Herbette has measured the distance, for the ACh receptor, from the binding site to the lipid bilayer polar head groups. Apparently it's not as great as one might think in terms of the ability of the drug to get to the site via the membrane rather than through the aqueous route.

Henningfield: Dr Stolerman has performed a valuable service for us. Dr Iversen opened our symposium with a discussion on drug dependence; this may include both tolerance and physical dependence, but the psychic processes are the most difficult and arguably one of the most important aspects to model. Dr Stolerman laid out several models that can be used to quantitate the mechanisms and correlates of so-called psychic drug action. The assays include drug self-administration and drug discrimination paradigms, as well as determining how the drug affects learned behaviour. These are the behavioural mechanisms by which effects at the neuronal level ultimately result in widespread morbidity and mortality, due either to the chemical itself or to toxic factors in the delivery system, as is the case with tobacco products.

Dr Stolerman has also described the importance of evaluating a wide range of drug doses. Humans are exquisitely sensitive to and in control of the dose level of nicotine. These observations emphasize the importance of carefully selecting and validating nicotine doses used in neuropharmacological preparations. These studies give us some means of judging what are those relevant doses.

References

Clarke PBS 1984 Chronic central nicotinic blockade after a single administration of the bisquarternary ganglion-blocking drug chlorisondamine. Br J Pharmacol 83:527–535

Covarrubias M, Steinbach JH 1990 Excision of membrane patches reduces the mean open time of nicotinic acetylcholine receptors. Pflugers Arch, in press

Feltz A, Trautmann A 1982 Desensitization at the frog neuromuscular junction: a biphasic process. J Physiol (Lond) 322:257–272

Kumar R, Reavill C, Stolerman IP 1987 Nicotine cue in rats: effects of central administration of ganglion-blocking drugs. Br J Pharmacol 90:239–246

Maiti A, Salles KS, Grassi S, Abood LG 1986 Barrel rotation and prostration by vasopressin and nicotine in the vestibular cerebellum. Pharmacol Biochem Behav 25:583–588

Mitchell SN, Brazell MP, Joseph MH, Alavijeh MS, Gray JA 1989 Regionally specific effects of acute and chronic nicotine administration on rates of catecholamine and 5-hydroxytryptamine synthesis in rat brain. Eur J Pharmacol 167:311–322

Porchet HC, Benowitz NL, Sheiner LB, Copeland JR 1987 Apparent tolerance to the acute effect of nicotine results in part from distribution kinetics. J Clin Invest 80:1466–1471

Reavill C, Stolerman IP 1990 Locomotor activity in rats after administration of nicotinic agonists intracerebrally. Br J Pharmacol 99:273–278

Stolerman IP, Reavill C 1989 Primary cholinergic and indirect dopaminergic mediation of behavioural effects of nicotine. Prog Brain Res 79:227–237

Structural and functional heterogeneity of nicotinic receptors

Jon Lindstrom, Ralf Schoepfer, William G. Conroy and Paul Whiting

The Salk Institute for Biological Studies, P.O. Box 85800, San Diego, CA 92138, USA

Abstract. Three gene families of the ligand-gated ion channel gene superfamily encode proteins which bind cholinergic ligands: (1) nicotinic acetylcholine receptors (AChRs) from skeletal muscle, (2) AChRs from neurons, and (3) neuronal α-bungarotoxin-binding proteins (αBgtBPs). AChRs from muscles and nerves function as ACh-gated cation channels, but αBgtBPs do not appear to function in this way. A family of neuronal AChR subtypes has been characterized using monoclonal antibodies and cDNA probes. Neuronal AChRs exhibit sequence homologies with muscle AChRs, but differ in subunit composition, pharmacological and electrophysiological properties, and, in some cases, apparent functional roles. The genes that encode the subunits of the various purified AChR subtypes have been determined in several cases. Histological localization of AChR subunit mRNAs by *in situ* hybridization and of subunit proteins by immunohistochemistry is being conducted with increasing resolution. The subunit structure of αBgtBP is uncertain, but cDNAs have been identified for two subunits. Sequences of these cDNAs reveal that αBgtBPs are members of the ligand-gated ion channel gene family, and suggest that they could function as gated cation channels. Biochemical and molecular genetic approaches to studies of neuronal AChRs and related proteins are merging to provide a detailed description of a complex family of AChRs widely dispersed throughout the nervous system, which are probably important to many activities of the nervous system, but whose functional roles are not yet well characterized.

1990 The biology of nicotine dependence. Wiley, Chichester (Ciba Foundation Symposium 152) p 23–52

Many of the critical membrane proteins which characterize neurons are encoded by genes that belong to one of three superfamilies. One of these is the ligand-gated ion channel gene superfamily. This includes three gene families encoding protein subunits which are the subjects of this review: (1) skeletal muscle nicotinic acetylcholine receptors (AChRs), (2) neuronal nicotinic AChRs, and (3) neuronal α-bungarotoxin-binding proteins (αBgtBPs). The ligand-gated ion channel gene superfamily includes not only these excitatory gated cation channels, but also such inhibitory gated anion channels as receptors for glycine and γ-aminobutyric acid, and, probably, other receptors such as those for excitatory amino acids (Lindstrom et al 1987, Barnard et al 1987). The potential-gated ion channel gene superfamily is distinct from the ligand-gated superfamily; it includes proteins such as the sodium channels responsible for action potential (Catterall 1988). All neurotransmitter receptors characterized at this time which are not ligand-gated ion channels are single subunit proteins which lack an intrinsic effector element and so must interact via GTP-binding proteins with effector enzymes that generate second messengers. Examples of receptors in the GTP-binding protein-coupled receptor gene superfamily include rhodopsin, muscarinic and adrenergic receptors (Peralta et al 1988). Ligand-gated ion channels such as nicotinic AChRs from muscles and nerves are suited for rapid signalling on the millisecond time scale and typically desensitize on prolonged exposure to agonists, whereas GTP-binding protein-coupled receptors are characterized by responses with longer latencies and longer durations.

Within each receptor gene family, cloning of subunit cDNAs has revealed multiple receptors present in various amounts in different tissues, developmental states and species. AChRs are formed from several homologous subunits of different types arranged together to form a multisubunit ion channel. AChR subtypes differ in the combination of subunits of which they are composed. Thus the nomenclature used to describe various AChR subtypes is a problem. This problem is more complicated because different rationales have been used for naming AChR subunits by various laboratories. In this paper types of AChR are referred to by the names of the genes that encode their subunits, where this is known. The nomenclature used for naming the subunits is explained subsequently. In the future, it may be possible to provide a rational nomenclature for all the subunits of the ligand-gated ion channel gene superfamily. The immediate problems are identifying: (1) what subunit genes exist, (2) what subunit protein combinations normally occur, and (3) what are the properties of these different receptors.

Molecular studies of nicotinic acetylcholine receptors

Studies in my laboratory of AChRs from muscles and electric organs led to the development of a large library of subunit-specific monoclonal antibodies (mAbs), some of which subsequently were found to identify homologous epitopes on neuronal AChRs and were then used to immunoaffinity purify these AChRs. Simultaneously, cDNAs for subunits of AchRs from electric organs and muscles were used by other laboratories to identify homologous cDNAs from neuronal cDNA libraries. Studies with mAbs and cDNAs proceeded in parallel. Libraries of mAbs to purified neuronal AChRs permitted purification and characterization of various neuronal AChR subtypes from different species, while cDNA probes based on the initial neuronal cDNAs isolated led to the identification of more neuronal cDNAs. There has now been a convergence and

cross-over of these approaches. This has led to the identification of the genes
which encode the component subunits of several different purified neuronal AChR
subtypes, and to the production of antibodies to bacterially expressed cDNA
fragments which are proving to be useful tools for biochemical studies. Over the
past few years these studies have resulted in an abundance of new information
about neuronal nicotinic AChRs, which will be briefly reviewed here. The limit on
references has necessitated compromises for which I apologize to interested readers.

A summary of the properties of purified neuronal AChR subtypes, the
subunits that compose them, and the genes that encode these subunits is given
in Fig. 1, with the muscle AChR subtypes for comparison. The following few
paragraphs explain this in more detail.

To understand neuronal nicotinic AChRs, it is important first to understand
some basic features of nicotinic AChRs from muscles and electric organs. AChRs
from *Torpedo* electric organs are composed of four kinds of subunits termed
α, β, γ and δ in order of increasing apparent molecular weight (Lindstrom
et al 1987). All of these subunits have similar, but distinct, amino acid sequences.
This same nomenclature has been applied to the subunits of AChRs from fetal
or denervated adult muscle, whereas synaptic AChRs from innervated adult
muscle are thought to differ by the substitution of ϵ subunits for the closely
related γ subunits of extrasynaptic AChRs of denervated muscle (Witzemann
et al 1987). It is not currently known whether this sort of developmental
alteration in subunit composition occurs in neuronal AChRs. In each electric
organ AChR there are two α subunits and one each of β, γ and δ subunits
arranged around a central cation channel like barrel staves, in the order $\alpha\beta\alpha\gamma\delta$
(Kubalek et al 1987). The α subunits are known to form the ACh binding sites,
because labelling of α subunits by MBTA [4-(N-maleimido)benzyltrimethyl-
ammonium] and αBgt is inhibited by ACh and cholinergic ligands. After
reduction of the disulphide bond which normally links the unique cysteine pair
α192,193 of α subunits, MBTA covalently reacts with these cysteines, showing
that they are near the ACh binding site (Kao et al 1984, Kao & Karlin 1986).
αBgt binds to short synthetic α subunit peptides which include this cysteine pair.
Another characteristic structural feature of muscle AChR α subunits is the main
immunogenic region. This conformation-dependent epitope includes amino acid
residues within the sequence α66-76 (Tzartos et al 1988, Das & Lindstrom 1989).
The function of this region is unknown.

The sequences of muscle AChR α subunits, which contain the ACh binding
site, are highly conserved through evolution (Fig. 2), more so than the sequences
of the other subunits which contribute to the structure of the AChR channel.
Nonetheless, it is evident that the structures of all the subunits that form the
muscle AChR gene family are highly conserved, and that the basic structure
of muscle nicotinic AChRs had developed more than 400 million years ago,
by the time marine elasmobranchs evolved, and has varied little since. This
contrasts sharply with neuronal nicotinic AChRs, whose subunits seem to have

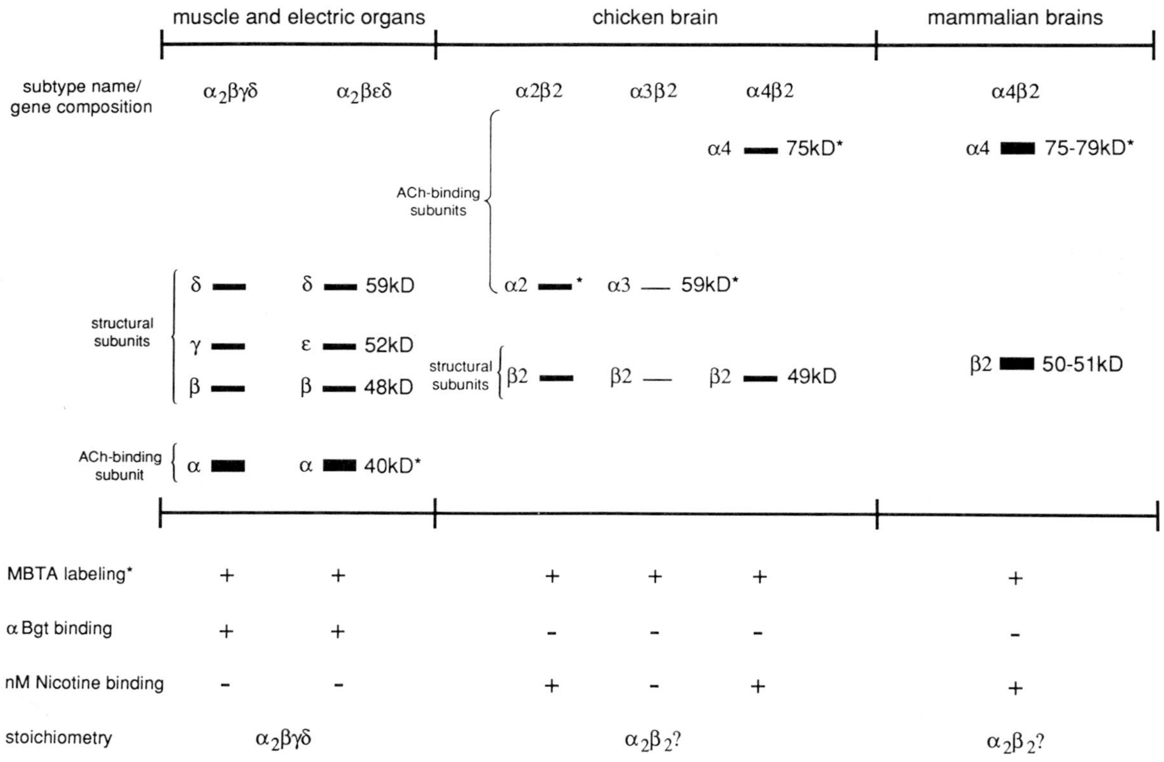

FIG. 1. Comparison of nicotinic AChR subtypes from muscles and brain. The thickness of the bars in the upper part of the figure represents the relative abundance of each subunit. *, subunits that can be specifically labelled with MBTA [4-(N-maleimido)benzyltrimethylammonium] and thereby identified as ACh-binding subunits.

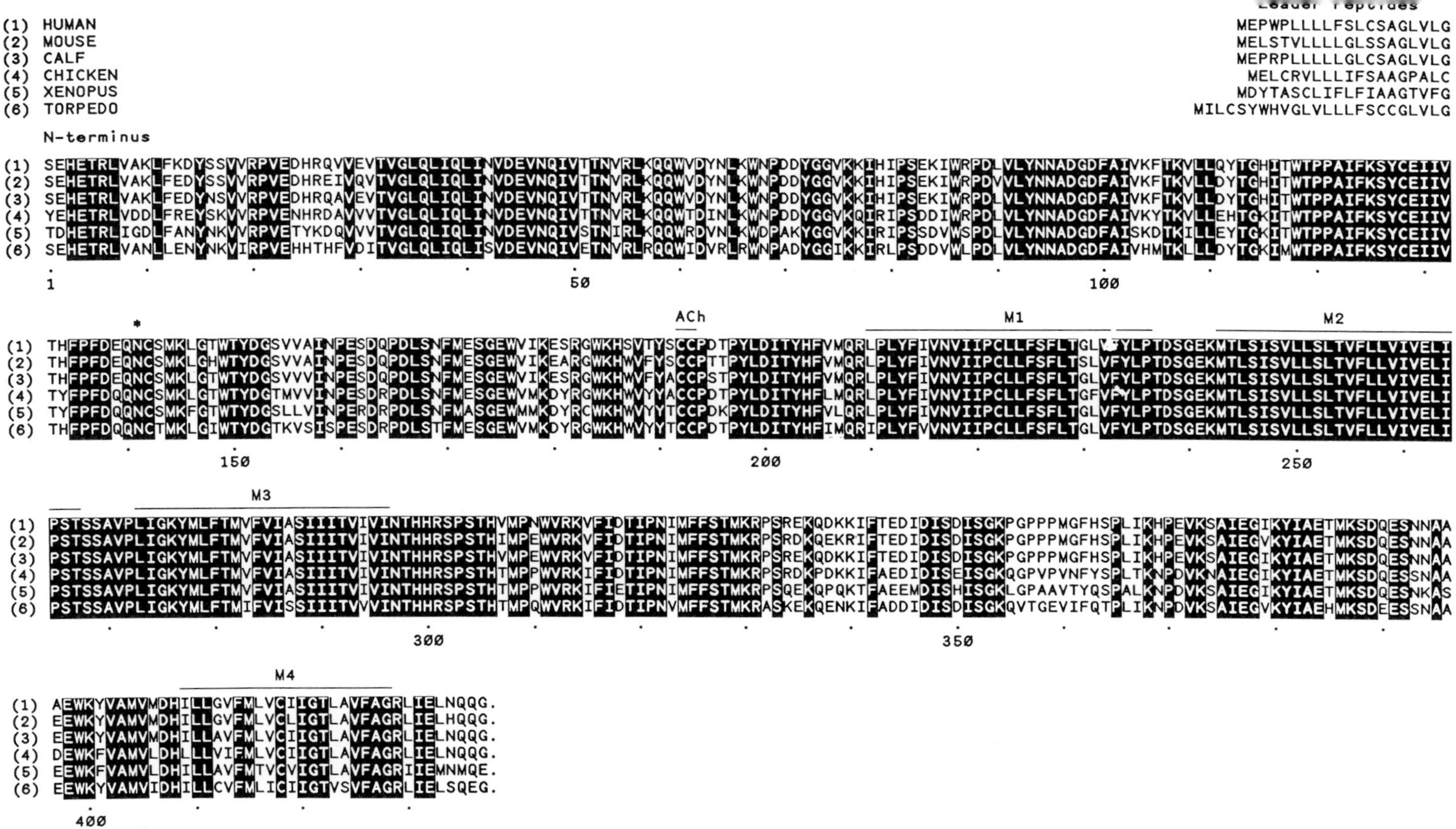

FIG. 2. Homologies between muscle-type AChR α subunits in various species. Human sequence taken from Schoepfer et al 1988b; mouse from Boulter et al 1987; calf from Noda et al 1983; chicken from Nef et al 1988; *Xenopus* from Baldwin et al 1988; *Torpedo* from Noda et al 1982. ACh, disulphide-linked cysteines near the ACh binding site; M1–M4, hydrophobic putative transmembrane sequences; *, putative N-glycosylation sites.

rapidly diverged as the central nervous system became more complex (Fig. 3). These subunits could then presumably form AChR subtypes with specialized functions.

The sequences of muscle α subunits shown in Fig. 2 reveal structural features characteristic of all members of the ligand-gated ion channel gene family. These include four hydrophobic, highly conserved sequences termed M1, M2, M3 and M4, which are thought to form α helical transmembrane domains; a pair of disulphide-linked cysteines at positions α128 and 142; and a long stretch of relatively poorly conserved sequence between M3 and M4, which is on the cytoplasmic surface of α subunits and appears to be rather loosely organized. The large cytoplasmic domain between M3 and M4 of each of the subunits of muscle AChRs contains several prominent epitopes that bind mAbs both in the native AChR and in denatured subunits (Ratnam et al 1986). The corresponding large putative cytoplasmic domains of other members of the gene family have proven to be good antigens for raising subunit-specific antibodies, some of which recognize native AChRs (Schoepfer et al 1989, R. Schoepfer & J. Lindstrom, unpublished). The putative transmembrane domain M2 appears to be most closely associated with the lining of the cation channel (Imoto et al 1988). The putative transmembrane domain M4 appears least conserved, and therefore functionally less critical, and therefore may be associated with membrane lipids. M1 is adjacent to the cysteine pair α192,193 unique to ACh-binding subunits, thus it may be involved in channel gating. M3 and/or other conserved sequences may be responsible for the specific association of multiple subunits to form the ion channel characteristic of this gene superfamily. Most or all of the N-terminal part of the α subunit preceding M1 is thought to be extracellular. This region includes such extracellular features as the main immunogenic region (α66-76), the N-glycosylation site (Asp α141), and the ACh-binding site (near Cys α192,193).

A series of neuronal cDNAs containing sequences homologous to those encoding muscle AChR subunits were identified by screening neuronal cDNA libraries, initially with muscle AChR α subunit cDNA probes under low stringency hybridization conditions. cDNAs encoding proteins that contained cysteines homologous to α192,193 were thought (correctly, as it turns out) to be ACh-binding subunits and termed 'α2, α3, α4, α5, . . .' in order of discovery (Boulter et al 1986, Goldman et al 1986, Wada et al 1988, Nef et al 1988). Other homologous neuronal cDNAs lacking these cysteines were termed 'β2, β3, . . .' or 'non-α', or simply 'structural subunits' (Schoepfer et al 1988a, Deneris et al 1988, 1989). Fig. 3 compares the deduced sequences of corresponding ACh-binding subunits from rats and chickens. Fig. 4 compares the deduced sequences of β2 structural subunits from chickens and rats. Although there is quite high sequence homology between corresponding subunits in different species, there is great diversity between subunits in the putative large cytoplasmic domain between M3 and M4. This may indicate that this sequence is important for defining the unique properties of each subunit, or that it is unimportant and therefore not tightly constrained by evolution, or a mixture of these two alternatives.

Neuronal nicotinic AChRs were first immunoaffinity purified from chicken brains using a mAb (mAb 35) to the main immunogenic region of electric organ AChRs (Whiting & Lindstrom 1986). As shown in Table 1, these neuronal AChRs consisted of only two kinds of subunits. We initially named these subunits, like those of muscle AChRs, α and β in order of increasing molecular weight. Now that it has been possible to identify the genes that encode these subunits, it has proven to be more convenient to name the subunits according to the genes that encode them, as shown in Fig. 1. The gene encoding the structural subunit of this AChR was identified as β2 by determining the N-terminal amino acid sequence of the purified subunit and comparing this with sequences deduced from cDNA clones (Schoepfer et al 1988a). The ACh-binding subunit of this AChR was identified by specific affinity labelling with [³H]MBTA (Whiting & Lindstrom 1987a). The gene encoding this ACh-binding subunit was determined by showing that an antiserum to a bacterially expressed cDNA fragment corresponding to the large putative cytoplasmic domain of the α2 sequence specifically bound to this subunit on Western blots (R. Schoepfer, B. Conroy, J. Lindstrom, unpublished). Curiously, mAb 35 and mAb 210, which are specific for the main immunogenic region on muscle AChR ACh-binding (α) subunits, bind to β2 structural subunits of neuronal AChRs (Whiting et al 1987a, Schoepfer et al 1989). In native neuronal AChRs they bind only to the α2β2 and α3β2 types and not to the α4β2 type, even though this uses the same β2 structural subunit. mAb 270, raised to purified neuronal AChRs, binds to β2 structural subunits in all of these AChR subtypes (Whiting et al 1987a). Apparently, the gene duplication processes that led to the evolution of these families of homologous subunits segregated the main immunogenic region and ACh-binding site together on α subunits of muscle AChRs, while in neuronal AChRs these two domains were segregated to different subunits. The assembly of α4 subunits with β2 subunits in the neuronal receptor occludes the epitope on β2 that cross-reacts with the main immunogenic region, but α2 and α3 subunits do not occlude this epitope. The α2β2 AChRs immunoisolated from detergent extracts of chicken brains exhibited high affinities for ACh and nicotine ($K_i = 1.1 \times 10^{-9}$M), much lower affinity for curare ($K_i = 1.1 \times 10^{-5}$M), and negligible affinity for αBgt (Whiting et al 1987a).

Recently, we found that preparations of AChR immunoaffinity purified from chicken brains using mAbs to the β2 structural subunit (e.g. mAb 270) contained small amounts of neuronal AChR subtype with α3 ACh-binding subunits (W. Conroy, R. Schoepfer, J. Lindstrom, unpublished). mAbs to a bacterially expressed cDNA fragment corresponding to the large putative cytoplasmic domain of α3 subunits faintly label on Western blots a band of the same apparent molecular weight as α2. α3-specific antibodies can deplete a negligible fraction

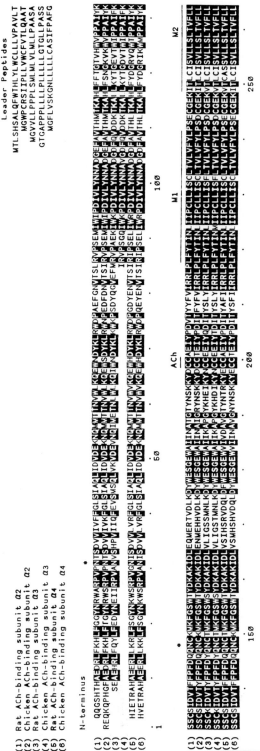

Leader Peptides

(1) Rat ACh-binding subunit α2 — MTLSHSALQFWTHLYLWCLLLVPAVLT
(2) Chicken ACh-binding subunit α2 — MGWPCRSIIPLLYWCFVTLQAAT
(3) Rat ACh-binding subunit α3 — MGVVLPPPLSWLWLVLMLLPAASA
(4) Chicken ACh-binding subunit α3 — GTGAPPPLLLPLLLLGTGLLPASS
(5) Rat ACh-binding subunit α4 — MGFLVSKGNLLLLLCASIFPAFG
(6) Chicken ACh-binding subunit α4

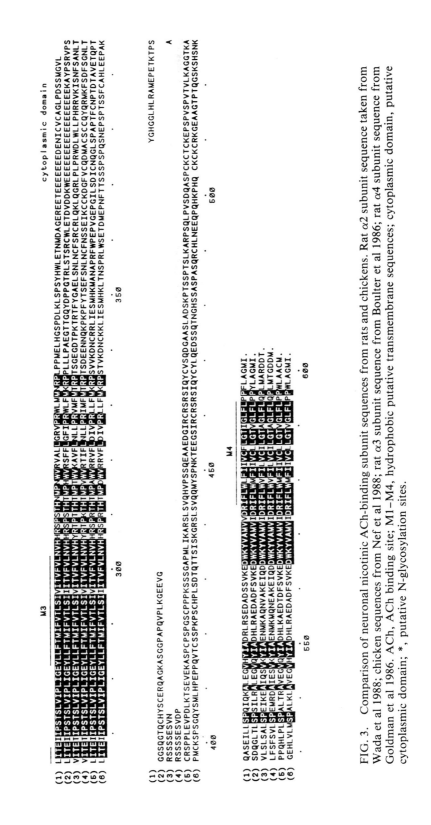

FIG. 3. Comparison of neuronal nicotinic ACh-binding subunit sequences from rats and chickens. Rat α2 subunit sequence taken from Wada et al 1988; chicken sequences from Nef et al 1988; rat α3 subunit sequence from Boulter et al 1986; rat α4 subunit sequence from Goldman et al 1986. ACh, ACh binding site; M1–M4, hydrophobic putative transmembrane sequences; cytoplasmic domain, putative cytoplasmic domain; *, putative N-glycosylation sites.

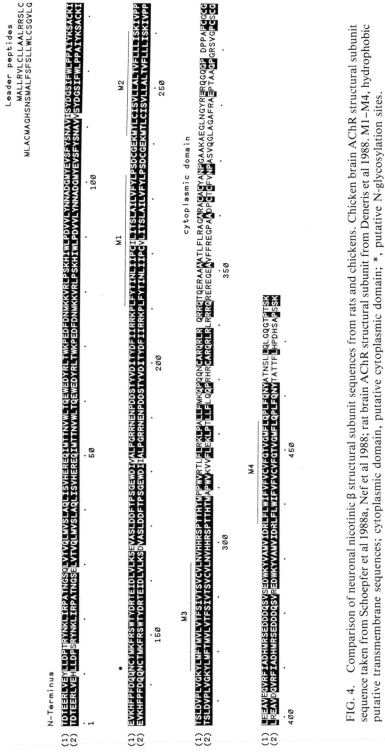

FIG. 4. Comparison of neuronal nicotinic β structural subunit sequences from rats and chickens. Chicken brain AChR structural subunit sequence taken from Schoepfer et al 1988a, Nef et al 1988; rat brain AChR structural subunit from Deneris et al 1988. M1–M4, hydrophobic putative transmembrane sequences; cytoplasmic domain, putative cytoplasmic domain; *, putative N-glycosylation sites.

of the high-affinity nicotine binding sites from extracts of chicken brains, but they can bind all of the AChRs in extracts of chicken ciliary ganglia and most of the AChRs in extracts of chicken retina (Schoepfer et al 1989, Whiting et al 1990, Boyd et al 1988). Northern blots of chicken brain RNA reveal substantial amounts of mRNA for β2 and α4 subunits and little mRNA for α3 subunits, whereas α3 and β2 mRNAs are abundant in retina and ganglia, but α4 mRNA is less abundant in retina and absent in ganglia. α3β2 AChRs are a minor subtype in brain, but a major one in retina and ganglia; this is a good example of the differential expression of AChR subtypes in various tissues and central nervous system regions. The AChRs in ciliary ganglia are pharmacologically similar to the predominant types in brain in not binding αBgt, but differ in having high affinity for neuronal Bgt and much lower affinity for nicotine.

A second major subtype of neuronal AChR was immunoaffinity purified from chicken brains using mAb 270 to structural subunits or mAbs to purified neuronal AChRs specific for α4 subunits, as shown in Fig. 1 (Whiting et al 1987a). This AChR is the most prominent subtype identified in mammalian brains. It is composed of β2 structural subunits and α4 ACh-binding subunits. As shown in Fig. 5, N-terminal sequencing of purified AChR subunits was used to identify the genes that encode its subunits (Schoepfer et al 1988, Whiting et al 1990). Note that apparently identical structural subunits are components of at least three different AChR subtypes which employ α2, α3 or α4 ACh-binding subunits (Fig. 1). The pharmacological properties of α4β2 AChRs immunoisolated from brain extracts closely resemble those of the α2β2 AChR; they have high affinity for nicotine ($K_i = 1.6 \times 10^{-9}$M), lower affinity for curare ($K_i = 3.7 \times 10^{-6}$M), and negligible affinity for αBgt.

A single AChR subtype was found to account for over 90% of the high affinity nicotine binding in extracts from rat brains (Whiting & Lindstrom 1987b). These α4β2 AChRs were immunoaffinity purified using mAb 270 raised against AChR from chicken brains. The genes encoding the subunits were identified by N-terminal sequencing of purified subunits, as shown in Fig. 5 (Whiting et al 1987b). The apparent molecular weights of the ACh-binding and structural subunits were 79 kDa and 51 kDa, respectively. This AChR, like α2β2 and α4β2 AChRs of chicken brains, exhibited high affinity for small cholinergic ligands (cytosine $K_i = 2.1 \times 10^{-9}$M), lower affinity for curare ($K_i = 1.3 \times 10^{-4}$M), and negligible affinity for αBgt.

α4β2 AChRs also appear to account for over 90% of the high affinity nicotine binding in extracts from bovine and human brains (Whiting & Lindstrom 1988). The 75 kDa ACh-binding subunit (which is specifically labelled with MBTA) and the 50 kDa structural subunit of immunoaffinity-purified bovine brain AChRs cross-react with subunit-specific mAbs raised to the α4 ACh-binding and β2 structural subunits of rat brain AChRs, respectively, thereby identifying the genes that encode these subunits. Like the corresponding AChR subtype

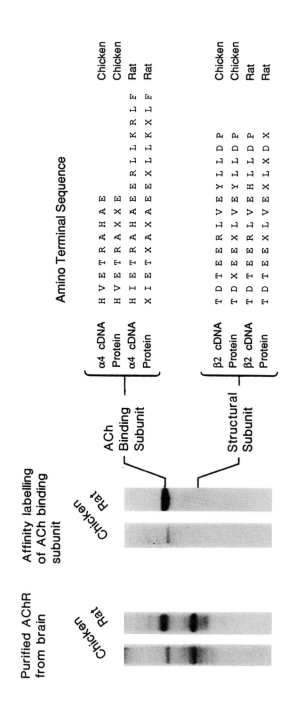

FIG. 5. Subunit structure of α4β2 AChRs from brains of chickens and rats. The first panel shows the band pattern of the silver-stained subunits of immunoaffinity-purified AChRs resolved by electrophoresis on acrylamide gels in SDS. The second panel shows the autoradiograph of AChRs affinity labelled with [^{3}H]MBTA before electrophoresis to identify the ACh binding subunits. The third panel compares the N-terminal amino acid sequences of the purified subunits with the N-terminal sequences deduced from the corresponding cDNAs to show how the genes encoding these subunits were identified. Data taken from Whiting et al 1987b, 1990, Whiting & Lindstrom 1987a, Schoepfer et al 1988a.

from other species, the $\alpha4\beta2$ AChRs extracted from bovine brain have high affinity for agonists (nicotine $K_i = 1.6 \times 10^{-8}$M in bovine and 6.5×10^{-9}M in human), lower affinity for curare ($K_i = 1.9 \times 10^{-5}$M in bovine and 4.7×10^{-5}M in human), and negligible affinity for αBgt.

Mammalian brains thus appear to express primarily $\alpha4\beta2$ nicotinic AChRs. However, they probably also express small amounts of other AChR subtypes, as indicated by the presence of small amounts of mRNA for $\alpha2$ and $\alpha3$ ACh-binding subunits detected in limited areas of rat brains by *in situ* hybridization (Wada et al 1989). Relatively large amounts of mRNA for $\alpha4$ ACh-binding subunits and $\beta2$ structural subunits were detected by *in situ* hybridization in extensive areas of rat brains.

By injecting synthetic mRNAs into *Xenopus* oocytes, where they are translated, functional ACh-gated cation channels have been obtained by combinations of $\beta2$ structural subunits with $\alpha2$, $\alpha3$ or $\alpha4$ ACh-binding subunits, as summarized in Table 1. This is consistent with biochemical evidence that these subunit combinations are characteristic of AChR subtypes found *in vivo*, and shows that these produce functional AChRs. It is also possible to produce at least partially functional AChRs in *Xenopus* oocytes using combinations of subunits which do not occur *in vivo*: $\beta2$ structural subunits have been reported to substitute for β subunits of muscle AChRs, and rat $\alpha4$ subunits alone have been reported to produce ACh-gated cation channels (Boulter et al 1987). Thus it is important to determine what subunit combinations actually occur *in vivo*, as we have done using immunological techniques. $\beta3$ subunits expressed in combination with $\alpha2$, $\alpha3$ or $\alpha4$ subunits have been reported not to produce functional channels, suggesting that $\beta3$ subunits might assemble with another ACh-binding subunit, be a subunit of an αBgtBP, or be a component of a receptor for another transmitter, among other possibilities (Deneris et al 1989).

TABLE 1   ACh-gated cation channel properties of AChRs expressed in *Xenopus* oocytes

AChR type	Blockage by αBgt	Blockage by neuronal αBgt	Primary conductance (pS)	Channel duration (msec)	Reference
$\alpha_2\beta\gamma\delta$ of bovine muscle	+	n.t.	40	7.6	Sakmann et al 1985
$\alpha2\beta2$ of rat neurons	–	–	33.6	2.9	Papke et al 1989
$\alpha3\beta2$ of rat neurons	–	+	15.4	4.0	Papke et al 1989
$\alpha4\beta2$ of rat neurons	–	+	13.3	2.16	Papke et al 1989
$\alpha4\beta2$ of chicken neurons	–	n.t.	20	n.t.	Ballivet et al 1988

n.t., not tested.

The subunit stoichiometry and organization of neuronal nicotinic AChRs has not been precisely determined, but evidence suggests that they differ from those of muscle AChRs. Fig. 6 compares the known organization of subunits within muscle AChRs, with the possible alternative subunit organizations within neuronal AChRs. It seems a reasonable hypothesis that neuronal AChR subunits are organized like barrel staves around a central cation channel with alternate ACh-binding and structural subunits, as are AChRs from *Torpedo* electric organ. It is known that there is more than one copy of each type of subunit in a neuronal AChR, because an AChR bound to an affinity column by a mAb specific for either subunit can then bind another [125I]labelled mAb of the

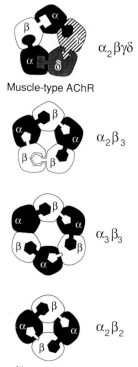

FIG. 6. Organization of subunits of nicotinic receptors around the central cation channel. The experimentally determined organization of subunits of *Torpedo* AChR subunits is depicted at the top of the diagram. Neuronal AChRs are shown as having the same pattern of alternating ACh-binding and structural subunits around a central ion channel as is observed for *Torpedo* $\alpha_2\beta\gamma\delta$ AChRs. Three possible arrangements of the two kinds of subunits that form neuronal AChRs are depicted. The $\alpha_2\beta_3$ or $\alpha_3\beta_2$ subunit stoichiometries have been eliminated by the observation that neuronal AChRs contain equal numbers of each subunit. The measured size of neuronal AChRs does not clearly distinguish between the alternative stoichiometries $\alpha_2\beta_2$ and $\alpha_3\beta_3$.

same specificity (Whiting et al 1987a). The observation of a Hill coefficient of 1.51 for ACh activation of $\alpha4\beta2$ AChRs expressed in *Xenopus* oocytes also suggests that there are about two $\alpha4$ subunits in each AChR (Ballivet et al 1988). Using a method in which the relative amounts of subunits in an AChR are quantitated by labelling denatured AChR with ^{125}I, the amount of ^{125}I in each subunit is measured and then corrections are made for differences in the number of tyrosines in each subunit, the correct stoichiometry was determined for *Torpedo* AChR: $\alpha_2\beta\gamma\delta$ (W. Whiting et al, in preparation). The same method applied to $\alpha4\beta2$ AChRs from brains of chickens, rats and cattle showed that in all three cases there were exactly equal amounts of both types of subunit. This means that neuronal AChRs cannot have the pseudopentagonal symmetry of muscle AChRs, i.e. they cannot have the stoichiometries $(\alpha4)_2(\beta2)_3$ or $(\alpha4)_3(\beta2)_2$. Circular arrangements of five subunits of two kinds suffer from the constraint that one of the subunits must bind uniquely both to the other type of subunit and to itself, an apparent barrier to efficient subunit assembly. The problem is to decide whether the stoichiometry is $(\alpha4)_2(\beta2)_2$ or $(\alpha4)_3(\beta2)_3$. Circular arrangements of equal numbers of two kinds of subunits in alternating order allow each subunit to interact uniquely with the other, an appealing concept for efficiently assembling unique closed arrays of subunits. On sucrose gradients using crude extracts, these AChRs co-sediment with monomers of *Torpedo* AChR. Sucrose gradient sedimentation is not a very precise measure of molecular weight. Also, the extensive putative cytoplasmic domain on $\alpha4$ subunits may significantly alter the shape and sedimentation properties of $(\alpha4)_n(\beta2)_n$ AChRs with respect to $\alpha_2\beta\gamma\delta$ AChRs. The approximate calculated molecular weight of glycosylated *Torpedo* AChR monomers labelled with αBgt is 303 kDa; whereas the corresponding calculated molecular weights are 263 kDa for rat $(\alpha4)_2(\beta2)_2$ and 394 kDa for rat $(\alpha4)_3(\beta2)_3$. These results are marginally more consistent with the idea that neuronal AChRs have the subunit stoichiometry $\alpha_2\beta_2$. This use of minimum number of subunits to satisfy the observed properties of equal numbers of at least two subunits of each kind and the theoretical requirement for barrel staves enclosing a central channel is aesthetically appealing. The observation that neuronal AChRs tend to exhibit smaller conductances than do muscle AChRs (Table 1) is consistent with the idea that the four subunits of an $(\alpha4)_2(\beta2)_2$ AChR would form a smaller channel than would the five subunits of an $\alpha_2\beta\gamma\delta$ AChR or the six subunits of an $(\alpha4)_3(\beta2)_3$ AChR. $\alpha_2\beta_2$ is certainly the simplest way to accommodate equal numbers and at least two copies of each subunit in an AChR. In unusual circumstances, such as *Xenopus* oocytes, where AChR synthesis may be driven by unusual amounts and ratios of subunit mRNAs, subunits may sometimes associate in abnormal stoichiometries (Papke et al 1989).

Neuronal AChR proteins have been localized histologically using [^{3}H]ACh, [^{3}H]nicotine, [^{125}I]mAbs, or mAbs indirectly localized with enzymes or fluorescence (Clarke et al 1985, Jacob et al 1986, Keyser et al 1988, Sargent et al 1989, Swanson et al 1987, Watson et al 1988). The mRNAs that encode these proteins have been localized by *in situ* hybridization with [^{35}S]cRNA (antisense RNA) (Wada et al 1989). Sometimes the mRNA in the cell bodies can be far from sites of AChR protein localization. For example, in all retinal systems that have been studied using mAbs to AChRs (i.e. fish, frogs, chicken and rats), AChRs made in the cell bodies of retinal ganglion cells are exported to pre- or extrasynaptic parts of the central projections of their axons (Keyser et al 1988, Sargent et al 1989, Swanson et al 1987), where they are found at high densities, for example, in the superior colliculus (Clarke et al 1985, Swanson et al 1987). These AChRs, and many others in the central nervous system, may act in presynaptic locations to modulate transmitter release or in extrasynaptic locations perform functions even further removed from the classic postsynaptic role of $\alpha_2\beta\epsilon\delta$ AChRs in muscle or $\alpha3\beta2$ AChRs in ganglia. There is evidence that nicotinic AChRs can enhance release of ACh and γ-aminobutyric acid from synaptosomes immunoisolated using mAb 270 (J. Irons et al, unpublished). It has also been reported that growth of projections from retinal ganglion cells in culture is affected by nicotinic AChRs (Lipton et al 1988).

$\beta2$ structural subunits have been localized in many areas of the rat central nervous system using either mAb 270 or antisense $\beta2$ RNA (Swanson et al 1987, Wada et al 1989). These results suggest that nicotinic AChRs constitute part of a major excitatory pathway in the central nervous system. $\alpha4$ ACh-binding subunit mRNA is nearly as widespread as that of $\beta2$, but mRNAs for $\alpha2$ and $\alpha3$ ACh-binding subunits are more restricted in their distribution. The binding pattern in rat brain of mAb 270 parallels that of [^{3}H]ACh or [^{3}H]nicotine and differs from that of [^{125}I]αBgt (Clarke et al 1985, Swanson et al 1987). The pattern of mAb 270 binding is more restricted and somewhat different from the binding pattern of probes for $\beta2$ mRNA. Nicotinic AChRs are especially concentrated in the lateral spiriform nucleus and optic tectum of chicken brains, for example. In rat brain, the areas with high concentrations of nicotinic AChRs include the superior colliculus, medial habenula and interpeduncular nucleus.

Good cellular resolution of AChRs in chicken retina has been achieved using mAbs 210 and 270 to $\beta2$ structural subunits (Keyser et al 1988). Ganglion cells, displaced ganglion cells and amacrine cells were labelled.

Some immunoelectron microscopic localization of nicotinic AChRs has been done. In chicken ciliary ganglion cells, they were localized on the cell surface, at synapses and intracellularly using mAb 35 to structural subunits (Jacob et al 1984, 1986). Frog retinotectal projections were labelled at extrasynaptic sites with another mAb to the main immunogenic region (Sargent et al 1989).

Molecular studies of neuronal α-bungarotoxin-binding proteins

Rat brains contain about twice as many binding sites for αBgt as for nicotine (Whiting & Lindstrom 1987b). The relatively large amount of these proteins suggests that they may be important, but their function is not known. The αBgtBPs on chicken ganglionic neurons or rat PC12 cells do not appear to function as ACh-gated cation channels (Patrick & Stallcup 1977). In chicken ciliary ganglia, αBgtBPs, unlike $\alpha3\beta2$ AChRs, are not located at synapses, but instead are found on pseudodendrites (Jacob et al 1984). The ability of αBgtBPs to bind small cholinergic ligands and αBgt, and to react with MBTA (after reduction) suggests that αBgtBPs may be members of the AChR gene family. However, their endogenous ligand, if any, remains unknown. It has been suggested, for example, that the endogenous ligand of the αBgtBP could be blood-borne thymopoietin (Quik et al 1989). The subunit composition of αBgtBPs has not been clearly established. Further evidence that αBgtBPs might be members of the AChR gene family was provided by the observation that a partial N-terminal amino acid sequence of αBgtBP from chicken brain resembled that of AChRs (Conti-Tronconi et al 1985).

Recently, using oligonucleotide probes based on this reported N-terminal sequence, we have been able to clone and sequence cDNAs for two closely related subunits of αBgtBPs (R. Schoepfer et al, unpublished). The authenticity of these clones was established by demonstrating that antisera and mAbs raised to unique putative large cytoplasmic domains of these subunits bound to [^{125}I]αBgt-labelled αBgtBP extracted from chicken brains. Antibodies to the subunit designated αBgtBP $\alpha1$ recognized about 75% of the labelled protein, while antibodies to the αBgtBP $\alpha2$ subunit recognized less than 20% of the total, suggesting there may be different subtypes of these proteins analogous to the different subtypes of neuronal AChRs. These subunits were designated as α because they contain a cysteine pair homologous to $\alpha192, 193$, suggesting that they may be ligand-binding subunits. The deduced amino acid sequences prove that they are members of the ligand-gated ion channel family. Their sequences are rather distantly related to those of AChRs from both nerve and muscle, but they contain all of the primary features of subunits in this family, including hydrophobic sequences homologous to M1, 2, 3 and 4 and cysteines homologous to $\alpha128$ and 142. There is nothing apparent in the available sequences of the two subunits to suggest that these could not function as ligand-gated cation channels.

Thus, the cDNA and mAb tools are now available to permit the purification and characterization of the subunit structure of αBgtBP subtypes using methods similar to those applied to neuronal nicotinic AChRs. Using existing cell lines that express αBgtBP and combinations of expressed αBgtBP subunit cDNAs, it may be possible to identify the functional activity of these molecules. Finally, it should be possible to return to tissue and whole animal studies to discover the functional roles of these dark horses of the AChR gene family.

Conclusions

Immunochemical and molecular genetic approaches to studies of muscle nicotinic AChRs, neuronal nicotinic AChRs and neuronal αBgtBPs are converging to provide a detailed description of a complex family of AChRs. Neuronal AChRs and neuronal αBgtBPs are widely dispersed throughout the nervous system, and are probably important to many of its activities, but their functional roles are not yet well characterized.

The heterogeneity of receptor types identified by molecular techniques in these gene families and others suggest that a new pharmacological nomenclature will have to be developed in which receptor types will be distinguished by the combination of subunit gene products which compose them, rather than just by their pharmacological properties or tissue location.

Acknowledgements

This work was supported by grants from the NIH (NS 11323), the Muscular Dystrophy Association, the Alexander Onassis Public Benefit Foundation, the U.S. Army (DAMD17-86-C-6148), the Council for Tobacco Research-USA, Inc., and the California Chapter of the Myasthenia Gravis Foundation.

References

Ballivet M, Nef P, Couturier S et al 1988 Electrophysiology of a chick neuronal nicotinic acetylcholine receptor expressed in *Xenopus* oocytes after cDNA injection. Neuron 1:847–852

Baldwin TJ, Yoshihara CM, Blackmer K, Kinter CR, Burden SJ 1988 Regulation of acetylcholine-receptor transcript expression during development in xenopus-laevis. J Cell Biol 106:469–478

Barnard E, Darlison M, Seeburg P 1987 Molecular biology of the GABA$_A$ receptor: the receptor/channel superfamily. Trends Neurosci 10:502–509

Boulter J, Evans K, Goldman D et al 1986 Isolation of a cDNA clone coding for a possible neural nicotinic acetylcholine receptor α subunit. Nature (Lond) 319:368–374

Boulter J, Connolly J, Deneris E, Goldman D, Heinemann S, Patrick J 1987 Functional expression of two neuronal nicotinic acetylcholine receptors from cDNA clones identifies a gene family. Proc Natl Acad Sci USA 84:7763–7767

Boyd R, Jacob M, Couturier S, Ballivet M, Berg D 1988 Expression and regulation of neuronal acetylcholine mRNA in chick ciliary ganglia. Neuron 1:495–502

Catterall W 1988 Structure and function of voltage-sensitive ion channels. Science (Wash DC) 242:50–61

Clarke P, Schwartz R, Paul S, Pert C, Pert A 1985 Nicotinic binding in rat brain: autoradiographic comparison of [^{3}H]acetylcholine, [^{3}H]nicotine, and [^{125}I]αbungarotoxin. J Neurosci 5:1307–1315

Conti-Tronconi B, Dunn S, Barnard E et al 1985 Brain and muscle nicotinic acetylcholine receptors are different but homologous proteins. Proc Natl Acad Sci USA 82:5208–5212

Das M, Lindstrom J 1989 The main immunogenic region of the nicotinic acetylcholine receptor. Interaction of monoclonal antibodies with synthetic peptides. Biochim Biophys Res Comm 165:865–871

Deneris E, Connolly J, Boulter J et al 1988 Primary structure and expression of β2: a novel subunit of neuronal nicotinic acetylcholine receptors. Neuron 1:45–54

Deneris E, Boulter J, Swanson L, Patrick J, Heinemann S 1989 β$_3$: A new member of nicotinic acetylcholine receptor gene family is expressed in brain. J Biol Chem 264:6268–6272

Goldman D, Simmons D, Swanson L, Patrick J, Heinemann S 1986 Mapping of brain areas expressing RNA homologous to two different acetylcholine receptor α subunit cDNAs. Proc Natl Acad Sci USA 83:4076–4080

Imoto K, Busch C, Sakmann B et al 1988 Rings of negatively charged amino acids determine the acetylcholine receptor channel conductance. Nature (Lond) 335: 645–648

Jacob MH, Berg DK, Lindstrom J 1984 A shared antigenic determinant between the electrophorus acetylcholine receptor and a synaptic component on chick ciliary ganglion neurons. Proc Natl Acad Sci USA 81:3223–3227

Jacob MH, Lindstrom JM, Berg DK 1986 Surface and intracellular distribution of a putative neuronal nicotinic acetylcholine receptor. J Cell Biol 103:205–214

Kao P, Karlin A 1986 Acetylcholine receptor binding site contains a disulfide crosslink between adjacent half-cystinyl residues. J Biol Chem 261:8085–8088

Kao P, Dwork A, Kaldamy R et al 1984 Identification of the α subunit half-cystine specifically labeled by an affinity reagent for the acetylcholine receptor binding site. J Biol Chem 259:11662–11665

Keyser KT, Hughes TE, Whiting PJ, Lindstrom JM, Karten HJ 1988 Cholinoceptive neurons in the retina of the chick: an immunohistochemical study of the nicotinic acetylcholine receptors. Vis Neurosci 1:349–366

Kubalek E, Ralston S, Lindstrom J, Unwin N 1987 Location of subunits within the acetylcholine receptor: analysis of tubular crystals from *Torpedo marmorata*. J Cell Biol 105:9–18

Lindstrom J, Schoepfer R, Whiting P 1987 Molecular studies of the neuronal nicotinic acetylcholine receptor family. Mol Neurobiol 1:218–337

Lipton SA, Frosck MP, Phillips MD, Tauck DL, Aizenman E 1988 Nicotinic antagonists enhance process outgrowth by rat retinal ganglion cells in culture. Science (Wash DC) 239:1293–1296

Nef P, Oneyser C, Alliod C, Couturier S, Ballivet M 1988 Genes expressed in the brain define three distinct neuronal nicotinic acetylcholine receptors. EMBO (Eur Mol Biol Organ) J 7:595–601

Noda M, Takahashi H, Tanabe T et al 1982 Primary structure of α-subunit precursor of *Torpedo californica* acetylcholine receptor deduced from cDNA sequence. Nature (Lond) 299:793–797

Noda M, Furutani Y, Takahashi H et al 1983 Cloning and sequence analysis of calf cDNA and human genomic DNA encoding α-subunit precursor of muscle acetylcholine receptor. Nature (Lond) 305:818–823

Papke R, Boulter J, Patrick J, Heinemann S 1989 Single-channel currents of rat neuronal nicotinic acetylcholine receptors expressed in *Xenopus laevis* oocytes. Neuron 3:589–596

Patrick J, Stallcup W 1977 α-bungarotoxin binding and cholinergic receptor function on a rat sympathetic nerve line. J Biol Chem 252:8629–8633

Peralta E, Winslow J, Ashkenazi A, Smith D, Ramachandran J, Capon D 1988 Structural basis of muscarinic acetylcholine receptor subtype diversity. Trends Pharmacol Sci Suppl (Feb):6–11

Quik M, Afar R, Audhya T, Goldstein G 1989 Thymopoietin, a thymic polypeptide, specifically interacts at neuronal nicotinic α-bungarotoxin receptors. J Neurochem 53:1320–1323

Ratnam M, Sargent PB, Sarin V et al 1986 Location of antigenic determinants on primary sequences of subunits of nicotinic acetylcholine receptor by peptide mapping. Biochemistry 25:2621–2632

Sakmann B, Methfessel C, Fukuda K et al 1985 Role of acetylcholine receptor subunits in gating of the channel. Nature (Lond) 318:538–543

Sargent PB, Pike SH, Nadel DB, Lindstrom JM 1989 Nicotinic acetylcholine receptor-like molecules in the retina, retinotectal pathway, and optic tectum of the frog. J Neurosci 9:565–573

Schoepfer R, Whiting P, Esch F, Blacher R, Shimasaki S, Lindstrom J 1988a cDNA clones coding for the structural subunit of a chicken brain nicotinic acetylcholine receptor. Neuron 1:241–248

Schoepfer R, Luther M, Lindstrom J 1988b The human medulloblastoma cell line TE671 expresses a muscle-like acetylcholine-receptor. Cloning of the alpha subunit cDNA. FEBS (Fed Eur Biochem Soc) Lett 226:235–240

Schoepfer R, Halvorsen S, Conroy WG, Whiting P, Lindstrom J 1989 Antisera against an acetylcholine receptor $\alpha 3$ fusion protein bind to ganglionic but not to brain nicotinic acetylcholine receptors. FEBS (Fed Eur Biochem Soc) Lett 257:393–400

Schoepfer R, Conroy W, Whiting P, Gore M, Lindstrom J cDNA clones define brain α-bungarotoxin-binding proteins as members of the ligand-gated ion channel family, submitted.

Swanson LW, Simmons DM, Whiting PJ, Lindstrom JM 1987 Immunohistochemical localization of neuronal nicotinic receptors in the rodent central nervous system. J Neurosci 7:3334–3342

Tzartos S, Kokla A, Walgrave S, Conti-Tronconi B 1988 The main immunogenic region of human muscle acetylcholine receptor is localized within residues 63–80 of the α subunit. Proc Natl Acad Sci USA 85:2899–2903

Wada K, Ballivet M, Boulter J et al 1988 Functional expression of a new pharmacological subtype of brain nicotinic acetylcholine receptor. Science (Wash DC) 240:330–334

Wada E, Wada K, Boulter J et al 1989 The distribution of $\alpha 2$, $\alpha 3$, $\alpha 4$, and $\beta 2$ neuronal nicotinic receptor subunit mRNAs in the central nervous system: a hybridization histochemical study in the rat. J Comp Neurol 284:314–335

Watson JT, Adkins-Regan E, Whiting P, Lindstrom JM, Podleski TR 1988 Autoradiographic localization of nicotinic acetylcholine receptors in the brain of the zebra finch (peophila guttata). J Comp Neurol 274:255–264

Whiting PJ, Lindstrom JM 1986 Purification and characterization of a nicotinic acetylcholine receptor from chick brain. Biochemistry 25:2082–2093

Whiting P, Lindstrom J 1987a Affinity labeling of neuronal acetylcholine receptors localizes acetylcholine binding sites to their β subunits. FEBS (Fed Eur Biochem Soc) Lett 213:55–60

Whiting P, Lindstrom J 1987b Purification and characterization of a nicotinic acetylcholine receptor from rat brain. Proc Natl Acad Sci USA 84:595–599

Whiting PJ, Lindstrom JM 1988 Characterization of bovine and human neuronal nicotinic acetylcholine receptors using monoclonal antibodies. J Neurosci 8:3395–3404

Whiting P, Liu R, Morley BJ, Lindstrom J 1987a Structurally different neuronal nicotinic acetylcholine receptor subtypes purified and characterized using monoclonal antibodies. J Neurosci 7:4005–4016

Whiting P, Esch F, Shimasaki S, Lindstrom J 1987b Neuronal nicotinic acetylcholine receptor β subunit is coded for by the cDNA clone $\alpha 4$. FEBS (Fed Eur Biochem Soc) Lett 219:459–463

Whiting P, Schoepfer R, Conroy W et al 1990 Differential expression of nicotinic acetylcholine receptor subtypes in brain and retina, submitted.

Whiting W, Cooper J, Lindstrom J Neuronal nicotinic receptors are composed of equal numbers of acetylcholine-binding and structural subunits, in preparation

Witzemann V, Barg B, Nishikawa Y, Sakmann B, Numa S 1987 Differential regulation of muscle acetylcholine receptor γ and ϵ subunit mRNAs. FEBS (Fed Eur Biochem Soc) Lett 223:104–112

DISCUSSION

Lunt: In Bath we are very fortunate in having a collaboration with a group of protein molecular modellers who are interested in the rather speculative procedure of trying to predict a protein tertiary structure from primary sequence. One of the problems with looking at the structural organization of the receptors is a lack of quantitative structural data: the best we have are fairly low resolution electron diffraction patterns.

The modellers, David Osguthorpe and Vic Cockcroft, have searched crystallographic data bases for proteins with a bundle of four α helices. One such protein is myohaemerythrin, which has a bundle of four α helices of about the same dimensions that we would predict the nicotinic receptor to have. They have taken the primary sequence of the neuronal α subunit of the nicotinic receptor and substituted that onto the crystal structure for myohaemerythrin. This particular neuronal receptor is an insect α subunit that expresses a functional channel when injected into *Xenopus* oocytes, without a β-type subunit. It is a clone from locust that was isolated by John Marshall in a collaboration with Eric Barnard's laboratory in Cambridge.

The result of the modelling is quite interesting. When the α subunit sequence is substituted onto myohaemerythrin and we look at the four transmembrane helices, M1, M2, M3 and M4, M2 comes out lining the channel and that fits with what we know about the contribution of the helices to the channel properties. M4 lies on the outside of the bundle and seems to be the helix that interacts with the lipid phase.

We have constructed models with four and five subunits. The model with four subunits gives a smaller channel than that with five subunits. The channel with five is basically too big to show any discrimination; one couldn't control the size of that channel such as to close it fully. Four subunits give a channel that is much more the size that one would anticipate and that could effectively be closed. It's speculative, we don't have the hard structural data for the receptor, but as far as the packing of this neuronal sequence is concerned, the model suggests that four subunits fit better than five.

Colquhoun: The argument about conductance is not very compelling because the difference is not very big. The conductance for an extrajunctional type of muscle receptor is more or less the same as that for a sympathetic ganglion receptor.

Heinemann: The *Torpedo* receptor is the one for which we have the best structural data. Have you used *Torpedo* receptor sequences in your model?

Lunt: Not yet. So far this has only been done putting four or five identical subunits together. For the *Torpedo* receptor there is the added complication of different sequences for every subunit.

Collins: How consistent is the use of four transmembrane helices with the observation that in the *Torpedo* receptor, antibody raised against the C-terminal end binds to the cytostolic surface?

Lindstrom: There is some debate about this. Antibody data suggest that the C terminus is on the cytoplasmic surface (Ratnam et al 1986, Young et al 1985); however, data on accessibility to reducing agents from McCrea et al (1987) and DiPaola et al (1989) argue that it is on the extracellular surface.

Changeux: These computer experiments give models of the open channel. Then the subunits can be tilted to give the closed structure. What you are looking at is the structure of the maximally open channel.

Lunt: With five subunits it's very difficult to rearrange them in any way to give a completely closed channel.

Changeux: Unwin & Zampighi (1980) have shown for the gap junction channel that tilting of the 'connexons' yields a closed channel. You are using helices which are parallel to the axis of symmetry. If you tilt the subunits, the size of the channel changes.

Colquhoun: There is no reliable information on the physical size of an open or a closed channel.

Heinemann: In the brain we have identified seven genes that we call $\alpha 2$, $\alpha 3$, $\alpha 4$, $\alpha 5$, and $\beta 2$, $\beta 4$, $\beta 3$. We call the first set α subunits because they have adjacent cysteines analogous to the *Torpedo* Cys192,193. We have shown that $\alpha 4$ will form a functional receptor by itself, so it must be a ligand binding protein. We think these α subunits are all ligand binding subunits. In our terminology, $\alpha 1$ is the subunit in muscle. The β subunits are so called because $\beta 2$ and $\beta 4$ each substitute for $\beta 1$ to form a muscle-type receptor. Therefore they have a β function; they will not substitute for any of the other muscle subunits.

We think *Torpedo* and muscle receptors have a pentameric structure on the basis of work by Nigel Unwin, Arthur Karlin, Robert Stroud and many others. I think it's unlikely that the subunits would substitute for one another in a very different structure, therefore I think the neuronal receptors are probably also pentamers. The glycine receptor is another member of this family and Heinrich Betz and his collaborators have shown that it is a pentamer.

We can form functional nicotinic receptors by expressing these genes in *Xenopus* oocytes in various combinations. We have shown that except for $\alpha 4$, it is not possible to see any conductance when the α subunits are expressed alone. In the brain we think there are always two subunits, an α and a β, consistent with the data that Jon Lindstrom has shown. When we combine $\alpha 2$ with $\beta 2$ we get a functional receptor in oocytes. We can combine $\alpha 2$ or $\alpha 3$ or $\alpha 4$ with $\beta 2$ and make three different receptor subtypes; we can substitute $\beta 4$ for $\beta 2$ and make three more subtypes. So six different receptor subtypes can be made with these five gene products and each subtype has different characteristics.

In the case of $\alpha 5$ and $\beta 3$ we have not been able to show any function, even though structurally they are very homologous to the other subunits. However, $\alpha 5$ and $\beta 3$ are outliers, more related to each other and less to the other subunits. It is possible that $\alpha 5$ and $\beta 3$ are not nicotinic receptor subunits; they may recognize a different ligand which at present is unknown.

We have looked at the expression of these genes in the CNS. The mRNAs for $\alpha3$ and $\alpha4$ are expressed very widely, but $\alpha2$ and $\alpha5$ are expressed in much more localized regions. If you compare these patterns of expression with nicotine binding, in most places where we see high nicotine binding, one of the α genes is expressed. Of the β subunits, $\beta2$ is the most widely distributed; $\beta3$ and $\beta4$ are expressed much more locally.

These data show that the nicotinic receptors are expressed almost everywhere in the CNS, therefore you would expect to see many behavioural effects of nicotine and that is the case.

Iversen: Do you think that all six possible brain receptors actually exist?

Heinemann: We don't have any evidence directly related to this question.

Lindstrom: I would like to comment on the stoichiometry. You argued that because $\beta2$ and $\beta4$ can substitute in muscle-type ACh receptors expressed in *Xenopus* oocytes, the overall stoichiometry should be the same. However, β subunits in muscle-type ACh receptors are found between two α subunits (Kubalek et al 1987). Their role seems to be to separate two α subunits. In a neuronal receptor consisting of two subunits of each kind, that is precisely the role of β subunits; all you are doing is repeating the symmetry by putting a second β subunit in on the other side of those two α subunits.

Changeux: Recent results on the identification of the amino acids from the agonist binding site give some insight into the distinction between the ability to bind α-bungarotoxin and neural bungarotoxin. Affinity labelling studies (Dennis et al 1988, Galzi et al 1990) show that there are three loops involved in the structure of the binding site for cholinergic ligands and not only the two cysteines identified by Arthur Karlin and co-workers. The amino acids from the two other loops are evolutionarily conserved between the muscular and neuronal receptors that have been sequenced. Do you have any idea which domain of the α subunit contributes to the difference between α-bungarotoxin binding to muscle and neuronal receptors?

Lindstrom: There are several observations (e.g. Wolf et al 1988) which suggest that not all subtypes of neuronal ACh receptors bind neuronal α-bungarotoxin. The $\alpha3\beta2$ subtype binds it very well; the $\alpha4\beta2$ subunit binds it with much lower affinity. In our hands, and those of Halvorsen & Berg (1987), in detergent solution neither subtype binds it, so binding depends on conformation of the receptor. If you co-express $\alpha3$ and $\beta4$, the receptor does not bind αBgt, saying that β also contributes to the conformation required for binding (Duvoisin et al 1989).

Changeux: This is interesting, because it looks as if the pharmacology of the different combinations of subunits is quite different, at least for this toxin.

Heinemann: You are right, the $\alpha3\beta2$ receptor is blocked very efficiently by neuronal bungarotoxin, whereas $\alpha3\beta4$ is not. This says that $\beta4$ affects whether the toxin can pharmacologically block the receptor, but we have no toxin binding data.

Changeux: Did you look at the M2 with channel blockers such as chlorpromazine?

Lindstrom: Not yet. Rapier et al (1987) report that histrionicotoxin has similar effects on the cation channels of muscle and neuronal nicotinic receptors. From that they argue that the channels are basically similar.

Changeux: From the pharmacological point of view, it would be very important to have the two categories of pharmacological agents acting on the brain receptor. Since chlorpromazine has been shown to act as a blocker of the ACh gated ion channel in muscle, it would be interesting to know if it shows the same action on brain nicotinic receptors.

Wonnacott: We've looked at histrionicotoxin and it blocks presynaptic nicotinic receptors that mediate transmitter release in the brain, but not [³H]nicotine binding, i.e. its action is non-competitive.

Heinemann: Dr John Connolly in our group has looked at a derivative of chlorpromazine that is used clinically, and it blocks all the receptor subtypes tested.

Changeux: Does it also block the different combinations of subunits? This creates some interesting openings as far as the pharmacology of these receptors is concerned.

Heinemann: Dr John Connolly who worked in my lab studied the pharmacology and many of the agents that are thought to work against other ligand-gated channels also work against nicotinic neuronal subtypes, so these agents are clearly non-specific.

Schwartz: I have shown that non-competitive inhibitors of the nicotinic receptor also block the chloride channel associated with the γ-aminobutyric acid (GABA) receptor in brain. When you say that these agents are non-specific, in a sense it depends on their concentration, because those same compounds at high concentrations produce seizure activity or lower the seizure threshold in humans and animals. This specific action could be produced by block of the GABA-gated chloride channel.

Changeux: This is very interesting. The serine (or threonine) ring is also present in other ligand-gated ion channels.

A point about the stoichiometry: I am a little confused. Didn't you publish that the channel was a pentamer?

Lindstrom: The data we reported (Whiting et al 1987) did not allow us to determine the stoichiometry conclusively. Our current data suggest that there are equal numbers of α4 and β.

Changeux: Are you more confident about this labelling technique? It is a little difficult to accept that with one technique you obtain a tetramer and in the other a pentamer! There are examples from Aaron Klug's work on viruses that a given subunit can be included in an environment with either four or five subunits with a *quasi*-equivalence between subunits . . .

Lindstrom: I think it is possible that neuronal nicotinic receptor subunits are sufficiently different from muscle ones to aggregate with a different stoichiometry; but I could be wrong. I have shown the only data available.

Papke et al (1989) have injected *Xenopus* oocytes with different ratios of α2 and β2 mRNAs and observed receptors with different electrophysiological properties. They assume that these different amounts of subunits can assemble in different ways to give different functional receptors. So the stoichiometry may vary under some circumstances.

Colquhoun: Could I ask Dr Heinemann and Dr Lindstrom if they think there is a finite probability that there is a third sort of subunit which might help to resolve this argument?

Lindstrom: I think the probability that there is a third type of subunit is low. We've purified receptor subtypes from chicken brain, rat brain and bovine brain. All of these species give us two subunits, which when expressed in *Xenopus* oocytes produce functional receptors. Because we don't see them, and we don't seem to need them for functional receptors, I think it is unlikely that the receptors we have studied contain more than two kinds of subunits.

Colquhoun: But these receptors expressed in oocytes, although they are functional, probably have the wrong conductance. It is not yet clear that they are the real receptors.

Heinemann: I think the probability of additional subunits is reasonably high! The kind of genetic screening we have done to find these subunits has been very difficult because these genes are not closely related at the DNA level. We could have easily missed some that have diverged from the α and β subunits that we have found so far. Secondly, we have done some PCR experiments, which are much more sensitive, and we have evidence that there are more genes related to the nicotinic receptors, we just haven't characterized them yet. Thirdly, if you look at the history of the *Torpedo* receptor, where it was easy to purify the protein, it was difficult to figure out how many subunits there were from the protein chemistry. The protein chemistry in the CNS is much more difficult. It is a tremendous achievement of Jon's to find these subunits and I think there could easily be more subunits.

Changeux: Did you look at the N-terminal sequence of all the subunits that you have? Is there any homology of the N-terminal sequence in any of the α and β bands you are looking at? It is an average population of brain nicotinic receptors and there might be some dominant species. But, if there are several subunit genes, these subunits must contribute to the mass of the whole receptor population in the brain.

Lindstrom: They do, but there are dominant subtypes. In rat brain, receptors composed of α subunits purified by immunoaffinity with mAb 270 account for 90% of the high affinity nicotine binding sites. The β2 structural subunit, located both by *in situ* hybridization (Wada et al 1989) and by mAb 270 binding (Swanson et al 1987), is dominant.

If we look at the N-terminal sequence, whether we purify the receptor using a monoclonal antibody specific for the β2 subunit or one specific for the α4 subunit, we get a single sequence (Schoepfer et al 1988).

Grunberg: Jon, in your figure of chick and rat brain [^{3}H]nicotine cholinergic binding, you did not present data for nicotine as an antagonist in the rat brain, although you did show various doses of nicotine acting as an antagonist in the chicken brain. Is this because nicotine was not tried in that experiment or because nicotine did not antagonize in rat brain?

Lindstrom: It competes. Those experiments measured [^{3}H]nicotine binding. We have done that experiment, but the results weren't on the figure (Whiting & Lindstrom 1986, 1987).

Heinemann: We have found that nicotine activates all the nicotinic receptor subtypes tested so far: α2β2, a3β2, a4β2, a2β4, a3β4, a4β4.

Grunberg: The reason I ask is that for those of us interested in the neurobiology of dependence, the rat has provided a very good model.

Heinemann: The genes that we have identified are all rat genes.

Collins: Jon, you showed that there were greater concentrations of [^{3}H]nicotine binding in the neonatal chick brain than in the adult. Why are there two different nicotinic receptors (if you believe the bungarotoxin binding site is one) at higher concentrations in the neonatal brain than in the adult?

Lindstrom: One answer is programmed cell death, another is a parallel to what happens in muscle before innervation or after denervation where there are extrajunctional receptors all over the surface of the muscle and only receptors turning over very slowly at junctions thereafter.

Kellar: I would like to come back to the α3 subunit. This is found in ganglion cells and also in PC12 cells. There have been several unsuccessful attempts to bind nicotine and other ligands to those receptors. The α3 subunit also occurs in brain.

Heinemann: And in the adrenal gland.

Kellar: Is that the one receptor that might be different from the other receptors labelled by agonists?

Lindstrom: Receptors containing the α3 subunit seem to have much lower affinity for nicotine than do receptors containing the α4 or α2 subunits.

Heinemann: We shouldn't talk about just α subunits. We have evidence that the pharmacology can depend on which β subunit is associated with the α subunit.

Kellar: Is there a complex of α3 with any β that will bind nicotine with high affinity?

Heinemann: We haven't measured nicotine binding. To get back to the PC12 cells, by analysing the mRNAs, we know that α3 and α5 and also β2 and β4 are expressed in PC12 cells. We know from expression in oocytes that properties of the α3 receptor are very different depending on whether it is associated with β2 or β4. α3β4 gives a bursting pattern when it binds ACh, it opens and closes in bursts and stays open for a long period of time, whereas α3β2 does not. This work was done by Dr Roger Papke in our group.

Lindstrom: There seem to be more subtype mRNAs than we know what to do with. It could be that different subunit combinations are used at different developmental times in the same cell type.

Heinemann: Dr Irm Hermans-Borgmeyer in our group found that the mRNAs for some of the genes are expressed at very high levels in the embryo. It could be something to do with the way innervation is taking place. We have also cloned one of the glutamate receptors, which from the structure is a member of the same superfamily as the nicotinic receptors. The NMDA receptor is involved during development in setting up some of the neural networks.

Lindstrom: At the Society for Neuroscience Meeting in Phoenix, USA, 1989, Stuart Lipton (Abstract 263.6) presented very interesting results indicating that ganglion cells in culture express both NMDA receptors and nicotinic receptors on neurites. Agonists for either receptor cause the neurite to retract. This is an example of receptors at non-synaptic sites doing things you might not expect. Even though they have channels open for only milliseconds, they might affect developmental processes whose effects last a life time.

Awad: Since there are species and tissue-specific differences in the molecular structure of the nicotinic receptor, does the binding affinity of nicotine in the brain differ between species? I have found that the peripheral-type benzodiazepine binding sites show dramatic species-specific differences in their binding affinity (Awad & Gavish 1987).

Lindstrom: It's important when discussing neuronal nicotinic receptors not to move casually between species, especially if you are only making pharmacological measures. For example, snake muscle ACh receptors do not bind αBgt, whereas muscle-type ACh receptors from most other species do. This is not of great significance; there are a couple of amino acid differences in the binding sites of receptors from those species that are particularly relevant. It doesn't mean you are talking about a completely different kind of receptor. Similarly, we should not make too much of pharmacological differences of neuronal nicotinic receptors between species, but should classify receptors where possible in terms of genes that encode particular subunits, which is becoming feasible.

Collins: We have looked at [^{3}H]nicotine binding in mouse, rat and human and there is not a measurable difference in the binding affinities.

Awad: For peripheral-type benzodiazepine binding sites there is a K_d of 1 nM in rat tissues and more than 10 µM in calf tissues (Awad & Gavish 1987).

Collins: We find K_ds of 2–5 nM in human brain, rat brain and mouse brain.

Gray: Could somebody explain why there are different genes coding for different subunits that are all going to respond to ACh as a nicotinic receptor?

Lindstrom: The region in which the homologies diverge most dramatically is the region between the 3rd and 4th hydrophobic domains which, at least in muscle receptors, is on the cytoplasmic surface. This sequence is unique to each subtype. That could mean either that it is very important in defining the unique properties of these subtypes, or that it's very unimportant because there's little genetic constraint on the sequence. The cytoplasmic domain is the part of the receptor that is phosphorylated, which could affect its activation, the rate of desensitization, its association with peripheral postsynaptic membrane proteins, such as the 43 kDa protein, or its association with the cytoskeleton, which might localize the receptor to either specific presynaptic or postsynaptic localizations or affect transport of the receptor from the cell body to the periphery.

Wonnacott: The $\alpha2$ subunit is abundant in chick brain compared with the small amounts in rat brain which are very localized. Do you know the distribution in chick brain and possible functional significance? Could behavioural pharmacologists do anything with the chick to explore the significance of the abundance of this subunit?

Lindstrom: No one seems interested in using chick for behavioural studies.

Changeux: There is another set of interpretations that concerns the developmental aspects. If you want to have a given receptor gene expressed in a given cell in the brain, instead of re-using the same receptor gene for all different locations, it may be easier to duplicate that gene, add this receptor gene to the battery of genes already expressed in that cell, and have the differentiation controlled by a master gene.

Gray: I was very impressed by the restricted localization of the $\alpha2$ subunit to just a couple of nuclei in the rat brain. Is there any point to that localization, unless that receptor does something functionally different to the others that are not similarly localized?

Changeux: The regulatory sequences that control the expression of a given set of genes in a given neuron or set of neurons may share common elements. In addition, regulatory proteins acting on these DNA elements may specify this particular neuron.

Gray: Then these different genes may in no way relate to the different kinds of behavioural pharmacology in the adult animal that Ian Stolerman described.

Changeux: They may have evolved independently and just by chance possess different structural properties. On the other hand, it would be interesting for the pharmacologist to distinguish these different gene products in order to make reagents targeted to different areas of the brain.

Heinemann: I think we are over-emphasizing how similar these receptor proteins are. When you first see the sequence, you look for similarities and focus on this feature. As Jon said, the cytoplasmic region, which is likely to interact with cellular mechanisms, is totally different in the different subunits. $\alpha2$ in the cytoplasmic region has a PEST sequence that has been shown to confer instability in other proteins, so the $\alpha2$ receptor may be turning over very rapidly and might be used for specific transient functions.

We have done single channel recordings on many of the combinations and each combination has different biophysical properties. I think they should be regarded as different receptors that just happen to bind nicotine.

Schwartz: Similar problems have come up with the GABA receptor; people have identified different subtypes with different combinations of subunits. The pharmacology has been used to compare concentration–response curves of electrophysiological recordings and binding to look at the different sensitivities for all the combinations. We can now use selective benzodiazepines, which have different clinical properties, to separate effects on sedation from anticonvulsant effects, for example, and start to associate the different clinical effects with various benzodiazepine/GABA receptor subtypes.

Iversen: The molecular pharmacological studies done in the last few years have revealed a remarkable difference between the neural and brain-type nicotinic receptors and those in the periphery. They may be similar in their evolution, but their pharmacologies are very different, particularly in the sensitivity to nicotine, which is why smokers can smoke without incurring muscular paralysis via peripheral receptors!

References

Awad M, Gavish M 1987 Binding of [^{3}H]Ro 5-4864 and [^{3}H]PK 11195 to cerebral cortex and peripheral tissues of various species: species differences and heterogeneity in peripheral benzodiazepine binding sites. J Neurochem 49:1407–1414

Dennis M, Giraudat J, Kotzyba-Hibert F et al 1988 Amino acids of the *Torpedo marmorata* acetylcholine receptor α subunit labeled by a photoaffinity ligand for the acetylcholine binding site. Biochemistry 27:2346–2357

DiPaola M, Czajkowski C, Karlin A 1989 The sidedness of the COOH terminus of the acetylcholine δ subunit. J Biol Chem 264:15457–15463

Duvoisin R, Deneris E, Patrick J, Heinemann S 1989 The functional diversity of the neuronal nicotinic receptors is increased by a novel subunit: β4. Neuron 3:487–496

Glazi JL, Revah F, Black D, Goeldner M, Hirth C, Changeux JP 1990 Identification of a novel amino acid αTyr 93 within the active site of the acetylcholine receptor by photoaffinity labeling: additional evidence for a three loop model of the acetylcholine binding site. Submitted

Halvorsen S, Berg DK 1987 Affinity labeling of neuronal acetylcholine receptors with an α neurotoxin that blocks receptor function. J Neurosci 7:2547–2555

Kubalek E, Ralston S, Lindstrom J, Unwin N 1987 Location of subunits within the acetylcholine receptor: analysis of tubular crystals from Torpedo marmorata. J Cell Biol 105:9–18

McCrea PD, Popot JL, Engelman DM 1987 Transmembrane topography of the nicotinic acetylcholine receptor δ subunit. EMBO (Eur Mol Biol Organ) J 6:3619–3626

Papke R, Boulter J, Patrick J, Heinemann S 1989 Single-channel currents of rat neuronal nicotinic acetylcholine receptors expressed in Xenopus laevis oocytes. Neuron 3:589–596

Rapier C, Wonnacott S, Lunt G, Albuquerque E 1987 The neurotoxin histrionicotoxin interacts with the putative ion channel of the nicotinic acetylcholine receptors in the central nervous system. FEBS (Fed Eur Biochem Soc) Lett 212:292–296

Ratnam M, Le Nguyen D, Rivier J, Sargent PB, Lindstrom J 1986 Transmembrane topography of nicotinic acetylcholine receptor: immunochemical tests contradict theoretical predictions based on hydrophobicity profiles. Biochemistry 25:2633–2643

Schoepfer R, Whiting P, Esch F, Blacher R, Shimasaki S, Lindstrom J 1988 cDNA clones coding for the structural subunit of a chicken brain nicotinic acetylcholine receptor. Neuron 1:241–248

Swanson L, Simmons D, Whiting P, Lindstrom J 1987 Immunohistochemical localization of neuronal nicotinic receptors in the rodent central nervous system. J Neurosci 7:3334–3342

Unwin PNT, Zampighi G 1980 Structure of the junction between communicating cells. Nature (Lond) 545–549

Wada E, Wada K, Boulter J et al 1989 The distribution of $\alpha 2$, $\alpha 3$, $\alpha 4$ and $\beta 2$ neuronal nicotinic receptor subunit mRNAs in the central nervous system: a hybridization histochemical study in the rat. J Comp Neurol 284:314–335

Whiting P, Lindstrom J 1986 Pharmacological properties of immunoisolated neuronal nicotinic receptors. J Neurosci 6:3061–3069

Whiting P, Lindstrom J 1987 Purification and characterization of a nicotinic acetylcholine receptor from rat brain. Proc Natl Acad Sci USA 84:595–599

Whiting P, Esch F, Shimasaki S, Lindstrom J 1987 Neuronal nicotinic acetylcholine receptor β subunit is coded for by the cDNA clone $\alpha 4$. FEBS (Fed Eur Biochem Soc) Lett 219:459–463

Wolf KM, Ciarleglio A, Chiappinelli V 1988 Kappa-Bungarotoxin: binding of a neuronal nicotinic receptor antagonist to chick optic lobe and skeletal muscle. Brain Res 439:249–258

Young E, Ralston E, Blake J, Ramachandran J, Hall Z, Stroud R 1985 Topological mapping of acetylcholine receptor: evidence for a model with five transmembrane segments and a cytoplasmic COOH-terminal peptide. Proc Natl Acad Sci USA 82:626–630

Mechanism of action of the nicotinic acetylcholine receptor

Joe Henry Steinbach

Department of Anesthesiology and Department of Anatomy and Neurobiology, Washington University School of Medicine, 660 South Euclid Avenue, Saint Louis, MO 63110, USA

Abstract. Nicotinic acetylcholine receptors at peripheral synapses mediate rapid and effective excitatory synaptic transmission. The functional properties of peripheral and central nicotinic acetylcholine receptors are similar, yet in the central nervous system nicotinic receptors do not appear to occur postsynaptically at many excitatory synapses. Two properties of nicotinic receptors are that significant Ca^{2+} influx can occur through the receptor channel and that at low agonist concentrations steady activation of nicotinic receptors can occur. These are discussed in the context of presynaptic and postsynaptic localizations of nicotinic receptors.

1990 The biology of nicotine dependence. Wiley, Chichester (Ciba Foundation Symposium 152) p 53–67

This paper considers the question of how nicotinic acetylcholine receptors are activated, and what happens once they are.

What do nicotinic receptors do at the neuromuscular junction?

The nicotinic acetylcholine receptor (AChR) at the skeletal neuromuscular junction is involved in the rapid and essentially one-for-one transmission of a presynaptic action potential to cause an action potential in the muscle. We have a reasonably detailed picture of the activation properties of this type of receptor (Table 1, reviewed in Steinbach 1989). Binding of ACh is rapid and of relatively low affinity; high degrees of occupancy are likely to be achieved because of an extremely high ACh concentration transient in the cleft (probably about 10 times the dissociation constant). Channel opening is rare for unliganded or monoliganded AChR, but occurs at a high rate for diliganded AChR. The rates for channel opening and for ACh dissociation are approximately equal, so a diliganded AChR with a closed channel has a 50:50 or better chance of

TABLE 1   Conductance and burst duration for nicotinic AChR[a]

	Conductance (pS)	Burst (msec)[b]	Note
rat muscle junctional	62	2.3	e
rat muscle non-junctional	42	9.2	e
chick muscle	—[c]	4.5	e
rat sympathetic ganglion	35	11	f
rat parasympathetic	25, 50[d]	5, 30	g
rat chromaffin cell	25	10, 80	h
rat retinal ganglion	35	—	i
chick ciliary ganglion	25, 40	0.4, 1.3	j
chick sympathetic ganglion	20, 35, 50	3	k
Cloned mRNA expressed in *Xenopus* oocytes			
rat $\alpha2 + \beta2$	15, 34	4, 3	l
rat $\alpha3 + \beta2$	5, 15	1.6, 4	l
rat $\alpha4 + \beta2$	7	2	l
chick $\alpha4 + n\alpha$	20	—	m

[a]At -70 mV, room temperature. [b]Neglecting brief bursts. [c]Not reported. [d]Cells showing multiple functional classes of AChR. [e]Abstracted from Steinbach 1989. [f]Mathie et al 1987. [g]D. J. Adams, personal communication 1989. [h]Hirano et al 1987. [i]Lipton et al 1987. [j]Margiotta & Gurantz 1989. [k]L. Role, personal communication 1988. [l]Papke et al 1989. [m]Ballivet et al 1988.

opening its channel. Once open, the channel closing rate is much less than the opening rate, so the probability that a diliganded channel is open rather than closed is quite high, greater than 0.9. Channels open in 'bursts' of several openings separated by short closed intervals, because a closing is often followed by a reopening, given the relative rates for dissociation and channel opening mentioned above. Muscle AChRs desensitize in the continued presence of ACh, but no experiments have shown that desensitization occurs physiologically at normal neuromuscular junctions, where there is esterase activity. However, desensitization does occur at lower concentrations of agonist than does activation and the desensitized form has a higher affinity for ACh, so in the steady state an AChR with bound ACh is more likely to be desensitized than active over a wide range of ACh concentrations.

What are the physiological consequences of this pattern of gating? Muscle AChRs work rapidly and efficiently when given a brief transient of a high ACh concentration. They do not work well when presented with a low or maintained concentration of ACh. The postsynaptic current is large and brief. A rapid rising phase results from ACh diffusing and binding to AChR in a small disc of postsynaptic membrane, and to a lesser degree from a lag between binding and channel opening (reviewed in Salpeter 1987). The slower falling phase is largely determined by the channel burst duration, since rebinding of ACh is rare at junctions with normal levels of ACh esterase activity.

The open channel conducts those cations commonly found in physiological solutions relatively indiscriminately (K^+, Na^+, Mg^{2+}, Ca^{2+}). Divalent ions bind more tightly to sites in the channel than do monovalent ions. They can also reduce conductance by an ion screening effect in the channel 'vestibules'. Overall, divalent ions both permeate the channel and reduce the flux of monovalent ions (Dani 1988, 1989). The obvious physiological role of the ion fluxes is to depolarize the muscle fibre membrane, and this indeed appears to be the major role.

What are nicotinic receptors on neurons like?

In qualitative terms, nicotinic receptors on neurons and chromaffin cells are similar in function to those on muscle fibres. There are quantitative differences in channel burst duration and conductance, and the affinity for ACh may be lower, but overall the similarities are striking (Table 1 and references therein). Channel opening occurs preferentially after binding of more than one ACh molecule, since Hill coefficients are usually larger than one. As far as it has been examined, ion permeation appears generally similar and the reversal potentials in normal solutions are all near 0mV.

When mRNAs coding for receptor subunits are expressed in *Xenopus* oocytes the eggs develop depolarizing responses and inward currents to applied ACh, which have the appropriate pharmacology for nicotinic AChRs. Several combinations of subunit mRNAs have now been expressed in oocytes, and the results are shown in Table 1. One point of interest is that the results for neuronal nicotinic AChRs in cells do not correlate well with the results of expression of defined subunits (Table 1). This is in contrast to AChR from muscle or electroplax, which shows quite similar properties when expressed in oocytes and *in situ* (for example, Mishina et al 1986). There are two possible explanations: one is that additional neuronal subunits have yet to be tested (Isenberg & Meyer 1989, Boulter et al, cited in Papke et al 1989; M. Ballivet, personal communication 1988); the other is that the differences arise from post-translational effects, either in the oocyte or in the neurons.

All nicotinic receptors found on neurons or neuron-related cells show quite strong desensitization on prolonged applications of nicotinic agonists. The high affinity nicotine-binding site in brain (reflecting largely receptors composed of $\alpha4$ and $\beta2$ subunits; Whiting et al 1987, Schoepfer et al 1988) is a receptor which undergoes a large increase in agonist affinity upon desensitization. Other neuronal nicotinic AChRs do not undergo such a large change in affinity (Kemp & Morley 1986), and even muscle-type receptors show differences (desensitized receptors from *Torpedo* show high affinity, whereas those from *Electrophorus* or rat show lower affinity, see Karlin 1980).

What do nicotinic AChRs on neurons do?

The results in Table 1 show that there are not overwhelming differences in the properties of various nicotinic ACh receptors. This suggests that the neuronal receptors should work in approximately the same fashion as those at the neuromuscular junction. They should mediate rapid excitatory transmission, and be driven by a large, brief increase in ACh concentration. This appears to be true for peripheral nicotinic synapses. However, in the brain rapid excitation is apparently subserved by the non-NMDA (N-methyl-D-aspartate) class of excitatory amino acid receptor in the vast majority of cases examined.

**Two additional properties of
nicotinic AChRs and one question of location**

There are two properties of nicotinic AChRs which suggest that these receptors could take part in other physiological interactions at synapses. The first is the ability of the nicotinic AChR channel to conduct Ca^{2+} ions. The second is that nicotinic AChRs can show steady-state activation at low agonist concentrations. Finally, if nicotinic AChRs in the central nervous system (CNS) were located presynaptically, the physiological consequences of receptor activation might be altered or enhanced by the small size of the presynaptic bouton.

Ca^{2+} flux

Although the AChR channel is viewed as a non-selective cation channel, the Ca^{2+} flux through an open channel is not very different from that through a voltage-gated Ca^{2+} channel for equal driving force. For the channel on BC_3H1 cells (from a mouse brain tumour), which have a mammalian muscle-type receptor, the inward Ca^{2+} current at negative membrane potentials is about 2% of the total current, which is equivalent to a conductance of 0.8 pS (J. Dani, personal communication 1989). The neuronal nicotinic AChR found on rat parasympathetic ganglion cells has the same or higher Ca^{2+} permeability (D. J. Adams, personal communication 1989) as does the receptor expressed in *Xenopus* oocytes injected with rat $\alpha3$ and $\beta2$ subunit mRNAs (J. Dani, personal communication 1989). In comparison, the conductance of voltage-gated Ca^{2+}-selective channels is about 0.5–1 pS in physiological solutions (Fenwick et al 1982, Hess et al 1986). AChR channels open at negative membrane potentials, at which the driving force for Ca^{2+} is maximal, in contrast to voltage-gated Ca^{2+} channels. However, Ca^{2+} channels have a much more positive reversal potential so they will conduct inward Ca^{2+} current at potentials positive with respect to 0mV, whereas AChR channels will pass little inward Ca^{2+} current at potentials positive with respect to their reversal potential.

The consequences of this hypothetical Ca^{2+} influx cannot be assessed, since the detailed location, density and activation properties of the receptors are unknown. However, it might well affect presynaptic processes such as facilitation and potentiation of release, as well as general properties such as Ca^{2+}-dependent membrane conductances or enzymic activities.

Persistent activation

Katz & Miledi (1977) first demonstrated a persistent, very small depolarization at neuromuscular junctions treated with antiesterases, which apparently results from the continuous application of a low concentration of ACh to the postsynaptic membrane. The relevance of this observation in the present context is that it shows there can be a 'window current' at low concentrations of agonist—a persistent activation in the absence of complete desensitization. The size of this current will depend on the concentration dependences of the activation and steady-state desensitization curves for the particular receptor. Lipton (1988) has made similar observations for rat retinal ganglion cells in culture.

Presynaptic localization

The physiological effects of receptor activation need to be assessed in light of the small size of the bouton and attached small diameter fibre, which constitute the 'postsynaptic' element of a presynaptically located receptor. The membrane properties of boutons are not known, but if we assume that a 'typical' bouton is a sphere 2 μm in diameter and the attached axon is an infinite cable 0.2 μm in diameter, then the input resistance of the bouton is approximately $3-10 \times 10^9$ ohm. A single channel providing an inward current of 1pA (for example, a muscle-type channel open at a membrane potential of $-25\,mV$) would depolarize the bouton by more than 1mV. Another way to state the same relationship is that the input conductance of the bouton is about $1-3 \times 10^{-10}\,S$, so the steady opening of 2–30 channels would shift the membrane potential halfway to the reversal potential.

An inward Ca^{2+} current of 1pA flowing for 10 msec carries about 30 000 Ca^{2+} ions, enough to raise the average intrabouton Ca^{2+} concentration to 12 μM. The rough estimates given earlier suggest that a total AChR-mediated current of 50pA would carry this much Ca^{2+} current, corresponding to the activation of 20–100 channels. It should be pointed out that this is 10% of the available extracellular Ca^{2+} (if we assume that the available extracellular volume contains 2 mM Ca^{2+} and is a shell 20 nm thick surrounding the bouton). Hence Ca^{2+} entry would result in a significant increase in intracellular Ca^{2+} and perhaps a significant depletion of extracellular Ca^{2+}.

Non-traditional nicotinic mechanisms in the CNS

This speculative discussion will point out some possible mechanisms by which nicotinic AChRs might work in a 'non-traditional' way in the CNS. The discussion will consider two pairs of alternatives: (1) should we view the mechanism of action as mediated by the traditional general cation conductance or by Ca^{2+} influx, and (2) should we view the localization as postsynaptic or presynaptic?

The consequences of the increase in conductance depend on the duration of action. A long-lasting depolarization (perhaps 30 msec, to $-30\,mV$) can result in gating of voltage-dependent conductances, including inactivation of Na^+- and some K^+- and Ca^{2+}-selective channels and opening of some K^+-selective channels. The net effect is likely to be a decrease in excitability by inactivation of inward-conducting channels. This could have major effects presynaptically by reducing the presynaptic action potential and Ca^{2+} current. Even if the steady depolarization is slight, random opening and closing of nicotinic AChR channels could provide a brief pulse of inward current large enough to bring a bouton to threshold for an action potential. For instance, a single muscle-type channel in a bouton with an input resistance of 10 Gohm would depolarize the bouton from $-60\,mV$ to $-50\,mV$ if it remained open longer than about 5 msec. A steady level of random channel activation could produce a randomly occurring background activity presynaptically.

Postsynaptically this mechanism would be less important if the receptors were located on the soma or proximal dendrites, since it appears that postsynaptic nicotinic effects in the CNS are unlikely to involve large conductance increases or depolarizations. However, for receptors on small diameter distal dendrites two possible effects can be envisaged. During the conductance increase, the currents from more distal inputs would be shunted and information lost. In addition, dendrites have a number of voltage- and Ca^{2+}-dependent currents (reviewed in Hounsgaard & Midtgaard 1989), which might be affected. If the depolarization lasted only a short time, it would have significantly smaller effects. The duration of the depolarization would depend on the time course of the transient increase in ACh concentration, on the channel burst duration and on the time constant of the membrane, none of which are known.

Ca^{2+} entry could have major effects, but they are even harder to predict. Simulations of the transient increase in intracellular Ca^{2+} concentration after gating of Ca^{2+} channels show very large spatial and temporal gradients (reviewed in Smith & Augustine 1988). It seems likely that a nicotinic AChR channel would produce a similar pattern. Depending on the duration of influx and the location of sites of action (e.g. Ca^{2+}-activated K^+-channels or release zones), very rapid, profound effects could result. Depending on the volume of the cytoplasmic compartment, the intracellular Ca^{2+} concentration could rise rather high for a prolonged period. The effects on membrane channels could include increased K^+ conductance, increased non-selective cation conductance and reduced Ca^{2+} conductance. Overall, it seems most likely that there would be an increase in resting outward current. This current would offset the nicotinic receptor current, and also would increase the membrane shunt. Presynaptically it would probably increase the probability of failure of action potentials to invade a bouton. Postsynaptically it would reduce excitatory input and shunt more distal inputs. Presynaptic effects on release would depend on the location of the channels; most likely, there would be enhanced facilitation. Other consequences of Ca^{2+} influx are too multifarious to enumerate; for example, one explanation for anticholinesterase-induced myopathy is that the enhanced Ca^{2+} influx at the neuromuscular junction stimulates Ca^{2+}-dependent proteases (Leonard & Salpeter 1979).

So what might happen in the presence of nicotine?

It is clear that we cannot give any answer here. It is not even certain whether we should be looking for mechanisms involving nicotinic presynaptic inhibition or postsynaptic excitation. In addition, it is unclear whether chronic nicotine intake results in persistent desensitization or persistent activation. If the high-affinity nicotine-binding component is the site of action, then desensitization seems most likely. In the case of other receptors, it is hard to know.

Summary and outlook

There are more uncertainties than data, but it is apparent that a relatively small number of nicotinic AChRs on presynaptic terminals could have effects on release. Unfortunately, it is not obvious whether the effects will be inhibitory or stimulatory because the sign of the effect depends on the properties of the receptors and other properties of the terminal membrane and release mechanism. One problem is that the effects may not be very robust, which makes it difficult to find a suitable synapse to study. It is clear that analysis of the functioning of the brain nicotinic AChR must take place at two levels. We need more information about the biophysical properties of receptors of defined structure. Even more, though, we need clear examples of CNS synapses where the physiological effects of receptor activation can be examined in detail.

Acknowledgements

I thank D. J. Adams, M. Ballivet, J. Boulter, J. Dani, J. Margiotta, R. Papke and L. Role for discussion of unpublished results and C. Ifune, C. Lingle and E. McCleskey for general discussions. Work in my lab is supported by grant NS 22356.

References

Ballivet M, Nef P, Couturier S et al 1988 Electrophysiology of a chick neuronal nicotinic acetylcholine receptor expressed in Xenopus oocytes after cDNA injection. Neuron 1:847–852

Dani J 1988 Ionic permeability and the open channel structure of the nicotinic acetylcholine receptor. In: Pullman A et al (eds) Transport through membranes: carriers, channels and pumps. Kluwer Academic Publishers, p 297–319

Dani J 1989 Site-directed mutagenesis and single-channel currents define the ionic channel of the nicotinic acetylcholine receptor. Trends Neurosci 12:125–128

Fenwick EM, Marty A, Neher E 1982 Sodium and calcium channels in bovine chromaffin cells. J Physiol (Lond) 331:599–635

Hess P, Lansman JB, Tsien RW 1986 Calcium channel selectivity for divalent and monovalent cations. J Gen Physiol 88:293–319

Hirano T, Kidokoro Y, Ohmori H 1987 Acetylcholine dose-response relation and the effect of cesium ions in the rat adrenal chromaffin cell under voltage clamp. Pfluegers Arch Eur J Physiol 408:401–407

Hounsgaard J, Midtgaard J 1989 Dendrite processing in more ways than one. Trends Neurosci 12:313–315

Isenberg KE, Meyer GE 1989 Cloning of a putative neuronal nicotinic acetylcholine receptor subunit. J Neurochem 52:988–991

Karlin A 1980 Molecular properties of nicotinic acetylcholine receptors. In: Cotman CW et al (eds) The cell surface and neuronal function. Elsevier Science Publishers, Amsterdam, p 191–260

Katz B, Miledi R 1977 Transmitter leakage from motor nerve endings. Proc R Soc Lond B Biol Sci 196:59–72

Kemp G, Morley BJ 1986 Ganglionic nACHRs and high-affinity nicotinic binding sites are not equivalent. FEBS (Fed Eur Biochem Soc) Lett 205:265–268

Leonard JP, Salpeter MM 1979 Agonist-induced myopathy at the neuromuscular junction is mediated by calcium. J Cell Biol 82:811–819

Lipton SA 1988 Spontaneous release of acetylcholine affects the physiological nicotinic responses of rat retinal ganglion cells in culture. J Neurosci 8:3857–3868

Lipton SA, Aizenman E, Loring RH 1987 Neural nicotinic acetylcholine responses in solitary mammalian retinal ganglion cells. Pfluegers Arch Eur J Physiol 410:37–43

Margiotta J, Gurantz D 1989 Changes in the number, function and regulation of nicotinic acetylcholine receptors during neuronal development. Dev Biol 135:326–339

Mathie A, Cull-Candy SG, Colquhoun D 1987 Single-channel and whole-cell currents evoked by acetylcholine in dissociated sympathetic neurons of the rat. Proc R Soc Lond B Biol Sci 232:239–248

Mishina M, Toshiyuki T, Keiji I et al 1986 Molecular distinction between fetal and adult forms of muscle acetylcholine receptor. Nature (Lond) 321:406–410

Papke RL, Boulter J, Patrick J, Heinemann S 1989 Single channel currents of rat neuronal nicotinic acetylcholine receptors expressed in *Xenopus laevis* oocytes. Neuron 3:589–596

Salpeter MM 1987 The vertebrate neuromuscular junction. Alan R. Liss, New York, p 1–54

Schoepfer R, Whiting P, Esch F, Blacher R, Shimasaki S, Lindstrom J 1988 cDNA clones coding for structural subunit of a chicken brain nicotinic acetylcholine receptor. Neuron 1:241–248

Smith SJ, Augustine GJ 1988 Calcium ions, active zones and synaptic transmitter release. Trends Neurosci 11:458–464

Steinbach JH 1989 Structural and functional diversity in vertebrate skeletal muscle nicotinic acetylcholine receptors. Annu Rev Physiol 51:353–365

Whiting P, Esch F, Shimasaki S, Lindstrom J 1987 Neuronal nicotinic acetylcholine receptor β-subunit is coded for by the cDNA clone α_4. FEBS (Fed Eur Biochem Soc) Lett 219:459–463

DISCUSSION

Lindstrom: There is evidence from a number of quarters that many of these neuronal nicotinic receptors are presynaptic, so the mechanisms could be very important. Calcium influx through receptor channels may have effects in addition to facilitating transmitter release. For example, Stuart Lipton has described nicotinic receptors on nerve growth cones and shown that adding ACh causes retraction of the processes. He showed evidence that this was mediated largely by calcium passage through these receptors.

Other ion fluxes could also be important. Wong & Gallagher (1989) found ACh-gated K^+ channels in rat brains. They showed that these receptors were blocked by neuronal bungarotoxin (Bgt). They didn't test whether they were blocked by α-bungarotoxin (αBgt). This sort of K^+ channel in αBgt-binding proteins could have escaped detection, since it's an inhibitory channel.

Steinbach: One additional possibility is that nicotinic receptors directly mediate postsynaptic inhibition. Cells in the dorsolateral septal nucleus in rats show a hyperpolarization in response to nicotinic agonists, without any preceding depolarization (Wong & Gallagher 1989). This response differs from that reported by McCormick & Prince (1987) in medial habenular cells, in which a membrane hyperpolarization followed a nicotinic depolarization, and apparently was elicited by the initial depolarization. Nicotine has also been reported to reduce the frequency of extracellularly recorded action potentials of cerebellar Purkinje cells (de la Garza et al 1987). However, we have seen no effect of ACh on Purkinje cells in cell cultures (J. Zempel & J.H. Steinbach, unpublished observations).

The mechanism of this nicotinic postsynaptic inhibition in vertebrate cells is not clear; for example, it is possible that a Ca^{2+} influx could activate a K^+ conductance (Tokimasa & North 1984). However, there are inhibitory responses on invertebrate neurons that are apparently directly mediated by nicotinic receptors (Kehoe 1972). The cloned vertebrate neuronal nicotinic ACh receptor subunits all result in expression of channels with reversal potentials near 0mV, so none of them could directly mediate inhibition.

Kellar: What would happen to your calculations if the receptors were not on the axon terminal but were on the cell body?

Steinbach: If they were postsynaptically localized on the cell body, the effects would be qualitatively similar but quantitatively close to negligible, particularly at a low density ($100/\mu m^2$). If they were on distal dendrites, which have an average diameter of less than a micron, then the consequences would be similar to those of presynaptic receptors. The electrical characteristics are similar to those of presynaptic boutons, and the small volume of a section of dendrite might result in appreciable changes in intracellular Ca^{2+} concentrations.

Changeux: Meyer Jackson has shown that ACh channels may open spontaneously in the absence of ACh. Such recordings can be used to assay the ratio between the sensitized and resting states. Has this been shown for the neuronal receptor?

Steinbach: We have not confirmed Meyer Jackson's results. He is using primary rat myotubes and we use mouse BC_3H1 cells, but they both express muscle α, β, δ γ subunits in their ACh receptors.

Changeux: The results may vary with the allosteric constant. Is the allosteric constant for the brain receptor the same as that for the muscle receptor? In muscle, the receptor is stabilized in the 'resting', activatable conformation so that the neuromuscular junction is almost 100% efficient in transmitting nerve impulses. In the brain, there may be cholinergic synapses that are not 100% efficient. On the other hand, they may be preferentially stabilized in a desensitized conformation with a relatively low transmission efficiency. They may be subject to 'sensitization' by allosteric effectors. For the NMDA receptor, glycine is an allosteric activating effector, for the GABA receptor, benzodiazepines are activating.

Steinbach: PC12 cells don't show spontaneous openings (C. Ifune, J. H. Steinbach, unpublished observations). I don't think such openings occur in peripheral-type neuronal nicotinic receptors, is that right?

Colquhoun: We see no obvious spontaneous openings in rat or frog endplates, or in sympathetic neurons. If they are there, their rate must be much lower than that Jackson sees.

Steinbach: An implication of Lipton's (1988) paper on release of ACh in retinal cultures is that there is a very low spontaneous rate of opening for the nicotinic receptor channels of neonatal rat ciliary ganglion cells, although he does not explicitly address this point. That's the extent of our knowledge about central nicotinic receptors. I am not convinced that spontaneous openings are relevant for any nicotinic receptors.

Changeux: Do you think that in nicotinic synapses in the brain the receptor is in a state that has low efficiency? Are there regulatory systems that activate them, by analogy with the other receptors (NMDA, GABA) that I mentioned earlier?

Steinbach: I think that's probably right. There may not even be a nicotinic synapse in the sense of physically defined presynaptic and postsynaptic elements with a close morphological relationship to each other. It may be a much more diffuse entity. If the nicotinic response were elicited by receptor working at relatively low concentrations of agonists, it would no longer be necessary to have as defined a synaptic structure. That would also make it physiologically harder to look at, because the strong synapses are the ones that you notice; weak synapses could remain undetected for a long time.

Colquhoun: Why do you say it might be that way? The only one that has been characterized is the Renshaw cell synapse, which is supposed to be a classical fast one.

Steinbach: I don't have a reason, except for the fact that nicotinic receptors are found in regions such as the cortex, where it is not clear to me that strong nicotinic effects have been shown that would reflect a ganglionic-type synapse. Perhaps there doesn't have to be a ganglionic-type synapse for the receptors to be physiologically apparent.

Colquhoun: Until recently, when people talked about central cholinergic mechanisms they always meant muscarinic. But if you ask the people who deal with that subject whether they think the fibres that release ACh, which undoubtedly has muscarinic effects, are there solely to have slow effects or whether these fibres also release a fast transmitter, they have no idea.

Steinbach: So do you think fast nicotinic transmission might be widespread in the CNS, we just don't know about it yet?

Colquhoun: I see no evidence that bears on this in one way or the other, except perhaps the Renshaw cell.

Grunberg: This conference is about the biology of nicotine dependence and not the biology of cholinergic action. Therefore, if we take the kind of approach that you have done, but consider that in the human or animal self-administering nicotine there are elevated tonic levels during the day plus bursts in specific regions of the brain, could you speculate about the effects of these phenomena in terms of physiological function.

Steinbach: The difficulty is that there are very few data on nicotine as a desensitizing agent. If you apply 100 μM nicotine to any neuron that's been studied by recording postsynaptically, it desensitizes. For PC12 cells, where nicotine action has been studied by radioactive Na^+ flux, nicotine is somewhat better at desensitizing than ACh (Boyd 1987). There the EC_{50} of nicotine is about 3μM.

Grunberg: But you are still talking about *in vitro* preparations.

Steinbach: A problem with determining brain levels of nicotine in smokers is that they consist of peaks and troughs. The peak of nicotine in the brain lasts for a few minutes. That's an infinite amount of time with respect to many of these desensitization processes, particularly at 37 °C. The peak concentration is probably several hundred nanomolar. My bet is that during the peak time there is an initial phase of excitation, if the nicotine enters the brain quickly enough, followed by some desensitization. At some time during the trough in brain nicotine concentration, the receptor may or may not recover from that desensitization. I don't know whether the net effect during the trough would be tonic activation of brain receptors or whether everything would stay desensitized.

Gray: I keep hearing about desensitization of the nicotinic receptor. Then there are behavioural effects such as those Ian Stolerman described earlier, which people talk about in terms of tolerance. Tolerance in locomotion, for example, meant that what was initially a locomotor depressant effect turns into a locomotor activational effect as you give chronic nicotine. That is only tolerance if you choose to interpret it that way. I am not sure I know of any good behavioural examples that are quite clearly desensitization or tolerance.

We have been looking at noradrenaline release in the rat hippocampus. We give a dose of 0.8 mg/kg nicotine systemically and measure release by an *in vivo* dialysis probe. We see (S. N. Mitchell, M. P. Brazell, personal communication) a pulsatile release of noradrenaline followed by a 30% elevation of the baseline that lasts for 100–120 minutes. A second systemic injection elicits another pulse release of the transmitter which is as big as the first; so we see no desensitization. Both the elevated baseline and the second response are inhibited by mecamylamine, so they are mediated by nicotinic receptors.

London: We find evidence for desensitization at a receptor binding level (Takayama et al 1989). Incubation with concentrations of ATP up to 1 mM increases the affinity for ACh recognition sites, assayed with [³H]methyl-cabrabmyl choline. This observation suggests desensitization. An involvement of ATP in desensitization is consistent with what we know about phosphorylation reactions. In contrast, concentrations of ATP greater than 1 mM enhance the binding of probes such as [³H]mecamylamine and [³H]chlorpromazine, which recognize the inside of the channel. It therefore appears as though higher concentrations of ATP may be involved in resensitization.

Russell: I thought that one of the areas affected by Alzheimer's disease was the nucleus basalis, which contains cholinergic neurons sensitive to nicotine, presumably at a postsynaptic level; and that the projections of these neurons to the cortex release ACh, which might act on muscarinic or nicotinic receptors there. But the cell bodies of the nucleus basalis have nicotinic receptors and is there not evidence of loss of these receptors in Alzheimer's disease? Giving nicotine to patients with Alzheimer's disease can enhance their performance. Is this not an example of a postsynaptic nicotinic receptor in the CNS?

Steinbach: It is an interesting example. The problem is the definition of a 'postsynaptic' response. People have identified nicotinic responses and then conclusively shown that there's no effect of nicotinic antagonists on synaptic transmission in that pathway, for example in the interpeduncular nucleus (Brown et al 1984). Some of those initial correlations have ended up showing that nicotinic synaptic transmission doesn't exist!

Clarke: It's true that David Brown failed to find nicotinic cholinergic transmission in the interpeduncular nucleus. But four studies in rat brain have at least given us preliminary evidence for nicotinic cholinergic transmission. Synaptically driven neuronal responses have been recorded either at the single cell level or as population spikes, and these synaptic responses appeared to possess nicotinic pharmacology, as far as was studied. These include the medial habenula; there is a paragraph in the paper by McCormick & Prince (1987) where they describe short latency excitatory responses of single neurons to local application of ACh and nicotinic agonists.

Similar responses were observed when these cells were driven trans-synaptically by electrical stimulation of the stria medullaris, a mixed nerve pathway that carries the cholinergic input to the medial habenula. Some of my own work on the dopamine cells of the substantia nigra suggests that these neurons receive a nicotinic cholinergic input from the pedunculopontine nucleus (Clarke et al 1987). Again, some earlier work on the cerebellum (McCance & Phillis 1968) indicates a probable nicotinic cholinergic input to this structure.

Steinbach: We tested cultured cerebellar Purkinje cells and could find no effects of ACh (J. Zempel, J. H. Steinbach, unpublished). There's also the example of vasopressin-secreting neurons in the supraoptic nucleus (Cobbett et al 1986).

Clarke: And Misgeld et al (1980) have identified fast postsynaptic responses in rat neostriatum which have a nicotinic pharmacology.

Steinbach: Egan & North (1986) didn't show any effect on synaptic transmission in that system, they only showed a post synaptic response.

Kellar: That's correct. That was a recording from locus ceruleus.

Clarke: The examples I gave were all synaptically driven responses.

London: Concerning Alzheimer's disease and presynaptic versus postsynaptic nicotinic receptors, it's true that cell bodies in the nucleus basalis are cholinergic. Several laboratories have shown decreases in nicotinic receptors in the cerebral cortex and in the hippocampus, using [^{3}H]nicotine or [^{3}H]ACh as ligands (Nordberg & Winblad 1986, Kellar et al 1987, London et al 1989). We found this decrement in nicotinic binding in the brains of patients who died of Alzheimer's disease, which also showed a loss in choline acetyltransferase activity—a presynaptic cholinergic marker (Waller et al 1986). This association suggests that the loss of nicotinic receptors reflects a presynaptic deficit.

Grunberg: Clearly we are speculating when we try to relate behavioural studies to results obtained at the molecular level. We know of some marked and different behavioural reactions to nicotine, such as its effects on craving and satisfaction, which are affected by things such as what time of day the nicotine is taken. We know about actions of the drug that are different under different conditions—stress, physical or psychological. It would be fascinating for the molecular biologists to help those of us who are interested in the process of dependence to consider preparations which aren't designed solely to understand the general physiological mechanism but also take into account controls and groups receiving nicotine repetitively over long periods. It would be useful if the cells from animals chronically exposed to nicotine could be examined.

Steinbach: One of the things I hoped to learn at this meeting was whether people had identified proximal sites of action for at least one effect of nicotine. At the moment I am completely perplexed when presented with a title like that of my paper (Mechanism of action of the ACh receptor) in the context of this meeting. It is not clear what is the physiological role of nicotinic receptors in the brain. However, it would be a great help if I knew cell A is where you look for an effect of nicotine that starts in a second and lasts for a minute.

Gray: Of course understanding the way nicotine and ACh act at the synaptic level will be a critical part of our final understanding, but you cannot approach concepts like craving or memory without asking how the complete neuronal system works. This system consists of many different neuronal mechanisms, only some of which depend on nicotinic cholinergic transmission.

References

Boyd ND 1987 Two distinct phases of desensitisation of acetylcholine receptors of clonal rat PC12 cells. J Physiol (Lond) 389:45–67

Brazell MP, Mitchell SN, Gray JA 1989 Nicotine stimulated dopamine synthesis, release and metabolism in vivo. Br J Pharmacol 96:339

Brown DA, Docherty RJ, Halliwell JV 1984 The action of cholinomimetic substances on impulse conduction in the habenulointerpeduncular pathway of the rat in vitro. J Physiol (Lond) 353:401–409

Clarke PBS, Hommer DW, Pert A, Skirboll LR 1987 Innervation of substantia nigra neurons by cholinergic afferents from the pedunculopontine nucleus in rats: neuroanatomical and electrophysiological evidence. Neuroscience 23:1011–1020

Cobbett P, Mason WT, Poulain DA 1986 Intracellular analysis of control of rat supraoptic neurone activity in vitro by acetylcholine. J Physiol (Lond) 371:216P

de la Garza R, McGuire TJ, Freedman R, Hoffer BJ 1987 The electrophysiological effects of nicotine in the rat cerebellum: evidence for direct postsynaptic actions. Neurosci Lett 80:303–308

Egan TM, North RA 1986 Actions of acetylcholine and nicotine on rat coeruleus neurons in vitro. Neuroscience 19:565–571

Kehoe J 1972 Three acetylcholine receptors in Aplysia neurones. J Physiol (Lond) 225:115–146

Kellar KJ, Whitehouse PJ, Martino-Barrows AM, Marcus K, Price DL 1987 Muscarinic and nicotinic cholinergic binding sites in Alzheimer's disease cerebral cortex. Brain Res 436:62–68

Lipton S 1988 Spontaneous release of acetylcholine affects the physiological nicotinic responses of rat retinal ganglion cells in culture. J Neurosci 8:3857–3868

London ED, Ball MJ, Waller SB 1989 Nicotinic binding sites in cerebral cortex and hippocampus in Alzheimer's dementia. Neurochem Res 14:745–750

McCance I, Phillis JW 1968 Cholinergic mechanisms in the cerebellar cortex. Int J Neurophysiol 7:447–462

McCormick DA, Prince DA 1987 Acetylcholine causes rapid nicotinic excitation in the medial habenular nucleus of Guinea Pig, in vitro. J Neurosci 7:742–752

Misgeld U, Weiler MH, Bak IJ 1980 Intrinsic cholinergic excitation in the rat neuro-striatum: nicotinic and muscarinic receptors. Exp Brain Res 39:401–409

Nordberg A, Winblad B 1986 Reduced number of [^{3}H]nicotine and [^{3}H]acetylcholine binding sites in the frontal cortex of Alzheimer brains. Neurosci Lett 72:115–119

Takayama H, Majewska MD, London ED 1989 ATP: an allosteric modulator of the nicotinic receptor in brain. Soc Neurosci Abstr 15:64

Tokimasa T, North RA 1984 Calcium entry through acetylcholine-channels can activate potassium conductance in bullfrog sympathetic neurones. Brain Res 295:364–367

Waller SB, Ball MJ, Reynolds MA, London ED 1986 Muscarinic binding and choline acetyltransferase in postmortem brains of demented patients. Can J Neurol Sci 13:528–532

Wong LA, Gallagher JP 1989 A direct nicotinic receptor-mediated inhibition recorded intracellularly in vitro. Nature (Lond) 341:439–442

Modulation of nicotine receptors by chronic exposure to nicotinic agonists and antagonists

Allan C. Collins, Ratan V. Bhat, James R. Pauly and Michael J. Marks

Institute for Behavioral Genetics, School of Pharmacy, and Department of Psychology, University of Colorado, Campus Box 447, Boulder, Colorado 80309, USA

Abstract. Although numerous studies have demonstrated that chronic nicotine treatment often results in tolerance to this drug, the mechanisms that underlie this tolerance are not well defined. Recent evidence suggests that chronic nicotine treatment results in an up-regulation of brain nicotinic receptors, but the majority of these receptors may be desensitized or inactivated, thereby explaining tolerance. There is evidence that while all mouse strains show increased receptor numbers following chronic nicotine treatment, some mouse strains develop maximal changes in [^{3}H]nicotine binding before any tolerance is detected. Other strains show a high correlation between increase in receptor number and tolerance. Studies with several other nicotinic agonists indicate that up-regulation of nicotinic receptors can occur without changes in drug sensitivity. Similarly, chronic antagonist treatment can also elicit changes in receptors without affecting sensitivity to nicotine. Some of these discrepancies may be due to genetically influenced interactions between the adrenal steroid, corticosterone (CCS), and the nicotinic receptors. The addition of CCS *in vitro* inhibits binding to nicotinic receptors, and chronic CCS treatment results in decreases in the number of brain nicotinic receptors measured by [^{125}I]bungarotoxin binding. Either of these biochemical measures may explain why altering CCS concentrations *in vivo* results in altered sensitivity to nicotine. It may be that both changes in the number of receptors and altered steroid interactions with the nicotinic receptors explain tolerance to nicotine.

1990 The biology of nicotine dependence. Wiley, Chichester (Ciba Foundation Symposium 152) p 68–86

Chronic drug treatment often results in alterations in the intensity of response to the drug; either reduced (tolerance) or enhanced (supersensitivity) response may be seen. The development of tolerance to nicotine's noxious effects might play a critical role in facilitating the continued use of tobacco. The individuals who develop tolerance to nicotine's noxious effects may be those who progress from experimentation to chronic use. We know very little about the development of tolerance to nicotine in humans, but tolerance to nicotine has been studied in animals. For example, an acute injection of nicotine elicits depressed locomotor activity in the rat (Stolerman et al 1973, Clarke & Kumar 1983) and mouse (Hatchell & Collins 1977), but this effect decreases with chronic treatment.

Nicotine tolerance and receptor up-regulation

Although it is well established that chronic nicotine treatment results in tolerance to the drug, only minimal information is available concerning potential explanations for this tolerance. However, a number of studies have indicated that chronic treatment with nicotine elicits an increase in the number of brain nicotinic receptors.

Studies with the rat

Chronic nicotine injection, once or twice daily for seven days, results in an increase in the number of rat brain [^{3}H]acetylcholine (ACh) binding sites (Schwartz & Kellar 1983, 1985). This increase in binding coincides with development of nicotine-induced increases in locomotor activity (Ksir et al 1985, 1987). We examined the time course of tolerance development and loss in Sprague-Dawley rats using a chronic injection procedure (1.6 mg/kg twice daily) (Collins et al 1988). We attempted to correlate alterations in sensitivity to nicotine with alterations in $(-)$[^{3}H]nicotine binding (note that [^{3}H]ACh and [^{3}H]nicotine bind to the same site in rat and mouse brain [Marks et al 1986c, Martino-Barrows & Kellar 1987]). Tolerance to nicotine's depressant effects on locomotor activity and body temperature paralleled increases in [^{3}H]-nicotine binding, but tolerance lasted more than the seven days required for nicotine binding to return to control levels in five of the six brain regions. These results suggest that increases in [^{3}H]ACh/[^{3}H]nicotine binding may underlie the development of tolerance to nicotine's depressant effects in the rat, but the retention of tolerance may involve factors other than receptor changes.

Studies with the DBA/2 inbred mouse strain

Although we have detected the development of tolerance to nicotine in the mouse using chronic injection techniques (Hatchell & Collins 1977), we have been unable to elicit changes in receptor numbers by this means (unpublished data). Consequently, we have chosen to treat mice with nicotine using chronic infusion methodologies. The technique consists of implanting a cannula in the animal's jugular vein, as first described by Barr et al (1979). Chronic nicotine infusion is normally continued for 7–10 days. Two hours after infusion is stopped the animals are injected with either saline or a dose of nicotine ranging from 0.5–2.5 mg/kg; the effects of these injections on a battery of behavioural and physiological measures are determined between 1–15 minutes after injection. The binding of [^{3}H]nicotine and [^{125}I]bungarotoxin in membranes prepared from 6–8 brain regions is measured using methods described previously (Marks & Collins 1982).

In our first study (Marks et al 1983), we reported that chronic infusion of DBA/2 mice with 0.2, 1.0 or 5.0 mg/kg/h nicotine resulted in tolerance to nicotine's effects on rotarod performance, heart rate and body temperature and in increases in [^{3}H]nicotine binding in nearly all brain regions; significant increases in binding were elicited in some brain regions with the 0.2 mg/kg/h nicotine dose. Increases in [^{125}I]bungarotoxin binding were also observed, but these were restricted to the hippocampus and midbrain and were detected only in animals that had been treated with the 5 mg/kg/h dose. These changes reflected changes in maximal binding (B_{max}), since K_D values were not altered by chronic nicotine infusion. Thus, chronic nicotine treatment results in an increase in [^{3}H]nicotine binding at lower doses and in [^{125}I]bungarotoxin binding at higher doses. Subsequent studies used nicotine infusion doses of 8 mg/kg/h (Marks et al 1985), 3 mg/kg/h (Marks & Collins 1985, Marks et al 1986a), and 2, 4 and 6 mg/kg/h (Marks et al 1986b). These experiments also demonstrated that chronic nicotine treatment resulted in tolerance to several actions of nicotine and that increases in [^{3}H]nicotine and [^{125}I]bungarotoxin binding also occurred. Tolerance increased along with infusion dose such that at the highest infusion doses ED_{50}-like values were twice those obtained in control animals. [^{3}H]Nicotine binding increased in nearly every brain region studied; maximal changes (50–100% increases in B_{max} values) were elicited by the 2 mg/kg/h nicotine dose. [^{125}I]Bungarotoxin binding increased in only some brain regions (cortex, midbrain and hippocampus), but these effects were relatively small (20–30%) and were detected only at nicotine doses that exceeded 2 mg/kg/h.

The time courses of tolerance acquisition and loss have also been examined. In the first of these studies (Marks et al 1985), DBA/2 mice were chronically infused with nicotine (4 mg/kg/h) for 1–12 days. The development and loss of tolerance were measured, as were changes in the binding of [^{3}H]-nicotine and [^{125}I]bungarotoxin in six brain regions. The development and loss of tolerance to nicotine's effects on Y-maze activities, body temperature and heart rate paralleled the up-regulation and return to control, respectively, of [^{3}H]nicotine binding. Significant increases in the binding of [^{125}I]bungarotoxin were also observed in cortex and hippocampus, but these changes were achieved within two days and did not parallel tolerance development. In a subsequent study (Miner & Collins 1988), we determined that acquisition of tolerance to nicotine's seizure-inducing effects closely paralleled the up-regulation of [^{125}I]bungarotoxin binding, but the latter returned to control levels before tolerance to nicotine-induced seizures was lost.

Genetics of tolerance and receptor up-regulation

The studies of nicotine tolerance, described to this point, used the DBA/2 strain. The results obtained with this strain suggested that receptor up-regulation may play an important role in regulating the development of tolerance to nicotine. However, studies with several other mouse strains (Marks et al 1986a,b, Collins & Marks 1989) have demonstrated that while all mouse strains show increases in [^{3}H]nicotine and [^{125}I]bungarotoxin binding after chronic infusion of nicotine, tolerance does not always parallel receptor changes. Some strains, such as the C57BL/6 and DBA/2, develop measurable tolerance to nicotine infused in very low doses, whereas other strains, such as the C3H, fail to develop measurable tolerance until the nicotine infusion rates exceed 2 mg/kg/h. C3H mice are not tolerant to nicotine at chronic infusion doses that have elicited maximal, or near maximal, changes in [^{3}H]nicotine binding. These results indicate that changes in receptor numbers are not necessarily the cause of tolerance to nicotine.

Mechanisms of receptor up-regulation

The observation that chronic treatment with the nicotinic agonist, nicotine, results in an increase in nicotinic receptors was unexpected, because many studies have demonstrated that agonist treatment of receptors for other drugs generally results in decreases in receptors, whereas chronic antagonist treatment generally elicits receptor up-regulation. With this in mind, we (Marks et al 1983) and Schwartz & Kellar (1983) argued that nicotinic receptor up-regulation may occur because nicotine treatment results in a short-lived receptor activation followed by a longer-term desensitization. Chronic nicotine administration may cause prolonged desensitization, or even inactivation, of the nicotinic receptors which may result in either an increase in the rate of receptor synthesis or a decrease in the rate of receptor catabolism. Although there seems to be an increase in the absolute number of receptors, it is possible that there is a decrease in the number of activatable receptors, thereby explaining development of tolerance.

Chronic antagonist treatment

The desensitization model predicts that chronic treatment with a nicotinic antagonist, such as mecamylamine, should also result in receptor up-regulation. However, Schwartz & Kellar (1985) failed to observe an effect of chronic mecamylamine or dihydro-β-erythroidine injections on nicotinic receptors. Mecamylamine also did not block the up-regulation elicited by chronic nicotine injection. Therefore, Schwartz & Kellar (1985) suggested that agonist activity was required to up-regulate the receptor.

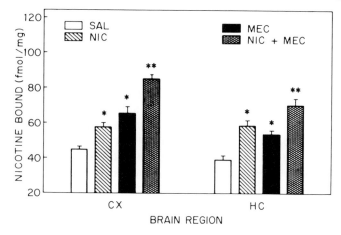

FIG. 1. Effects of chronic nicotine and mecamylamine infusion on [³H]nicotine binding. C57BL/6 mice were infused with saline, nicotine, mecamylamine, or nicotine plus mecamylamine for 10 days. Binding was measured in cortex (CX) and hippocampus (HC) 48 hours after infusion was stopped. Each bar represents the mean ± SEM of six animals. *, $P < 0.05$; **, $P < 0.01$ when compared to control binding.

Because chronic antagonist injections do not readily allow the continuous blockade of receptors, we infused C57BL/6 mice chronically with saline (controls), mecamylamine (3 mg/kg/h), nicotine (3 mg/kg/h), or nicotine plus mecamylamine for 10 days. The mice were challenged with saline or 1 mg/kg nicotine 48 hours after chronic infusion had been stopped; this time was chosen to allow complete elimination of the mecamylamine. Animals infused chronically with nicotine were tolerant to the drug, but none of the other treatment groups showed an altered response to it. Thus, chronic mecamylamine infusion did not elicit an altered response to nicotine, but when co-infused with nicotine it blocked the expected tolerance to nicotine. As noted in Fig. 1, chronic nicotine infusion resulted in increases in [³H]nicotine binding in both the cortex and the hippocampus. However, unlike the results reported by Schwartz & Kellar (1985), chronic mecamylamine infusion also resulted in increases in [³H]nicotine binding. When the two drugs were infused together, an even greater increase in binding was seen. Scatchard analyses indicated that these treatments resulted in changes in the B_{max} for [³H]nicotine binding; K_D values were unchanged. These results clearly demonstrate that nicotinic receptor antagonists can elicit increases in [³H]nicotine binding, but receptor changes need not alter the sensitivity (tolerance) to nicotine.

The mecamylamine–nicotine co-infusion yielded a surprising result. The nicotine dose that was used in these studies (3 mg/kg/h) is supramaximal; further increases in nicotine dose do not normally elicit further increases in binding. However, the addition of mecamylamine resulted in an additive increase in

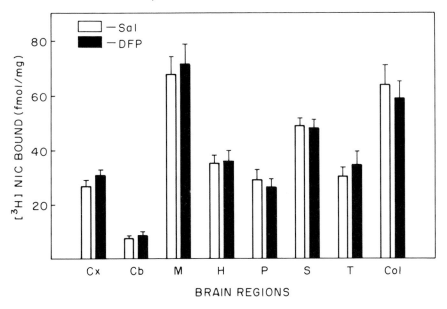

FIG. 2. Effects of chronic vehicle or diisopropyl fluorophosphate (DFP) injections on [³H]nicotine binding. C57BL/6 mice were injected every other day with saline or 2 mg/kg DFP for 21 days. Each bar represents mean ±SEM for eight animals. The brain regions studied were cortex (Cx), cerebellum (Cb), midbrain (M), hindbrain (H), hippocampus (P), striatum (S), hypothalamus (T) and colliculi (Col).

[³H]nicotine binding. This finding may mean that mecamylamine and nicotine affect different receptor populations. It should also be noted that co-treatment with mecamylamine blocked the development of tolerance to nicotine. This result also suggests that increases in binding do not necessarily result in tolerance to nicotine.

Effects of acetylcholinesterase inhibitors on nicotinic receptors

If receptor desensitization is a prerequisite for receptor up-regulation, agonists that vary in affinity for the [³H]nicotine binding site(s) should vary in their relative ability to elicit receptor up-regulation. Chronic treatment with agonists such as ACh, which has very low affinity for the receptor, might be relatively ineffective in eliciting receptor changes, whereas high affinity agonists, such as cytisine, might be very potent in this regard. Schwartz & Kellar (1985) explored this possibility by examining the effects of chronic injection with the irreversible acetylcholinesterase (AChE) inhibitor, diisopropyl fluorophosphate (DFP), on brain [³H]ACh binding. Chronic DFP treatment induced a decrease in [³H]ACh binding. Costa & Murphy (1983) have reported a similar change in

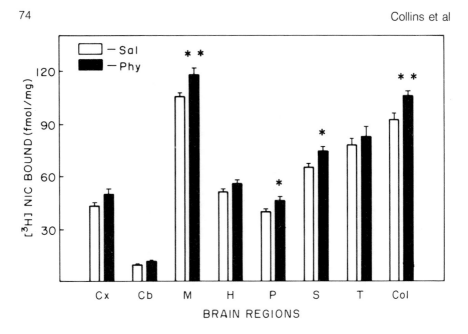

FIG. 3.   Effects of chronic physostigmine infusion on brain [³H]nicotine binding.
C57BL/6 mice were infused continuously with physostigmine (0.1 mg/kg/h) for 10 days.
Nicotine binding was measured two hours after infusion was stopped. Each bar represents
the mean ± SEM of six animals. The brain regions are designated as for Fig. 2. *,$P < 0.05$
when compared to control.

rat brain [³H]nicotine binding after chronic disulfoton treatment. These
findings might mean that low affinity agonists do not elicit receptor desensitization and that the neuron responds to excess stimulation by ACh by decreasing
receptor synthesis. In contrast, a recent report by De Sarno & Giacobini
(1989) indicated that chronic intracerebroventricular injection of the reversible
AChE inhibitor, physostigmine, resulted in an increase in [³H]nicotine
binding in rat brain. This result is puzzling, since both DFP and physostigmine
should increase synaptic ACh levels.

In an attempt to resolve this controversy, we treated C57BL/6 mice chronically
with DFP and physostigmine. Chronic DFP treatment was achieved by injecting
the animals with a 2 mg/kg dose of DFP every other day for 21 days, whereas
the animals were treated chronically with physostigmine by continuous i.v.
infusion (0.1 mg/kg/h) for 10 days. These treatment protocols resulted in
comparable inhibition of AChE activity (DFP, 44–66% in eight brain regions;
physostigmine, 65% in whole brain). However, different effects on [³H]-
nicotine binding were obtained. Fig. 2 demonstrates that chronic DFP treatment
did not alter [³H]nicotine binding in any of the eight brain regions studied,
but this treatment did elicit a reduction in muscarinic receptors (data not shown).

TABLE 1 Effects of chronic drug treatment on [^{3}H] nicotine binding

Chronic infusion	Cortex	Midbrain	Hindbrain
Saline	29.4 ± 1.9	82.9 ± 1.8	41.0 ± 1.4
Nicotine	47.2 ± 2.9^a	106.4 ± 3.4^a	57.8 ± 2.0^a
Anabasine	42.8 ± 2.6^a	105.7 ± 4.6^a	56.9 ± 3.1^a
Lobeline	33.3 ± 1.8	84.7 ± 2.7	42.6 ± 6.1

Each value represents mean $\pm$ the standard error nicotine binding (fmoles/mg protein), $n = 8$–12. Animals were infused with saline (controls) or the indicated drug (18.5 µmoles/kg/h) for 10 days. [a]$P < 0.01$ when compared to the saline-infused control value.

In contrast, chronic physostigmine treatment resulted in an increase in [^{3}H] nicotine binding in four of these brain regions (Fig. 3). Because we have failed to detect chronic DFP-induced changes in [^{3}H] nicotine binding using several other treatment protocols and two other inbred mouse strains, we are at a loss to explain our inability to reproduce the results obtained in rats. Nonetheless, the observation that chronic physostigmine treatment results in receptor up-regulation argues that ACh can, at high levels, produce receptor desensitization.

Effects of other cholinergic agonists

Schwartz & Kellar (1985) have reported that chronic injection of rats with the high affinity nicotinic agonist, cytisine, results in increases in [^{3}H] ACh binding. Cytisine has greater affinity for the nicotine/ACh binding site than does nicotine (Marks & Collins 1982). In an attempt to determine whether chronic administration of agonists with lower affinity for the receptor also elicits up-regulation, we examined the effects of chronic treatment with the nicotinic agonists, lobeline and anabasine. These compounds effectively compete with nicotine for its binding site (lobeline $IC_{50} = 0.075$ µM; anabasine $IC_{50} = 0.35$ µM). Table 1 presents the effects of chronic i.v. infusion (10 days) with equimolar doses (18.5 µM) of nicotine, lobeline and anabasine on [^{3}H] nicotine binding in three brain regions. Consistent with our previously reported results, nicotine infusion resulted in significant increases in binding in all three brain regions. Similarly, anabasine elicited increases in binding in all of the regions, but lobeline was without effect in any of the regions. These results suggest that no clear relationship between affinity for the nicotine binding site and agonist-induced changes in the receptor exists; if affinity predicted ability to up-regulate receptors, lobeline should have been more effective than anabasine.

The chronic infusion of anabasine elicited increases in [^{3}H] nicotine binding, but this increase in receptors was not sufficient to change the response to either anabasine or nicotine. This finding also argues that tolerance to nicotine involves more than changes in receptor numbers.

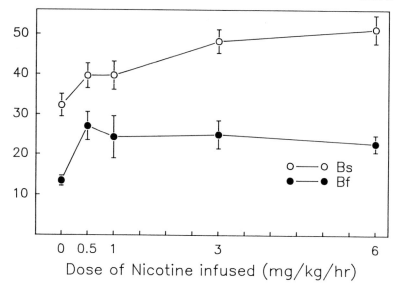

FIG. 4. Effects of chronic nicotine infusion on the fast and slow phases of nicotine binding. C57BL/6 mice were infused with saline or nicotine for 10 days. Fast binding (Bf) and slow binding (Bs) were estimated from association curves. Each point represents the mean ±SEM of three determinations.

Kinetic analysis of receptor desensitization

Lippiello et al (1987) reported that although nicotine appears to bind to a single class of sites, the association kinetics are biphasic. An initial rapid binding process and a slower binding process were detected. The rate and proportion of binding attributable to the slower process were dependent on the nicotine concentration; as the concentration of nicotine added to the incubations was increased, the rate of the slower binding process increased while the fraction of binding attributable to this process decreased. These investigators hypothesized that the initial, rapid phase of binding represented binding to a desensitized form of the receptor, and that the slower phase was due to binding to a lower affinity, activatable form of the receptor, which alters its conformation after binding to yield the high affinity, desensitized state. Consistent with this model, the kinetics of dissociation is characterized by a single rate constant.

If chronic agonist treatment alters the ratio of activatable:desensitized receptors, this alteration may result in tolerance to nicotine. To determine if chronic nicotine changes this ratio, we infused C57BL/6 mice for 10 days with saline and nicotine (0.5, 1.0, 3.0 and 5.0 mg/kg/h). Two hours after infusion was stopped the animals were sacrificed, their brains removed, the membrane fraction prepared and the association kinetics of [^{3}H] nicotine (20 nM) binding was measured. The association curves were fitted to a two-site model using a least squares method and the amounts of fast phase binding (Bf) and slow phase binding (Bs) were estimated. These values are presented in Fig. 4. Surprisingly, both Bf and Bs increase with chronic infusion, but Bf increases more rapidly at lower doses. Thus, low doses of nicotine increase the number of desensitized receptors, but the number of activatable receptors also seems to change. However, this result must be viewed with some suspicion because we do not know the rate of resensitization of the receptors; i.e. we do not know whether the fast-binding form is converted back to the slow-binding form, and, if so, what the rate of this process might be. If this occurred in less time than was required to remove the brains and prepare the membranes for assay, the results presented in Fig. 4 would not represent a valid estimate of the *in vivo* Bf:Bs ratio. Clearly, additional studies are required to resolve these issues. In particular, studies of changes in the Bf:Bs ratio must be done in mouse strains that differ in the relationship between tolerance development and receptor up-regulation.

Steroid interactions with the nicotinic receptors

Many smokers increase their tobacco use when placed in a stressful environment (Hall & Morrison 1973, Parkes 1983). In addition, tobacco use may increase the release of adrenal steroids. Because recent studies have demonstrated that certain steroids alter GABA receptor binding and function (Majewska 1987), we are investigating the potential effects of adrenal steroids on response to nicotine and on nicotinic receptor binding.

Effects of steroids on sensitivity to nicotine

The initial study that suggested that steroids may influence sensitivity to nicotine (Pauly et al 1988) determined whether adrenalectomy and steroid replacement altered sensitivity to nicotine in C3H mice. Adrenalectomy caused dramatic increases in sensitivity to the effects of nicotine on Y-maze activities, acoustic startle response, heart rate and body temperature. The effects of adrenalectomy could be reversed if the animals were provided with replacement steroid. Furthermore, control animals were made resistant to nicotine if they were treated chronically with corticosterone (CCS). Adrenalectomy did not alter brain [^{3}H] nicotine binding; [^{125}I] bungarotoxin binding was elevated, but only in the hippocampus. These results suggest that CCS may have an anti-nicotine effect.

In a subsequent study (Pauly et al 1990), we determined whether other mouse strains also exhibit increased sensitivity to nicotine after adrenalectomy. A summary of these results is presented in Table 2. A surprising result was obtained; after adrenalectomy some mouse strains, such as the C57BL/6 and

TABLE 2   Effects of adrenalectomy on sensitivity to nicotine

Mouse strain	Startle response	Y-maze rears	Y-maze crosses	Heart rate	Body temperature
A	0	0	0	+	0
BUB	+	0	0	0	0
C3H	+	+	+	+	+
C57	0	0	0	+	0
DBA	0	0	0	+	+
LS	0	+	+	+	+
SS	0	0	0	0	+

+ indicates that adrenalectomy resulted in increased sensitivity to nicotine; 0 indicates that it had no effect.

DBA/2, showed minimal changes in sensitivity to nicotine; others, such as the C3H and LS, were more sensitive to all of the nicotine effects.

The possibility that CCS might exert its anti-nicotine actions by inhibiting binding to the brain nicotinic receptors was examined by measuring binding, *in vitro*, in the presence of various concentrations of CCS. The effects of CCS on [³H]nicotine binding in four brain regions obtained from C3H mice are presented in Fig. 5. CCS inhibited binding in all of the brain regions, but 100% inhibition was never attained. Similar effects of CCS on [¹²⁵I]bungarotoxin binding were found (data not shown).

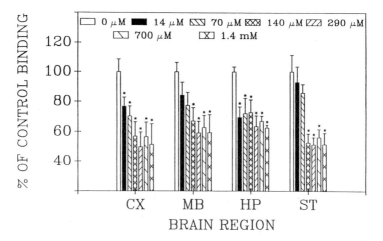

FIG. 5.   Inhibition of [³H]nicotine binding by corticosterone. Corticosterone (CCS) was added to the standard nicotine binding assays at the designated concentrations. Inhibition is presented in terms of % ± SEM of control binding. Inhibition was measured in cortex (CX), midbrain (MB), hippocampus (HP) and striatum (ST). *, $P < 0.05$ when compared to control.

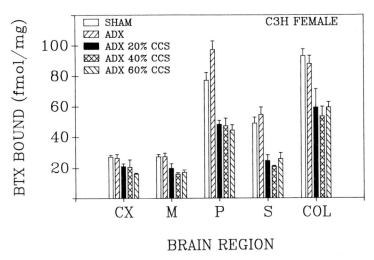

FIG. 6. Effects of adrenalectomy (ADX) and chronic corticosterone (CCS) treatment on brain [^{125}I] bungarotoxin (BTX) binding. C3H female mice were adrenalectomized and treated chronically with a cholesterol pellet or pellets containing 20%, 40% or 60% CCS. Binding was measured seven days after ADX. Sham-operated animals were the controls. Each bar represents the mean ± SEM of 6–10 determinations. Binding was measured in cortex (CX), midbrain (M), hippocampus (P), striatum (S) or colliculi (COL).

Chronic treatment with corticosterone

We have also been examining the effects of chronic CCS treatments on brain nicotinic receptor binding. Chronic CCS treatment has been achieved by preparing pellets containing mixtures of cholesterol and CCS. These pellets are implanted subcutaneously for seven days. This treatment has no effect on [^{3}H] nicotine binding, but chronic CCS treatment has a marked effect on [^{125}I] bungarotoxin binding. Fig. 6 presents the effects of adrenalectomy and treatment with 20, 40 and 60% CCS-containing pellets on [^{125}I] bungarotoxin binding in five brain regions. Adrenalectomy elicited an increase in binding only in the hippocampus. CCS treatment reduced binding in all of the brain regions assayed, but a dose–response relationship was not evident. We are currently studying the effects of lower doses and longer treatment times. Scatchard analyses indicated that this reduction in binding is due to a reduction in B_{max}; K_D values were not altered by chronic CCS treatment.

It is important to note that the chronic CCS-treated animals were tolerant to nicotine. This tolerance might be due to CCS-induced inhibition of [^{3}H] nicotine binding, or to the reduction in [^{125}I] bungarotoxin binding. Further studies are required to resolve this issue.

Conclusions

The studies reported here demonstrate that chronic nicotine treatment results in increases in both [^{3}H]nicotine and [^{125}I]bungarotoxin binding. These increases in binding are dose and time dependent. Although studies using a single strain of mouse, the DBA/2, suggest that changes in receptors may explain tolerance to nicotine, studies with other strains indicate that additional factors are involved. One such factor might involve steroid interactions with the nicotinic receptors. Those mouse strains that show a high correlation between receptor changes and tolerance (e.g. the C57BL/6 and DBA/2 strains) also show minimal changes in sensitivity to nicotine after adrenalectomy or CCS administration. On the other hand, the C3H strain is markedly affected by adrenalectomy and shows little correlation between chronic nicotine-induced receptor changes and tolerance development.

The observation that chronic mecamylamine treatment induces an up-regulation of nicotinic receptors supports the notion that nicotine-induced receptor desensitization is responsible for chronic nicotine-induced receptor changes. Since not all nicotinic agonists elicit receptor changes, it does not seem likely that receptor up-regulation can be predicted by the affinity of the agonists.

While receptor up-regulation might be due to desensitization of the receptor, our studies of the effects of chronic nicotine infusion on the association of [^{3}H]nicotine binding failed to provide the expected results: an increase in Bf and a decrease in Bs was expected, but both Bf and Bs increased after chronic nicotine infusion. However, because these assays were done a minimum of two hours after the tissue had been removed from the animal, we do not believe that the results presented here conclusively demonstrate that the expected change in the Bf:Bs ratio was achieved *in vivo*. Studies of the rate of conversion of the fast-binding form back to the slow-binding form must be done so that the results reported here can be interpreted properly. We suspect that an assay of receptor function might provide results that are less ambiguous.

The observation that altering CCS levels alters the sensitivity of the mouse to nicotine may explain why people increase their use of tobacco when stressed. If cortisol, the human equivalent of CCS, also has anti-nicotine actions, it may be that humans increase their tobacco intake when cortisol levels are elevated in an attempt to overcome the partial receptor blockade induced by the steroid hormone.

Acknowledgements

Studies from the authors' laboratory were supported by grants from the National Institute on Drug Abuse (DA-06391 and DA-05131) and from the R. J. Reynolds Tobacco Company. A. C. C. is supported, in part, by a Research Scientist Development Award (DA-00116). The technical assistance of E. A. Ullman, S. Selvaag and S. Turner is sincerely appreciated.

References

Barr JE, Holmes DB, Ryan LM, Sharpless SK 1979 Techniques for the chronic cannulation of the jugular vein in mice. Pharmacol Biochem Behav 11:115–118

Clarke PBS, Kumar R 1983 The effects of nicotine on locomotor activity in nontolerant and tolerant rats. Br J Pharmacol 78:329–337

Collins AC, Marks MJ 1989 Chronic nicotine exposure and brain nicotinic receptors—influence of genetic factors. Prog Brain Res 79:137–146

Collins AC, Romm E, Wehner JM 1988 Nicotine tolerance: an analysis of the time course of its development and loss in the rat. Psychopharmacology 96:7–14

Costa LG, Murphy SD 1983 [^{3}H]nicotine binding in rat brain: alteration after chronic acetylcholinesterase inhibition. J Pharmacol Exp Ther 226:392–397

De Sarno P, Giacobini E 1989 Modulation of acetylcholine release by nicotinic receptors in the rat brain. J Neurosci Res 22:194–200

Hall GH, Morrison CF 1973 New evidence for a relationship between tobacco smoking, nicotine dependence and stress. Nature (Lond) 243:199–201

Hatchell PC, Collins AC 1977 Influences of genotype and sex on behavioral tolerance to nicotine in mice. Pharmacol Biochem Behav 6:25–30

Ksir C, Hakan RL, Hall DP, Kellar KJ 1985 Exposure to nicotine enhances the behavioral stimulant effect of nicotine and increases binding of [^{3}H]acetylcholine to nicotinic receptors. Neuropharmacology 24:527–531

Ksir C, Hakan RL, Kellar KJ 1987 Chronic nicotine and locomotor activity: influences of exposure dose and test dose. Psychopharmacology 92:25–29

Lippiello PM, Sears SB, Fernandes KG 1987 Kinetics and mechanism of L-[^{3}H]nicotine binding to putative high affinity receptor sites in rat brain. Mol Pharmacol 31:392–400

Majewska MD 1987 Steroids and brain activity: essential dialogue between brain and body. Biochem Pharmacol 36:3781–3788

Marks MJ, Collins AC 1982 Characterization of nicotine binding in mouse brain and comparison with the binding of alpha-bungarotoxin and quinuclidinyl benzilate. Mol Pharmacol 22:554–564

Marks MJ, Collins AC 1985 Tolerance, cross tolerance, and receptors after chronic nicotine or oxotremorine. Pharmacol Biochem Behav 22:283–291

Marks MJ, Burch JB, Collins AC 1983 Effects of chronic nicotine infusion on tolerance development and nicotinic receptors. J Pharmacol Exp Ther 226:817–825

Marks MJ, Stitzel JA, Collins AC 1985 Time course study of the effects of chronic nicotine infusion on drug response and brain receptors. J Pharmacol Exp Ther 235:619–628

Marks MJ, Romm E, Gaffney DK, Collins AC 1986a Nicotine-induced tolerance and receptor changes in four mouse strains. J Pharmacol Exp Ther 237:809–819

Marks MJ, Stitzel JA, Collins AC 1986b Dose-response analysis of nicotine tolerance and receptor changes in two inbred mouse strains. J Pharmacol Exp Ther 239:358–364

Marks MJ, Stitzel JA, Romm E, Wehner JM, Collins AC 1986c Nicotinic binding sites in rat and mouse brain: comparison of acetylcholine, nicotine, and alpha-bungarotoxin. Mol Pharmacol 30:427–436

Martino-Barrows AM, Kellar KJ 1987 [^{3}H]acetylcholine and [^{3}H](-)nicotine label the same recognition site in rat brain. Mol Pharmacol 31:169–174

Miner LL, Collins AC 1988 The effect of chronic nicotine treatment on nicotine-induced seizures. Psychopharmacology 95:52–55

Parkes KR 1983 Smoking as a moderator of the relationship between affective state and absence from work. J Appl Psychol 68:698–708

Pauly JR, Ullman EA, Collins AC 1988 Adrenocortical hormone regulation of nicotine sensitivity in mice. Physiol Behav 44:109–116

Pauly JR, Ullman EA, Collins AC 1990 Strain differences in adrenalectomy-induced alterations in nicotine sensitivity in the mouse. Pharmacol Biochem Behav 35:171–179

Schwartz RD, Kellar KJ 1983 Nicotinic cholinergic receptor binding sites in the brain: regulation in vivo. Science (Wash DC) 220:214–220

Schwartz RD, Kellar KJ 1985 In vivo regulation of [^{3}H]acetylcholine recognition sites in brain by nicotinic cholinergic drugs. J Neurochem 45:427–433

Stolerman LP, Fink R, Jarvik ME 1973 Acute and chronic tolerance to nicotine measured by activity in rats. Psychopharmacologia 30:329–342

DISCUSSION

Changeux: I would like to come back to the muscle nicotinic receptor as a model, although what is true for the muscle receptor may not be exactly correct for the brain nicotine receptor. First, there is a short-term regulation of receptors referred to as desensitization. Another kind of regulation, which has been analysed extensively in the case of the muscle nicotinic receptor, concerns its biosynthesis. During formation of the motor endplate, which lasts 10–20 days, several processes of receptor synthesis occur sequentially or concurrently.

You mentioned the paradox of a decreased response and an increased number of nicotine binding sites. This is also seen in the case of the muscle receptor in extrajunctional areas. At early stages of endplate development, the ACh receptor is present all over the muscle surface. When the junction becomes active, the receptors in the extrajunctional areas disappear as a result of a repression of gene transcription that is dependent on electrical activity. When transmission is blocked, e.g. by curare, the biosynthesis of receptor increases again.

I don't know if this is also true for the brain receptor. Infusion of ACh or nicotine is expected to desensitize the postsynaptic membrane and to yield a chronic block. The electrical activity of the postsynaptic cell is expected to decrease as a consequence of this and thereby derepress synthesis of the receptor.

Collins: We are addressing those kinds of issues in experiments underway in our laboratory.

Rose: Clinically, the two approaches often discussed for nicotine dependence, as well as for other drug dependences, are giving an agonist replacement and giving an antagonist to block reinforcement. Each has problems: giving nicotine alone, for instance, doesn't totally block the reinforcement of smoking a cigarette. On the other hand, if you give mecamylamine, you might induce aversive symptoms.

Would one get a better clinical effect by combining an agonist with an antagonist? For example, if you combined nicotine with mecamylamine, you could saturate the receptor system but the person would not be intoxicated with nicotine because the level of stimulation would be controlled, nor would they be in a state of withdrawal, because the blockade effect of mecamylamine would be balanced by the nicotine. If the person then smoked a cigarette, there would be no reinforcing effects.

Did you ever look at the effects of an acute dose of nicotine on animals that were receiving simultaneously nicotine and mecamylamine?

Collins: We have been using minimitters that consist of a tiny radiotransmitter. These give continuous data regarding either the animal's locomotor activity and body temperature, or locomotor activity and heart rate.

We have used the locomotor activity and body temperature one to determine the effects of mecamylamine and nicotine. Unfortunately, if we treat an animal with mecamylamine alone, we see profound effects in those two measures, so that experiment didn't work.

Stolerman: The findings with adrenalectomy encourage us to look again at stress-related phenomena in connection with nicotine dependence or addiction. I would be interested to see comparable data for a measure of response to nicotine that is more directly linked to drug seeking than is body temperature.

Secondly, there's a distinction we need to make with regard to tolerance, if we want to relate tolerance to desensitization phenomena. This is the difference between acute and chronic tolerance to nicotine, both of which have been demonstrated experimentally. Chronic tolerance, the effect produced by repeated administrations of nicotine or by long-term infusions, seems to take quite a long time to develop and to wear off. It seems unlikely that this relates to the desensitization that neurophysiologists talk about, which has a very short duration. Even the acute tolerance produced by single doses of nicotine, where the time course of offset and onset may be in minutes or at the most in hours, seems slow in relation to desensitization.

Collins: It is difficult to interpret experiments designed to relate acute tolerance to receptor desensitization. We need to re-evaluate those experiments in light of the corticosterone date that I presented. The technique involves pretreating the animal with a dose of nicotine, then challenging it with another dose of nicotine later and asking whether or not that pretreatment alters the sensitivity to nicotine. In many cases, you see a reduced response to nicotine. We also know that nicotine injection elicits the release of corticosterone.

A potential mechanism for this behavioural desensitization is that nicotine releases the corticosterone and the corticosterone partially blocks the receptor so there is an attenuated response to the challenge dose. Alternatively, it could be due to receptor desensitization.

Stolerman: When we reported those results (Stolerman et al 1973), we showed that there was a two hour delay between the administration of the nicotine and the peak of tolerance. We argued against the desensitization hypothesis, and I am encouraged by your results on steroids.

Collins: Corticosterone may not be the most important steroid in this regard. We are looking at various corticosterone metabolites; some metabolites may be much more potent than the parent compound.

London: Is the inhibition of the nicotinic receptor by corticosterone competitive or non-competitive?

Collins: Non-competitive.

London: What concentrations produce inhibition?

Collins: We have used concentrations in the bungarotoxin (Bgt) binding assay from as little as 1 µg/ml, which is equivalent to the concentration in an unstressed animal, all the way up to heroic concentrations. We see inhibition at greater than physiological concentrations. One problem is that all of our binding assays with Bgt binding have had bovine serum albumin added to decrease non-specific binding of the Bgt to glass. BSA has high affinity binding sites for steroids. Consequently, I haven't a clue what the real free concentration in the steroid was that was inhibiting our Bgt binding assay. All I can say is that steroids do inhibit Bgt binding non-competitively. They also non-competitively inhibit binding of [^{3}H] nicotine to brain membranes.

Kellar: The down-regulation of nicotinic binding sites during treatment with cholinesterase inhibitors is seen in rats using at least three different cholinesterase inhibitors.

Collins: I think we are seeing a species difference there.

Kellar: I don't think you would expect to see up-regulation of nicotinic receptors before tolerance, only after tolerance. There could be no temporal relationship at all. If up-regulation is due to inactivation of receptor function, that may go on for days before you see an up-regulation, so I think it's going to be very hard to see a temporal relationship in that situation. You may see it more easily in the recovery of function.

Svensson: We have seen evidence for tolerance development in the mesolimbic dopamine system with repeated nicotine administration. This tolerance appeared with intermittent administration of nicotine but not with continuous administration of nicotine by an osmotic minipump. It seems like it's neither the total exposure to nicotine nor the duration of the administration but rather a series of high peak concentrations that is important in the development of tolerance.

Iversen: What was the measure?

Svensson: These were biochemical measures of dopaminergic activity.

Collins: That's entirely consistent with a study where we compared pulse infusion of nicotine versus continuous infusion of the same dose. We got much more tolerance with pulse infusion, so we are seeing the same effect on behaviour as you are seeing biochemically.

Gray: I am worried about the way the word 'tolerance' has been thrown around, particularly in the context of the overall theme of this meeting, nicotine dependence. There is a general view that dependence on a drug is very closely related to the development of tolerance to the drug. This may be true in some cases. My worry is that it's been taken for granted that nicotine induces general tolerance. There are lots of reasons to think that's not true. I am pretty certain that in nicotine self-administration experiments with animals there is little evidence that the dose that animals choose to self-administer increases during the experiment, except perhaps during a very early period. The human smoker reaches their two pack-a-day stage, or whatever, then stays there for many years.

'Tolerance' is being used, among other things, to refer to the phenomenon originally described by Ian Stolerman—that an initial effect of locomotor depression changes later to an effect of locomotor increase. That is not tolerance, it is a changed response to the drug. Furthermore, loss of response after a few repeated administrations of the drug may not differ from, for example, the loss of response to an audible tone. It is a characteristic of most behavioural responses that they diminish with repeated elicitation.

To go back to the question of the reinforcing effects of the drug, which is probably what dependence is about, this is probably related to dopamine release in the nucleus accumbens. There is clear evidence that that does not change with 15 days of repeated injections of nicotine, as shown by Damsma et al (1989). I am worried that the word tolerance is being used as though this was a general phenomenon relating to nicotine.

Collins: You are probably right, but I would like to clear up a point with respect to our work. I don't think many people would question that if you have a shift to the right of the dose-response curve, for biochemical or behavioural responses, you have achieved a reduced response or sensitivity. This, in my opinion, is tolerance. Furthermore, we have strain differences on the degree of that shift. I believe that is tolerance, because it takes a greater challenge dose to elicit the effect seen in a naive animal.

However, I think you have an extremely important point that nicotine effects on dopamine release, if that's related to why an animal or a human likes nicotine, may not show development of tolerance. I have argued in other quarters that many of the things that we have been measuring in our behavioural tests are reasons why people would choose not to smoke rather than to smoke. In other words, our results may relate to tolerance to nicotine effects that would deter an individual from smoking.

Stolerman: The answer to Jeffrey Gray's question is straightforward. Dose-response studies show that, acutely, small doses of nicotine can increase locomotor activity and larger doses decrease it. One can find doses of nicotine that acutely decrease activity but after chronic administration they increase it (Stolerman et al 1974, Clarke & Kumar 1983). Other factors are involved, but this shift in the dose–response curve may be the most important. These findings in rats fit well with those of Dr Collins in mice (Marks & Collins 1985, Collins et al, this volume). Overall, there are clear indications of tolerance to the locomotor depressant effect. As with other drugs, the appearance of tolerance depends on the effect measured; Jeffrey Gray is surely right when he says there's no evidence for tolerance to the positive reinforcing effect of nicotine that maintains self-administration.

References

Clarke PBS, Kumar R 1983 The effects of nicotine on locomotor activity in non-tolerant and tolerant rats. Br J Pharmacol 78:329–337

Collins AC, Bhat RV, Pauly JR, Marks MJ 1990 Modulation of nicotine receptors by chronic exposure to nicotinic agonists and antagonists. In: The biology of nicotine dependence. Wiley, Chichester (Ciba Found Symp 152) p 68–86

Damsma G, Day J, Fibiger HC 1989 Lack of tolerance to nicotine-induced dopamine release in the nucleus accumbens. Eur J Pharmacol 168:363–368

Marks MJ, Collins AC 1985 Tolerance, cross tolerance, and receptors after chronic nicotine or oxotremorine. Pharmacol Biochem Behav 22:283–291

Stolerman IP, Fink R, Jarvik ME 1973 Acute and chronic tolerance to nicotine measured by activity in rats. Psychopharmacologia 30:329–342

Stolerman IP, Bunker P, Jarvik ME 1974 Nicotine tolerance in rats: role of dose and dose interval. Psychopharmacologia 34:317–324

Presynaptic nicotinic receptors and the modulation of transmitter release

Susan Wonnacott, Alison Drasdo, Elizabeth Sanderson and †Peter Rowell

Department of Biochemistry, University of Bath BA2 7AY, UK and †Department of Pharmacology and Toxicology, University of Louisville, Kentucky, USA

Abstract. Nicotine is increasingly recognized to promote transmitter release in the brain by a direct action on presynaptic terminals. Pharmacological evidence indicates that this action is mediated by nicotinic receptors. From their sensitivity to mecamylamine, neosurugatoxin and neuronal bungarotoxin these presynaptic receptors can be distinguished from α-bungarotoxin-sensitive muscle-type nicotinic receptors, and can be correlated with [^{3}H]nicotine binding sites in the brain. The release of many transmitters in different brain regions is susceptible to stimulation by nicotine, but this effect is not ubiquitous. However, lesioning and subcellular fractionation studies suggest that the majority of brain nicotinic receptors are located presynaptically, so that a direct influence of nicotine on transmitter release assumes considerable importance. Although the sensitivity of presynaptic receptors is such that they are likely to be partially activated by doses of nicotine obtained by smoking, the desensitization-induced up-regulation of nicotinic binding sites that follows chronic nicotine treatment raises questions about their functional status during tobacco usage. Chronic administration of the agonist (+)anatoxin-a also up-regulated [^{3}H]nicotine binding sites, and led to increased nicotine-evoked transmitter release *in vitro*. This could have implications for the involvement of these receptors during withdrawal.

1990 The biology of nicotine dependence. Wiley, Chichester (Ciba Foundation Symposium 152) p 87-105

The early studies of Armitage et al (1969) were among the first to show that nicotine can promote the release of neurotransmitters in the brain, in this case acetylcholine release in the cat cerebral cortex. More recent *in vitro* studies utilizing brain slices in the presence of tetrodotoxin (Giorguieff-Chesselet et al 1979) or isolated nerve terminals (Rowell & Winkler 1984, Rapier et al 1988) have indicated that nicotine can act directly on the presynaptic terminal to increase transmitter release, rather than achieving this effect by postsynaptic stimulation and the generation of action potentials. Pharmacological characterization of this phenomenon suggests that, at least at low nicotine concentrations, this action is mediated by nicotinic acetylcholine receptors. The widespread distribution of these receptors presynaptically would permit the direct interaction of nicotine with diverse neurotransmitter and hormone systems in the central nervous system (CNS), and might contribute to the development and maintenance of nicotine dependence. This paper discusses this thesis in the context of recent *in vitro* experimental results.

Nicotine-evoked transmitter release is mediated by presynaptic nicotinic acetylcholine receptors: pharmacological evidence

The involvement of nicotinic receptors in mediating the stimulation of transmitter release by nicotine was initially controversial. The most widely studied system, and the one that will be focused on in this paper, is the nicotine-evoked release of dopamine from dopaminergic nerve terminals in the striatum. Some groups working on this system have reported antagonism by nicotinic antagonists, while others found no inhibition by these agents (see Table 1). The Ca^{2+} independence of nicotine-evoked dopamine release also suggested that it occurred by a non-physiological mechanism (Marien et al 1983, Takano et al 1983). These issues can be clarified by reference to the nicotine concentrations used. Specific antagonism by nicotinic agents and Ca^{2+} dependence of nicotine-evoked transmitter release can be demonstrated at low micromolar concentrations of nicotine, whereas millimolar concentrations of the drug appear to exert non-specific effects. This conclusion is in agreement with Westfall et al (1989). The concentration dependence of nicotine's presynaptic actions will be discussed in a later section.

The sensitivity of nicotine-evoked dopamine release to mecamylamine and pempidine (Table 1) implicates a presynaptic nicotinic receptor of the ganglionic type. The question of subclassification of nicotinic receptors has assumed a new impetus, after evidence from molecular biological studies for the expression of multiple subtypes in the central and autonomic nervous systems (see Lindstrom et al, this volume). Naturally occurring neurotoxins can be particularly discriminating probes for receptor subtypes, showing marked specificity coupled with high potency. We previously reported that the rare shellfish toxin, neosurugatoxin, which inhibits ganglionic but not endplate nicotinic receptors (Hayashi et al 1984), potently inhibited dimethylphenylpiperazinium (DMPP)- and nicotine-evoked dopamine release from striatal synaptosomes (Rapier et al 1985, 1990), whereas the neuromuscular blocker α-bungarotoxin (αBgt) had little effect even at high concentrations (see Table 2). The slight (20%) decrease in nicotine-evoked dopamine release after exposure to αBgt may reflect contamination with minor components of the snake venom. Of particular interest is the related polypeptide called variously Bgt3.1, $\varkappa$-bungarotoxin or toxin F, and referred to henceforth as neuronal bungarotoxin (Lindstrom et al 1987). This name reflects its inhibitory action at neuronal nicotinic receptors, principally in autonomic ganglia where it has been most studied (Chiapinnelli 1985,

TABLE 1 Summary of the characteristics of nicotine-evoked dopamine release from rat striatal preparations

Reference	Preparation	Nicotine concentration (M)	Antagonists tested	Concentration (M)	Inhibition	Ca^{2+}-dependence
Arqueros et al (1978)	Slices	$5 \times 10^{-4} - 1 \times 10^{-2}$			No	
Giorguieff-Chesselet et al (1979)	Slices	10^{-6}	dTC pemp	5×10^{-6} 10^{-5}	Yes Yes	Yes
Sakurai (1982)	Synaptosomes	$2 \times 10^{-4} - 5 \times 10^{-4}$	dTC hex	10^{-4} 10^{-4}	No No	
Takano et al (1983)	Synaptosomes	5×10^{-4}				No
Connelly & Littleton (1983)	Synaptosomes	$10^{-4} - 10^{-2}$	pemp hex	2×10^{-4} 5×10^{-4}	Yes No	No
Marien et al (1983)	Slices	$10^{-4} - 3 \times 10^{-3}$	hex	3×10^{-4}	No	No
Westfall et al (1989)	Slices	$10^{-6} - 10^{-4}$ $10^{-4} - 10^{-3}$	mec dTC mec	10^{-5} 5×10^{-5} 10^{-4}	Yes Yes No	Yes No
Rapier et al (1988,1990)	Synaptosomes	$10^{-6} - 10^{-4}$	mec pemp NSTX DHβE αBgt	5×10^{-6} 5×10^{-6} 5×10^{-8} 5×10^{-7} 2.5×10^{-7}	Yes Yes Yes Yes No	Yes

dTC, d-tubocurarine; mec, mecamylamine; DHβE, dihydro-β-erythroidine; hex, hexamethonium; pemp, pempidine; NSTX, neosurugatoxin.

Loring & Zigmond 1988). We have examined the effect of purified neuronal Bgt on nicotine-evoked [³H]dopamine release from striatal synaptosomes. In agreement with Schulz & Zigmond (1989), neuronal Bgt was an effective inhibitor of this response (Fig. 1). The antagonism by neuronal Bgt was statistically significant, in contrast to the marginal effect of αBgt, tested in parallel at the same concentration (Table 2). A 20 minute washout after removal of neuronal Bgt failed to restore responsiveness to nicotine, in agreement with the slow recovery in chick ciliary ganglia (Lipton et al 1987).

How does the pharmacological specificity of the presynaptic action of nicotine compare with other data for nicotinic receptors? Two (α3β2 and α4β2) of the three putative neuronal nicotinic receptor subtypes characterized so far by functional expression in *Xenopus* oocytes (Boulter et al 1987) appear to be sensitive to neuronal Bgt, but not to αBgt. The α4β2 combination has been

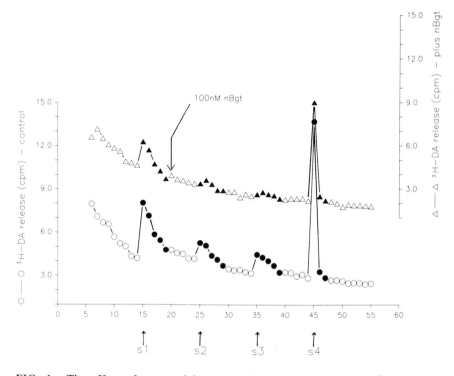

FIG. 1. The effect of neuronal bungarotoxin on nicotine-evoked [³H]dopamine release. Synaptosomes were prepared from rat striata, loaded with [³H]dopamine and perfused with Krebs' Ringer bicarbonate buffer as previously described (Rapier et al 1988). Following an initial stimulation (S₁) with 3µM nicotine, toxin was introduced into the buffer in the test chamber. Subsequent stimulations (S₂, S₃ = 3µM nicotine; S₄ = 20 mM KCl) were given in the presence (upper trace) or absence (lower trace) of neuronal Bgt.

TABLE 2   Comparison of effects of α-bungarotoxin and neuronal bungarotoxin on nicotine-evoked [³H]dopamine release

Toxin	Concentration	S_2 % control (toxin-free) response	S_3 % control (toxin-free) response
αBgt	0.1 μM	78.2 ± 18.7	84.3 ± 15.2
nBgt	0.1 μM	49.3 ± 12.2[b]	45.2 ± 8.9[a] washout[c]
nBgt	0.25 μM	58.2 ± 9.9[a]	47.3 ± 12.1[a]

Rat striatal synaptosomes were perfused as described in legend to Fig. 1. Following an initial stimulation (S_1) with 3μM nicotine, toxin was added to the perfusion buffer at the concentration indicated. Subsequent stimulations (S_2 and S_3) with 3μM nicotine were given after 20 and 50 minutes, respectively. Responses were calculated as a fraction of S_1 and compared with control values. Results are the means ± SEM ($n=3$). αBgt, α-bungarotoxin; nBgt, neuronal bungarotoxin. [a]$P<0.05$. [b]$P<0.01$. [c]Toxin removed from perfusion buffer after S_2 followed by 20 minute washout.

equated with the high affinity [³H]nicotine binding site in the brain (Whiting et al 1987), and we have previously proposed (Wonnacott et al 1989, Rapier et al 1990) that this binding site is a good candidate for the presynaptic receptor on striatal synaptosomes. This is based on their common sensitivity to neosurugatoxin and high stereoselectivity for (−)nicotine. One anomalous observation is the failure of neuronal Bgt to inhibit [³H]nicotine binding in competition assays (A. Drasdo & S. Wonnacott, unpublished, Wolf et al 1988). Although a similar disparity in the actions of mecamylamine is explained by the proposition that this drug may be a non-competitive antagonist, acting at the level of the nicotinic ionophore, it is improbable that a large polypeptide such as neuronal Bgt could have a similar non-competitive mode of action. Nevertheless, as we shall discuss later, there is considerable evidence for the presynaptic localization of [³H]nicotine binding sites, consistent with their having a role in the regulation of transmitter release.

How widespread is the presynaptic nicotinic modulation of transmitter release in the brain?

The data discussed so far have concerned the nicotinic modulation of dopamine release in the striatum. We can now address the question, 'does nicotine influence the release of other neurotransmitters throughout the brain?' The answer is very clearly affirmative; nicotine has been shown to modulate the release of several neurotransmitters, including noradrenaline, dopamine, acetylcholine and 5-hydroxytryptamine in cortex, hippocampus, hypothalamus and nucleus accumbens (for review, see Rowell 1987). In each case, nicotine enhances transmitter release in the absence of any depolarizing stimulus. This is compatible with the involvement of nicotinic receptor–cation channel complexes, which produce local depolarization in response to agonist binding (see

Wonnacott et al 1989). The presence of a cation channel in neuronal nicotinic receptors is implicit in the molecular biology and functional expression data (Boulter et al 1987), and can be deduced from the sensitivity of nicotine-evoked release of dopamine in the striatum and of acetylcholine in the hippocampus to the nicotinic channel blocker, histrionicotoxin (Rapier et al 1987).

There is evidence, however, that presynaptic nicotinic receptors are not present on all nerve terminals. Using the non-hydrolysable nicotinic agonist methylcarbamylcholine, Lapchak et al (1989) reported that, in contrast to the sensitivity of acetylcholine release from cholinergic nerve terminals in the hippocampus, there was no effect on acetylcholine release in the striatum. We have observed a similar differential sensitivity of noradrenaline release from cortical and hippocampal synaptosomes; despite similar levels of [^{3}H]noradrenaline uptake and K$^+$-evoked [^{3}H]noradrenaline release in the two tissues, only cortical synaptosomes give a clear response to nicotine (Fig. 2). In contrast, we found acetylcholine and GABA release in the hippocampus to be sensitive to nicotine (Wonnacott et al 1989). Regional specificity in nicotine sensitivity, with respect to a given transmitter, may arise from the absence of appropriate synaptic connexions, e.g. axo–axonic cholinergic synapses, to

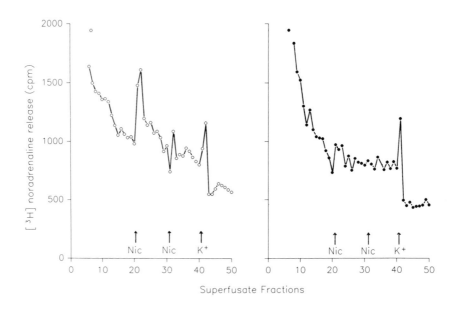

FIG. 2.   The effect of nicotine on noradrenaline release. Synaptosomes prepared in parallel from rat cortex (left panel) or hippocampus (right panel) were loaded with [^{3}H]noradrenaline. Perfusion was carried out essentially as previously described (Rapier et al 1988). Pulses of nicotine (10 μM) or KCl (20 mM) were delivered, and radioactivity released in consecutive 800 μl fractions was determined.

provide endogenous ligand for the receptor. As a consequence, the regional specificity will confer some degree of selectivity to the CNS responses to nicotine. In addition, there may be differences in sensitivity between nicotine-induced responses in different brain regions. This is discussed later.

For nicotine-evoked transmitter release in a given brain region, it is not yet known if all nerve terminals containing that transmitter have presynaptic nicotinic receptors. It is generally observed that the maximum release elicited by nicotine is some 3–5 times less than that achieved by other agents, such as KCl (Rowell 1987). This could reflect the lower efficacy of receptor-mediated release or, alternatively, could arise from the presence of nicotinic receptors on only 20–30% of the nerve terminals containing the transmitter in question.

How important are the presynaptic actions of nicotine, compared with postsynaptic mechanisms?

Although it is clear that nicotine can directly stimulate the release of neurotransmitters in many brain areas, this action will not have much physiological relevance if it is overshadowed by a major direct postsynaptic action of the drug. To address this question one can consider the relative disposition of pre- and postsynaptic nicotinic receptors in the brain, using radioligands such as [^{3}H]nicotine for their identification. Lesioning studies (Schwartz et al 1984, Clarke & Pert 1985) have shown losses of up to 40% of nicotinic ligand-binding sites in certain projection areas of dopaminergic or serotonergic neurons, consistent with the loss of presynaptic receptors on degeneration of the axon terminals. Postsynaptic receptors would be expected to proliferate after lesion. Because the brain areas examined will contain the terminals of non-dopaminergic or non-serotonergic neurons, which are spared by the lesions, many of the residual 60% of nicotinic ligand-binding sites may also be presynaptic.

A similar conclusion is reached for cholinergic synapses in the cortex and hippocampus from the consistent evidence of losses of nicotinic binding sites in Alzheimer's disease (for review, see Kellar & Wonnacott 1990). In contrast, the total population of muscarinic binding sites is little affected. Pharmacological differentiation of pre- and postsynaptic muscarinic receptors (M2 and M1 subtypes, respectively) indicates that only 10–20% are located on axon terminals, and these are also lost in Alzheimer's disease.

We have used a novel subcellular fractionation technique to explore the cellular distribution of ligand-binding sites. Non-equilibrium density gradient centrifugation on Percoll gradients (Dunkley et al 1988) separates synaptosomes from plasma membranes, thus achieving fractions enriched in pre- and postsynaptic elements, respectively. We have fractionated rat hippocampal tissue in this way. In contrast to the distribution of total muscarinic binding sites labelled by [^{3}H]quinuclidinyl-benzilate, which are enriched in the plasma membrane fractions, [³H]nicotine binding sites are clearly enriched in the synaptosome fractions (B. Thorne et al, unpublished). Although precise quantitation is not possible, this result confirms the notion implicit in the experimental and neurological degeneration examinations that the majority of [³H]nicotine binding sites are located presynaptically.

The heterogeneity of nicotinic receptor candidates emerging from molecular biology studies raises the possibility that high affinity agonist binding may characterize the presynaptic receptor, whereas postsynaptic nicotinic receptors may not be identifiable using these ligands. Certainly both $\alpha 3$ and $\alpha 4$ subunits are expressed in the substantia nigra and ventrotegmental areas, consistent with the disposition of two forms of receptor in the nigrostriatal and mesolimbic systems (Goldman et al 1987). As previously mentioned, the $\alpha 4$ gene product corresponds to the agonist-binding subunit of the [³H]nicotine binding protein (Whiting et al 1987), and is therefore a good candidate for the presynaptic nicotinic receptor. $\alpha 4$ is the most abundant nicotinic α subunit expressed in the brain (Goldman et al 1987), which again favours a predominantly presynaptic role for nicotinic receptors in the CNS. This conclusion is consistent with the meagre electrophysiological evidence for nicotinic receptors in the brain, since intracellular recording techniques can detect only somatic (postsynaptic) receptors. Thus, it may be concluded that a considerable proportion (and possibly the majority) of potential target sites for nicotine are located presynaptically, where they may directly influence transmitter release.

Are presynaptic nicotinic receptors physiologically relevant to the action of nicotine in tobacco smoking?

Having outlined the case for the preponderance of presynaptically located nicotinic receptors in the brain, we must consider the likelihood that they will be receptive to brain nicotine concentrations encountered during tobacco smoking, before any importance can be claimed for presynaptic nicotinic mechanisms in nicotine dependence. It is evident from Table 1 that nicotine concentrations used *in vitro* to characterize the presynaptic action vary widely between research groups. Very rarely has the concentration dependence of nicotine-evoked transmitter release been determined. However, we have previously reported (Rapier et al 1988) that the EC_{50} for nicotine-evoked dopamine release from striatal nerve terminals is 4μM (Fig. 3), and a very similar concentration dependence was found for [³H]GABA release from hippocampal nerve terminals. Notably, dopamine terminals in the nucleus accumbens appear to be more sensitive to nicotine, with an EC_{50} of 0.4 μM (Rowell et al 1987; Fig. 3).

Brain levels of nicotine during tobacco smoking have not been measured, but concentrations in the range 0.1–0.5 μM can be anticipated, on the basis of venous blood concentrations (see Rowell 1987, Benowitz, this volume).

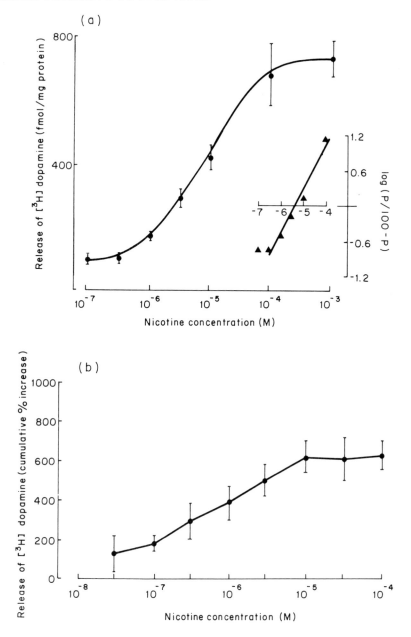

FIG. 3. Concentration dependence of nicotine-evoked transmitter release. (a) Nicotine-evoked [³H]dopamine release from striatal synaptosomes. EC_{50} for nicotine = 4μM. (From Rapier et al 1988.) (b) Nicotine-evoked [³H]dopamine release from minced nucleus accumbens. EC_{50} for nicotine = 0.4 μM (From Rowell et al 1987.)

Evidently such concentrations would be sufficient to stimulate presynaptic nicotinic receptors, without fully saturating them, and the mesolimbic system should be more sensitive. This is supported by *in vivo* studies: systemic administration of nicotine to rats increases the release of dopamine in the striatum (Imperato et al 1986, Damsma et al 1988) and in the nucleus accumbens (Imperato et al 1986), but the latter region is five times more sensitive to nicotine. In both tissues the effect of nicotine could be blocked by systemic administration of the centrally active antagonist, mecamylamine, in agreement with the *in vitro* studies discussed earlier in this paper. Thus, evidence is accumulating that the presynaptic stimulation of transmitter release may contribute to nicotine's effects on the brain, and the mesolimbic dopamine system may be particularly important (see Clarke, this volume). However, tobacco smoking is characterized by sustained blood nicotine levels and we must now consider the effect of constant nicotine exposure on presynaptic receptor function.

Chronic nicotinic agonist treatment and presynaptic receptors

It is well established that chronic treatment of rats with nicotine over a period of several days results, paradoxically, in the up-regulation of high affinity nicotinic agonist binding sites (Fig. 4; see Collins et al, this volume). Similar increases in [^{3}H]nicotine binding sites have been observed in the brains of human smokers (Benwell et al 1988). This has been attributed to the desensitization of the receptor by the continuous presence of agonist, such that the receptor is inactivated and more receptors are inserted into the membrane to compensate for the functional blockade (Schwartz & Kellar 1985). This raises several interesting questions. Firstly, is this phenomenon peculiar to nicotine, or is it produced by other nicotinic agonists? Secondly, what is the functional status of the increased number of receptors? If it is a compensatory change, it may maintain the same level of activity or produce a net increase or fail to compensate fully, resulting in a net loss of activity. Thirdly, what are the implications for the development of nicotine dependence and withdrawal symptoms?

We have addressed the first question by administering the nicotinic agonist (+)anatoxin-a to rats. From competition binding assays, this substance is 10 times more potent than nicotine (MacAllan et al 1988) and, as it is a secondary amine, it will readily penetrate the CNS. However, nothing is known about its metabolic half life. We administered a low dose (estimated 0.1 µmoles/day) by continuous infusion from implanted minipumps for seven days. Subsequently, [^{3}H]dopamine release and [^{3}H]nicotine binding were measured in striatal synaptosomes prepared from these animals (Table 3). There was a 30% increase in the number of binding sites in the treated preparation, compared with the control group that received an infusion of vehicle alone. This was paralleled by an increase in nicotine-evoked [^{3}H]dopamine release. There was clearly no

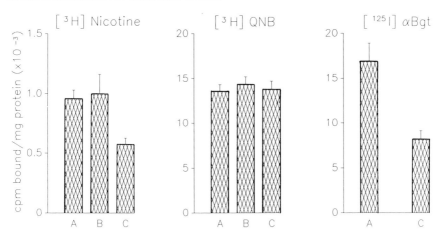

FIG. 4. Up-regulation of nicotinic binding sites by nicotine. Rats received a continuous infusion of nicotine (A, 2.4 mg/kg/day; B, 1.2 mg/kg/day) or saline (C) from implanted minipumps for nine days. Numbers of cholinergic binding sites in whole brain P_2 membranes were subsequently measured using [^{3}H]nicotine (20 nM), [^{3}H]quinuclidinyl-benzilate (QNB, 2 nM) and [^{125}I]α-bungarotoxin (αBgt, 5 nM). Results are means $\pm$ SEM ($n = 4$).

difference in K^+-evoked transmitter release between the two groups, and [^{3}H]dopamine uptake was unaltered. Comparison of the data from all the striatal synaptosome preparations demonstrates a positive correlation ($r = 0.64$) between the amount of nicotine-evoked [^{3}H]dopamine release and the number of [^{3}H]nicotine binding sites (Fig. 5). In contrast, there was no correlation between the number of binding sites and K^+-evoked release.

This study suggests that the up-regulation of nicotinic receptors is not unique to nicotine but may also be produced by other agonists. Thus, it may reflect a general property of the nicotinic receptor. Indeed, agonist-induced desensitization of the receptor is believed to be reflected in the high affinity binding of [^{3}H]acetylcholine, as well as [^{3}H]nicotine, a consequence of the prolonged exposure to the agonist during the *in vitro* binding assay (Schwartz & Kellar 1985). The increased number of receptors appears to be functionally competent *in vitro*, leading to increased transmitter release. This is in contrast to the results of Lapchak et al (1989), who observed a complete abolition of methylcarbamylcholine-evoked [^{3}H]acetylcholine release from hippocampal slices after chronic administration of nicotine to rats. However, there are differences between these studies. A fairly high nicotine dose (0.59 mg/kg) was given by twice-daily injections, compared with a low anatoxin-a concentration, and the brain slice preparation requires less time and washing than does the preparation of synaptosomes. Thus we may be seeing the recovery of function *in vitro* in the results presented in Table 3.

TABLE 3   Effects of chronic anatoxin-a treatment

	Control	Anatoxin-a treated	% Change
[³H]DA uptake (30 sec)	% total radioactivity		
	60.7 ± 3.6	57.9 ± 2.8	−4.7
[³H]DA release	%baseline release		
20mM KCl	241 ± 23	258 ± 18	+6.8
3µM nicotine	61 ± 5	87 ± 11	+42.0[a]
[³H]Nicotine binding sites	fmol/mg protein		
	25.2 ± 2.0	33.2 ± 2.5	+32.0[a]

Rats received a constant infusion of (+)anatoxin-a or saline for seven days from implanted minipumps. Synaptosomes were subsequently prepared from striata and assayed for [³H]dopamine (DA) uptake, [³H]dopamine release and [³H]nicotine binding sites. Results are the means ± SEM ($n = 12$ for each group). [a]$P < 0.05$.

What are the implications for nicotinic dependence? Because of the complexity of human smoking, where each puff of cigarette smoke delivers a bolus of nicotine superimposed on a sustained plasma nicotine concentration, the animal administration techniques (both injection and infusion) are crude representations of these conditions. Nevertheless, it is likely that nicotinic receptor numbers are increased in the brains of smokers as a result of persistent occupation and blockade by the maintained levels of nicotine. A fall in nicotine concentrations (following overnight abstinence and, more markedly, after quitting smoking) may allow the recovery of nicotinic receptor activity before receptor number returns to basal levels. This would produce an enhanced response (neurotransmitter release) to subsequent nicotine exposure (as in the first cigarette of the day) or to endogenous transmitter (contributing to withdrawal symptoms). The extent to which nicotine-evoked transmitter release contributes to positive reinforcement and the development of dependence, as opposed to the alternative view that chronic nicotine may suppress the normal nicotinic stimulation of transmitter release by endogenous acetylcholine, has still to be established.

Acknowledgements

Research carried out in the authors' laboratory was supported by MRC Project Grant No G8722675N to SW, and an NIH Visiting Fellowship to PR. Studies with anatoxin-a were carried out in collaboration with Dr E. X. Albuquerque. We are grateful to British American Tobacco Co Ltd for financial support, and to Dr Ralph Loring for providing neuronal bungarotoxin. A.D. and L.S. are supported by SERC postgraduate training awards.

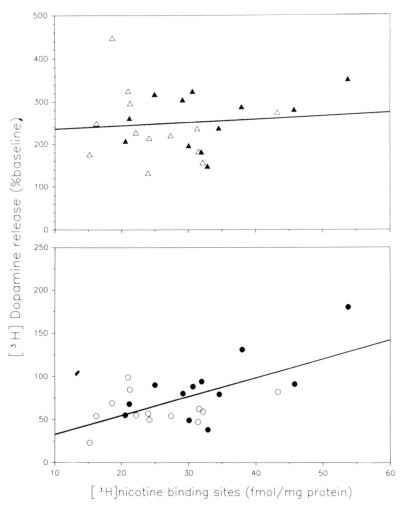

FIG. 5. Correlation between number of binding sites and evoked [³H]dopamine release. K⁺-evoked (upper panel) and nicotine-evoked (lower panel) [³H]dopamine release from striatal synaptosomes prepared from control (open symbols) or anatoxin-treated rats (filled symbols) are compared with the number of [³H]nicotine binding sites measured in the same preparations. Upper panel, r = 0.09; lower panel, r = 0.64.

References

Armitage AG, Hall GH, Sellars CM 1969 Effects of nicotine on electrocortical activity and acetylcholine release from cat cerebral cortex. Br J Pharmacol 35:152–160

Arqueros L, Nacuira D, Zunino E 1978 Nicotine-induced release of catecholamines from rat hippocampus and striatum. Biochem Pharmacol 27:2667–2674

Benowitz NL 1990 Pharmacokinetic considerations in understanding nicotine dependence. In: The biology of nicotine dependence. Wiley, Chichester (Ciba Found Symp 152) p 186–209

Benwell MEM, Balfour DJK, Anderson JM 1988 Evidence that tobacco smoking increases the density of $(-)[^3H]$-nicotine binding sites in human brain. J Neurochem 50:1243–1247

Boulter J, Connolly J, Deneris E, Goldman D, Heinemann S, Patrick J 1987 Functional expression of two neuronal nicotinic acetylcholine receptors from cDNA clones identifies a gene family. Proc Natl Acad Sci USA 84:7763–7767

Chiappinelli VA 1985 Actions of snake venom toxins on neuronal nicotinic receptors and other neuronal receptors. Pharmacol & Ther 31:1–32

Clarke PBS 1990 Mesolimbic dopamine activation—the key to nicotine reinforcement? In: The biology of nicotine dependence. Wiley, Chichester (Ciba Found Symp 152) p 153–168

Clarke PBS, Pert A 1985 Autoradiographic evidence for nicotine receptors on nigrostriatal and mesolimbic dopaminergic neurons. Brain Res 348:355–385

Collins AC, Bhat RV, Pauly JR, Marks MJ 1990 Modulation of nicotine receptors by chronic exposure to nicotinic agonists and antagonists. In: The biology of nicotine dependence. Wiley, Chichester (Ciba Found Symp 152) p 68–86

Connelly MS, Littleton JM 1983 Lack of stereoselectivity in ability of nicotine to release dopamine from rat synaptosomal preparations. J Neurochem 41:1297–1302

Damsma G, Westerink BHC, de Vries JB, Horn AS 1988 The effect of systemically applied cholinergic drugs on the striatal release of dopamine and its metabolites, as determined by automated brain dialysis in conscious rats. Neurosci Lett 89:349–354

Dunkley PR, Heath JW, Harrison SM et al 1988 A rapid Percoll gradient procedure for isolation of synaptosomes directly from an S1 fraction: homogeneity and morphology of subcellular fractions. Brain Res 441:59–71

Giorguieff-Chesselet MF, Kemel ML, Wandscheer D, Glowinski J 1979 Regulation of dopamine release by presynaptic nicotinic receptors in rat striatal slices: effect of nicotine in a low concentration. Life Sci 25:1257–1262

Goldman D, Deneris E, Luyten W, Kochhar A, Patrick J, Heinemann S 1987 Members of a nicotinic acetylcholine receptor gene family are expressed in different regions of the mammalian central nervous system. Cell 48:965–973

Hayashi E, Isogai M, Kagawa Y, Takayanagi N, Yamada S 1984 Neosurugatoxin, a specific antagonist of nicotinic acetylcholine receptors. J Neurochem 42:1491–1494

Imperato A, Mulas A, Di Chiara G 1986 Nicotine preferentially stimulates dopamine release in the limbic system of freely moving rats. Eur J Pharmacol 132:337–338

Kellar KJ, Wonnacott S 1990 Nicotinic cholinergic receptors in Alzheimer's disease. In: Wonnacott S et al (eds) Nicotine psychopharmacology: molecular, cellular and behavioural aspects. Oxford University Press, Oxford, p 341–373

Lapchak PA, Araujo DM, Quirion R, Collier B 1989 Effect of chronic nicotine treatment on nicotinic autoreceptor function and N-$[^3H]$methylcarbamylcholine binding sites in the rat brain. J Neurochem 52:483–491

Lipton SA, Aizeman E, Loring RH 1987 Neural nicotinic acetylcholine responses in solitary mammalian retinal ganglion cells. Pfluegers Arch 410:37–43

Lindstrom J, Schoepfer R, Whiting P 1987 Molecular studies of the neuronal nicotinic acetylcholine receptor family. Mol Neurobiol 1:281–337

Lindstrom J, Schoepfer R, Conroy WG, Whiting P 1990 Structural and functional heterogeneity of nicotinic receptors. In: The biology of nicotine dependence. Wiley, Chichester (Ciba Found Symp 152) p 23–52

Loring RH, Zigmond RE 1988 Characterization of neuronal nicotinic receptors by snake venom neurotoxins. Trends Neurosci 11:73–78

MacAllan DRE, Lunt GG, Wonnacott S, Swanson KL, Rapoport H, Albuquerque EX 1988 Methyllycaconitine and anatoxin-a differentiate between nicotinic receptors in vertebrate and invertebrate nervous systems. FEBS (Fed Eur Biochem Soc) Lett 226:357–363

Marien M, Brien J, Jhamandas K 1983 Regional release of [³H]dopamine from rat brain in vitro: effects of opioids on release induced by potassium, nicotine and L-glutamic acid. Can J Physiol Pharmacol 61:43–60

Rapier C, Harrison R, Lunt GG, Wonnacott S 1985 Neosurugatoxin blocks nicotinic acetylcholine receptors in the brain. Neurochem Int 7:389–396

Rapier C, Wonnacott S, Lunt GG, Albuquerque EX 1987 The neurotoxin histrionicotoxin interacts with the putative ion channel of the nicotinic acetylcholine receptors in the central nervous system. FEBS (Fed Eur Biochem Soc) Lett 212:292–296

Rapier C, Lunt GG, Wonnacott S 1988 Stereoselective nicotine-induced release of dopamine from striatal synaptosomes: concentration dependence and repetitive stimulation. J Neurochem 40:1123–1130

Rapier C, Lunt GG, Wonnacott S 1990 Nicotinic modulation of [³H]dopamine release from striatal synaptosomes: pharmacological characterisation. J Neurochem 54:937–945

Rowell PP 1987 Current concepts on the effects of nicotine in the central nervous system. In: Martin WR et al (eds) Tobacco smoking and health. Plenum, New York, p 191–207

Rowell PP, Winkler DL 1984 Nicotinic stimulation of [³H]acetylcholine release from mouse cerebral cortical synaptosomes. J Neurochem 43:1593–1598

Rowell PP, Carr LA, Garner AC 1987 Stimulation of [³H]dopamine release by nicotine in rat nucleus accumbens. J Neurochem 49:1449–1454

Sakurai Y, Takano Y, Kohjimoto Y, Honda K, Kamiya H 1982 Enhancement of [³H]dopamine release and its [³H]metabolites in rat striatum by nicotinic drugs. Brain Res 242:99–106

Schulz DW, Zigmond RE 1989 Neuronal bungarotoxin antagonises nicotinic function in rat caudate-putamen. Neurosci Lett 93:310–316

Schwartz RD, Kellar J 1985 In vivo regulation of [³H]acetylcholine recognition sites in brain by nicotinic cholinergic drugs. J Neurochem 45:427–433

Schwartz RD, Lehman J, Kellar KJ 1984 Presynaptic nicotinic cholinergic receptors labelled by [³H]acetylcholine on catecholamine and serotonin axons in brain. J Neurochem 42:1495–1498

Takano Y, Sakurai Y, Kohijimoto Y, Honda K, Kamiya HO 1983 Presynaptic modulation of the release of dopamine from striatal synaptosomes: differences in the effects of high K⁺ stimulation, methamphetamine and nicotinic drugs. Brain Res 279:330–334

Thorne B, Sanderson L, Wonnacott S, Dunkley P Isolation of hippocampal synaptosomes on percoll gradients: cholinergic and noradrenergic markers, submitted

Westfall TC, Mereu G, Vickery L, Perry H, Naes L, Yoon KP 1989 Regulation by nicotine of midbrain dopamine neurons. Prog Brain Res 79:173–185

Whiting P, Esch F, Shimasaki S, Lindstrom J 1987 Neuronal nicotinic acetylcholine receptor β-subunit is coded for by the cDNA clone α4. FEBS (Fed Eur Biochem Soc) Lett 219:459–463

Wolf KM, Ciarlegio A, Chiappinelli VA 1988 K-bungarotoxin: binding of a neuronal nicotinic receptor antagonist to chick optic lobe and skeletal muscle. Brain Res 439:249–258

Wonnacott S, Irons J, Rapier C, Thorne B, Lunt GG 1989 Presynaptic modulation of transmitter release by nicotinic receptors. Prog Brain Res 79:157–163

DISCUSSION

Colquhoun: Sue, the response in your system has a sharp peak then desensitizes quickly. In an endplate the response would come down rapidly (in seconds) at first, and then more slowly (minutes); after five minutes only 2% or so of the response would remain. If you plot the dose–response curves for the *peak* response, it would be the usual sigmoid curve; for the *equilibrium* response (after 5–10 minutes contact), it would again be a completely monotonic normal-looking dose–response curve but it would have a much lower maximum and it would be shifted to the left. There is a greater inhibition because of all that desensitization; in another sense it's more potent because the EC_{50} is shifted to the left.

If you don't take care to measure these things either at equilibrium or instantly, but measure somewhere in between, then the dose–response curve will be a mixture of these two, and won't tell you anything. When people ask whether the sensitivity would be compatible with effects from smoking, for example, you have to consider which of these dose–response curves you are talking about, or indeed are you talking about the undefined area in between.

Schwartz: I have been working on the the GABA receptor and have tried to correlate functional responses, such as ion flux, with binding properties. The problem is, and this may also be true for the nicotinic system, that we often do binding studies under very different conditions from those we use for functional studies: 0 °C in membrane homogenates versus 30 or 37 °C in cells, for example.

I use a preparation in which I can assay functional responses and binding in the same preparation under the same conditions. This gives very different results in terms of the pharmacology and the regulation of the receptor than those reported in the literature using binding assays done at 0 °C with 90 min incubation times. That may add to the complexity that we see in terms of multiple responses or differences in sensitivity in binding assays versus functional assays.

Wonnacott: What are the typical differences in sensitivity between functional blockade and binding in muscle?

Heinemann: There is a discrepancy between the labs working on this. In chicken, Mark Ballivet found that $\alpha4\beta2$ is not blocked by neuronal Bgt. We find that $\alpha4\beta2$ is blocked but by higher concentrations; also it's reversible, whereas the $\alpha3\beta2$ block is not. We should be a little cautious. We have some evidence that the block of $\alpha4\beta2$ might be due to another toxin that is present as a contaminant.

Wonnacott: Our toxin was from Ralph Loring.

Collins: Susan's results and those I presented earlier (Collins et al, this volume) show that if you treat an animal chronically with nicotine, stop the treatment and give the animal a chance to clear the nicotine, then remove the brain and try to measure the amount of desensitization, minimal evidence for receptor desensitization is obtained. However, this result may be a consequence of the receptor resensitizing during the time taken to do the experiments. Susan pointed out that in tissue slices things can be done more rapidly and that should facilitate those studies.

I would be remiss if I didn't emphasize that our steroid data could just as easily be explained by the fact that the nicotine stimulated a steroid release, and the blockade seen in a tissue slice may be due to steroid-induced desensitization or receptor blockade.

Benowitz: In synaptosome preparations, nicotine can be washed out and we might not see any functional antagonism. But *in vivo* studies show that there is tolerance of some sort that persists for about a week. Is there any evidence of persistent high affinity binding of nicotine in the brain that might last for days? Is that what you would postulate to explain the long duration of tolerance?

Collins: We don't know whether the binding sites that we are measuring are really receptors, they could just be proteins that bind nicotine. We need to do additional experiments to investigate the relationship between changes in these binding sites and physiological response. From our own data I am not sure we can determine this relationship simply by looking at the binding kinetics and making predictions about function. We need some additional tools. Shelley Schwartz should do some more nicotine-induced ion fluxes, we need something like that to sort out the relationship between binding and function.

Wonnacott: The problem is that to measure binding you have to soak the tissue in the agonist for long periods, so again you are going to distort the situation.

Collins: But that's at cold temperatures, Susan. We can get equilibrium binding in three minutes at 37 °C.

Wonnacott: That may be too long.

Schwartz: Concerning the long-term effects, in collaboration with Ted Slotkin at Duke we have treated pregnant rats with nicotine (2 mg/kg/day infusion). We can produce the same up-regulation of nicotinic binding sites in the mothers and in the fetus. After birth, the neonate is no longer exposed to nicotine but there is a persistent up-regulation of nicotinic sites through the period after weaning. That's using very low concentrations of nicotine, which correspond to smoking less than one pack of cigarettes per day in humans.

West: I heard recently about a technique called *in vivo* receptor binding. Would that help us understand some of these anomalies?

London: [³H]Nicotine can be used to label the sites *in vivo* in the mouse (Broussolle et al 1989). We have also done some studies with [¹¹C]nicotine. The problem is to estimate non-specific binding accurately. Agonists are far better than antagonists at interacting with nicotinic ACh recognition sites. Therefore, to estimate non-specific binding, potential inhibitors of *in vivo* [³H]nicotine binding would be needed at concentrations that would also produce toxicity. Ian Stolerman's work, however, suggests that we could use lobeline to estimate non-specific binding. Lobeline is somewhat toxic, but it is not as toxic as nicotine, cytisine or other agonists.

We have also pretreated animals with mecamylamine. This allows us to increase the dose of agonist to estimate non-specific binding. Nonetheless, *in vivo* binding is fraught with such difficulties in quantitation that at this point it can't be used to answer mechanistic questions.

Kellar: There is another method to address this point, namely *in vivo* release. There's no question that there is an increased number of binding sites. You can see it in slices, you can see it in homogenates. The question Susan Wonnacott raised is, is there a change in the function? If so, is there a change that you see both *in vivo* and *in vitro*, or both in slices and in cell preparations where phosphatases and other enzymes are working?

Wonnacott: The problem is that one uses an *in vitro* method to focus on a particular area, in this case the presynaptic locus. That kind of interpretation is sometimes more difficult using the *in vivo* methods, especially if you are giving systemic nicotine and you don't know which pathways might be provoking the response.

Gray: Susan, you showed a nice correlation between the number of nicotine binding sites and dopamine release. You also mentioned that in the nucleus accumbens you can get the same response to a lower dose of nicotine. Is there a higher density of nicotine receptors in the accumbens than in the striatum, and might this account for the different doses?

Clarke: I don't know the answer, but I doubt whether a difference in B_{max} is going to explain the difference in ED_{50}.

Wonnacott: I wouldn't have thought it would. If you determined dose-response curves, they should be the same in the two tissues, but the responses in the nucleus accumbens would be bigger all the way along.

Kellar: Not if there are many spare receptors. If there are 80% spare receptors, then you could get a nearly 10-fold difference.

Collins: We looked at the relationship between the response to nicotine, as measured in several different ways, and the number of nicotinic receptors. There is a correlation between receptor numbers and ED_{50}, which is really unexpected—we would have expected a correlation between receptor numbers and maximal response. We also found a correlation between nicotine binding sites in the striatum and locomotor activity of 0.64, almost exactly the same value as you got in your release studies!

Balfour: It is true that acute nicotine stimulates corticosterone production, but does the chronic administration of nicotine maintain corticosterone at the high level? If not, doesn't that dismiss that as a possible modulator of the changes of animals treated chronically with nicotine?

Collins: The data are incomplete. With our infusion methodology in rats we see an increase in corticosterone and then it returns towards control over our infusion time. We have no knowledge of what happens during withdrawal. We do see elevated concentrations of corticosterone throughout our infusion period.

Balfour: In our own studies in rats, habituation to the effects of nicotine on plasma corticosterone develops rapidly and after only five injections no response to nicotine is observed (Benwell & Balfour 1979).

References

Benwell MEM, Balfour DJK 1979 Effects of nicotine administration and its withdrawal on plasma corticosterone and brain 5-hydroxyindoles. Psychopharmacology 63:7–11

Broussolle EP, Wong DF, Fanelli RJ, London ED 1989 In vivo specific binding of [³H]*l*-nicotine in the mouse brain. Life Sci 44:1123–1132

Collins AC, Bhat RV, Pauly JR, Marks MJ 1990 Modulation of nicotine receptors by chronic exposure to nicotinic agonists and antagonists. In: The biology of nicotine dependence. Wiley, Chichester (Ciba Found Symp 152) p 68–86

General discussion I

Inactivation of nicotinic cholinergic receptors

Kellar: Professor Gray asked earlier whether or not there is tolerance to nicotine. Is it possible to correlate changes in receptors with *in vivo* function? We have studied this in a neuroendocrine model. We inject rats with nicotine i.v, collect blood samples and measure hormone concentrations; I would like to describe our results with prolactin.

If you inject a rat with nicotine, there is a 5–6-fold increase in prolactin in the serum 10 minutes after the injection. If you give a second injection one hour later, there is no response. Other prolactin releasers, such as morphine, serotonin agonists, thyrotropin releasing hormone (TRH), all release prolactin at this point. If you do the second injection of nicotine 24 hours after the first, the animal responds again. So there is a recovery from one dose of nicotine within one day. Bert Sharp of Minnesota has shown that this diminished response can be seen for at least six hours after a single injection. If you have injected 30–100 µg/kg of nicotine, there is still plenty of nicotine circulating. Therefore, this may be acute desensitization. Within 24 hours, which would represent 10–12 half lives, the function of the receptor is restored. The dose–response curve for desensitization is interesting because the receptor seems to be desensitized at a lower dose of nicotine than is needed to provoke prolactin release. The ED_{50} for prolactin release is approximately 100 µg/kg of nicotine. The ED_{50} for desensitization is about 25 µg/kg.

We then gave nicotine chronically for 10 days, and looked at what happens at certain times after the last injection of nicotine. In control animals that received water for 10 days there was a normal response. The animals that received nicotine for 10 days showed no response to nicotine, even eight days after the last injection. There is an increased number of nicotine receptors at this point. By 14 days after the last injection, there is some prolactin release and at 21 days the response is the same as in control animals. This is the same time course that we get for return of receptors to control levels after elevation by 50–80%. This suggests that the change in the number of receptors is a response to the lack of activation of the receptor; the cell senses that, and thus sees the nicotine as an antagonist, and up-regulates the receptors. We don't know what kind of nicotinic receptor this one is. Is it a strange receptor or is nicotine strange? We think it's the nicotine that is strange.

The complementary experiment is to give diisopropyl fluorophosphate (DFP), a cholinesterase inhibitor, for 10 days. In the control animals nicotine releases prolactin, as do morphine, serotonin agonists or TRH. After chronic administration of DFP, which down-regulates the receptors by more than 50%, the response to nicotine is diminished with no effect on the response to the other agents. This is not the same as what we saw with chronically administered nicotine. After chronic DFP, there is still a significant release of prolactin in response to nicotine, but it is diminished compared to that of controls (about twofold increase compared to fivefold increase). With chronic administration of nicotine there was inactivation—no response at all. The decreased response after DFP correlates very nicely with the down-regulation of receptors. It is the response to ACh; by inhibiting cholinesterase, we have increased the amount of ACh in the synapse; therefore there is a normal down-regulation of receptors. So the receptor is acting normally; the only thing different about the receptor is that it doesn't know we call nicotine an agonist.

Changeux: Your finding of a higher affinity for desensitization than for prolactin release agrees with what is known about the peripheral nicotinic receptor. You can even desensitize these receptors by low concentrations of agonist without activating them.

Stolerman: Several characteristics of the tolerance that you found with nicotine parallel those of tolerance to the locomotor depressant effect. One parameter you didn't give was the nature and extent of the shift in the dose–response curve; for the locomotor effect this is 2–3-fold to the right.

Kellar: We have not found any dose of nicotine that can increase prolactin after chronic injections of nicotine. This is not a shift in the dose–response curve, it is *inactivation*. However, our experiments are limited; we can only go up to about 200 µg/kg. (This is nicotine bititrate dihydrate, so in terms of the free base the concentration would be about one third of that.) Above those doses, nicotine induces convulsions in the animals.

Wonnacott: Could you pursue that *in vitro*? Treat the animals chronically with nicotine *in vivo*, then look at responses to high doses of nicotine *in vitro*?

Kellar: Not to release prolactin, because the releasing inhibitory factor, dopamine, would not be present. We are doing it with corticotropin releasing factor (CRF). We have done similar experiments with adrenocorticotropic hormone (ACTH) release *in vivo* and get similar results.

Rose: Do you have any mechanism that accounts for why the response takes 14 days to come back? Is the receptor in a desensitized state all that time or has it been taken out of action somehow?

Kellar: I think the renewed response is due to the synthesis of new receptors that have never been exposed to nicotine. In the meantime the increased number of binding sites represents inactive receptors that are being degraded by normal turnover mechanisms—that's what I would suspect.

Rose: In other words, there aren't any functional nicotine receptors that have seen nicotine during the chronic nicotine administration.

Kellar: That's right. With regard to this response there are no functional receptors that remain after the chronic administration of nicotine.

Clarke: Have you done a test to show that this is a central effect of nicotine?

Kellar: Yes, the response is blocked by mecamylamine but hexamethonium is about 10–20 times less potent, suggesting that the response is hypothalamic. We can put nicotine into the lateral ventricle of the brain, at doses that when given parentally do not cause release (1 µg or less), and it will release prolactin. That effect is blocked by mecamylamine.

Clarke: Although most people use hexamethonium as the control for the peripheral effects of nicotine and although hexamethonium and mecamylamine are equipotent in the cat, this has not been looked at very carefully in the rat. There is some evidence that hexamethonium is only about 1/20th as potent as mecamylamine in the periphery of the rat (Romano 1981). So maybe hexamethonium is not a great antagonist, even in the periphery, in the rat.

Russell: This is a remarkable effect, that a modest dose of nicotine appears to inactivate the prolactin response for about 14 days, and that recovery is dependent on the synthesis of new receptors. What is happening then in human smokers who are taking nicotine all the time? If smokers abstain from nicotine for 24 or 48 hours, there is a measurable prolactin release when they smoke. Even when they are chronically smoking, their prolactin levels are slightly lower, but not much lower. Does this mean that smokers are producing new functional receptors at a terrific pace to replace the ones that are being inactivated?

Kellar: You have to be careful; we use prolactin because it is convenient. There are several ways of releasing prolactin, this is one pathway that we can define at least part of. In humans, you have to be careful not to overinterpret the data with regard to the effect of nicotine on prolactin levels. There is evidence that smokers have more difficulty nursing babies, I don't know whether that is related to the effect I have described here.

Collins: You discussed heterologous desensitization and suggested that it doesn't occur in this system, i.e. that there is release by other prolactin releasing compounds. Have you any idea what the neuronal network might be in terms of the nicotine system versus the opiate system versus dopamine agonists?

Kellar: We know that with regard to prolactin there is a cholinergic neuron that acts on an opiate neuron. This releases, we believe, β endorphin onto an opiate receptor. This in turn releases serotinin onto a serotonin 1A receptor, which then disinhibits dopamine and releases prolactin. We don't know that there are not other synapses in between these! But, dopamine is the final mediator, because bromocriptine will reverse all of this.

Gray: Where is the starting ACTH neuron?

Kellar: Excellent question, we don't even know that it is in the hypothalamus. We are trying to find out. The serotonin and the dopamine synapses involved in prolactin release are in the hypothalamus—that's been shown by John Willoughby's lab in Australia. He injects a serotonin 1A agonist into the basal hypothalamus and gets release of prolactin. We don't know what the inputs are to the cholinergic neuron; we don't know whether there are even more synapses in between, but we do know this is the order of these synapses.

Collins: Does that mean that an animal that is tolerant to opiates will be cross tolerant to nicotine?

Kellar: I can't say tolerant. A morphine blocker, naltrexone, will block the effects of nicotine on prolactin release. But mecamylamine will not block the effects of morphine. We do see some tolerance to morphine, as other people have, but we haven't pursued that.

Location and function of nicotinic receptors in cultured cortical neurons

Lippiello: Our laboratory has been interested in two things: the cellular localization of nicotinic receptor sites in the CNS and the functional properties of those sites. We are using primary cultures of fetal rat cortical neurons and have been able to identify high affinity nicotine binding sites on these cells. These sites have all the characteristics of putative nicotinic receptors described in adult brain; their binding affinities and pharmacological specificity are essentially the same. The density of sites in these cells is around 20 fmoles/mg protein, which if you assume homogeneous distribution across the cells, is equivalent to about 1000 sites per cell. We have been examining potential probes for identifying where these sites are located on the cells. The approach we are now using is based on anti-idiotypic antibodies. John Langone (Baylor College) has produced anti-idiotypes against anti-nicotine antibodies. We screened a number of these anti-idiotypic antibodies, looking at their ability to inhibit nicotine binding and to label neuronal cells by indirect immunofluorescence. Two clones (420G11, 422F11) very effectively inhibit [^{3}H]nicotine binding to either solubilized receptors or intact cells. They also specifically label around 20% of the cells, as indicated by immunofluorescent staining. The immunofluorescent labelling can be blocked by nicotine; it is not blocked by α- or $\varkappa$-(neuronal) bungarotoxin, however.

We also tried to stain the cells with antibodies against choline acetyltransferase. Fetal cortical neurons do not appear to have detectable enzyme; this may suggest that fetal cortex contains few, if any, intrinsic cholinergic neurons. We have no evidence that these cells form synaptic contacts in culture. Nicotinic sites identified by the anti-idiotypes probably represent cell surface sites located diffusely across the surface of the cells.

The most intense labelling by the anti-idiotypes is on very thick dendritic processes, and to a lesser extent cell bodies, of pyramidal and bipolar neurons. The labelling is specific to neuronal cell types, since we don't see any labelling of glial cultures. We are fairly confident that the sites represent cell surface receptors. Interestingly, the anti-idiotypes do not show appreciable labelling over the first few days in culture. After about a week in culture one sees very nice staining. If the cells are permeabilized with saponin during the first few days in culture, the labelling appears primarily in cell bodies. So we think there may be a developmental change during the first week in culture related to the expression of these sites on the cell surface. We also believe that the anti-idiotypes are binding to high affinity nicotinic receptor sites, since the labelling cannot be blocked with α-bungarotoxin. However, we can't rule out a low affinity nicotine binding site or an α subunit that doesn't bind nicotine or bungarotoxin.

We have also been looking at the possible functional significance of these sites. To do this, we load the cells with fura-2, which is a calcium-sensitive dye, and use video microscopy and image analysis techniques to analyse nicotine-evoked changes in calcium flux. In agreement with the antibody labelling experiments, about 10–20% of the cells are responsive to nicotine in the calcium flux assay. Within about six seconds there is a significant response to nicotine which amounts to a twofold increase in intracellular calcium. Resting calcium levels are usually about 30–50 nM in these cells. By comparison, K^+ increased calcium levels to around 200–300 nM. Interestingly, about 20–30 seconds after the addition of nicotine, intracellular calcium returns to near resting levels. This may be an indication of desensitization of the calcium response. However, we haven't been able to link this phenomenon directly to nicotine-gated ion channels at this point.

Collins: What concentrations of nicotine do you use?

Lippiello: We typically use 50 nM to 1 µM. The experiments shown here were done at 0.5 µM. We have detected responses to as little as 50 nM. We have some evidence that the magnitude of the calcium response may depend on the resting potential of the cells. When we treat the cells with K^+, allow the calcium to return to resting levels, and then add nicotine, we see an enhanced response— about twice that seen without K^+. Dr Sam Deadwyler (Wake Forest University) is also doing some patch studies on these cells, and he sees a nicotine-evoked inward current, blockable with d-tubocurarine, that seems to desensitize in less than a minute.

We can block the calcium response with decamethonium, but mecamylamine seems to give less consistent results for some reason, at least with this cell preparation.

Pretreatment with 5–10 mM K^+ gives a nicotine response that is comparable to the response seen with depolarizing concentrations of K^+, so there appears to be some kind of synergism involved. One can also clamp the membrane potential at different levels, and the magnitude of nicotine-evoked electro-physiological responses is also affected. I'm not sure exactly what this means. In general, from what we have seen so far, the sites we are studying may represent high affinity postsynaptic receptors in the cortex, which are primarily modulatory in nature.

Gray: Would one expect responses as long as that, if the cells were hooked up in a normal wiring pattern in the cortex? It would take 26 seconds to get back to baseline. We were talking earlier about very fast nicotinic responses in the neuromuscular junction. Would calcium affect the function of the cell for that length of time in a wired-up neuron?

Lippiello: That's a good question. We would like to co-culture these cells with cells from other parts of the brain and possibly get them to form some synaptic connections. The sites we are looking at in our fetal cortical cultures are probably similar to those on immature muscle. They tend to be spread diffusely over the surface of the cells; we don't see much evidence for patches of sites.

Heinemann: Are the cells that are labelled with the anti-idiotypic antibodies the same cells that respond to nicotine?

Lippiello: The bipolar and pyramidal neurons that stain with the anti-idiotypes are morphologically the same as those responding in the calcium flux experiments. We are now trying to do the functional assay and then post-label the cells with the anti-idiotypes to confirm their identity.

Heinemann: Is binding of the antibody blocked by nicotine?

Lippiello: Yes, it takes a lot of nicotine to do that. One explanation is that there are also some low affinity nicotine sites present on these cells, in addition to the well-defined high affinity sites.

Schwartz: Do you think that one of the problems with these kinds of functional assays in an adult rat may be related to the way that mRNAs for receptors appear in fetal tissue then disappear, relatively speaking, in the adult?

Lippiello: Yes. Our system may enable us to assess developmental changes *in vitro*. We also have the capability to look at any two parameters, such as membrane potential and calcium flux, at the same time. We have some new probes for Na^+ and K^+ that we are testing for ion specificity.

Schwartz: In relation to what Joe Henry Steinbach said about what are the nicotinic receptors doing in the CNS, maybe we should be looking at the system as a modulatory system rather than a primary neurotransmission system. Your technique might be a good way of getting at that. This calcium flux technique has been worked out very nicely in cells for the glutamate system, for example. Maybe the way to look at this functionally in the adult is to look at modulation of glutamate neurotransmission by nicotinic compounds.

Lippiello: We think that may be the case. The magnitude of the nicotine-evoked calcium response is fairly modest compared to other things that cause extracellular calcium influx. Because pretreatment with K^+ tends to enhance the nicotinic response, it looks as though nicotinic effects may be primarily sub-threshold. However, as the resting potential becomes less negative, you may get to a point where there are enough nicotinic sites to fire the cell, resulting in a larger calcium response.

Clarke: Assuming this is receptor desensitization that you see, does receptor function come back in the prolonged presence of agonist?

Lippiello: We are trying that right now. The problem is to be sure that you washed out all the nicotine before re-stimulating the cells.

Clarke: In the prolonged presence of nicotine do you see another wave of activation? Let's say the receptors all desensitize for one minute and then all re-sensitize, have you noticed any further agonist response?

Lippiello: The cells are exposed to nicotine for a maximum of 2–3 minutes. During that continuous exposure there are no additional responses. We haven't looked at longer times.

Clarke: Is this definitely influx of calcium or could it have been relocalization from internal stores?

Lippiello: We don't know. This is all very preliminary.

Lunt: Have you used your anti-idiotype to map receptor localization in tissue sections?

Lippiello: John Langone has been doing that.

Lunt: Does it correlate with the sorts of patterns we are seeing using other ligands?

Lippiello: Yes. But my understanding is that it is difficult to label fixed tissue slices with the anti-idiotypes. Even in our cultured cells it takes an hour or more to label at room temperature, so I suspect there may be limited accessibility of the antibodies to the receptor sites.

References

Romano C 1981 Nicotine action on rat colon. J Pharmacol Exp Ther 217:828–833

Regulation of endocrine function by the nicotinic cholinergic receptor

K. Fuxe, L. F. Agnati*, A. Jansson, G. von Euler, S. Tanganelli, K. Andersson and P. Eneroth**

Department of Histology and Neurobiology, Karolinska Institutet, Box 60400, S-104 01 Stockholm, Sweden; **Department of Applied Biochemistry, Huddinge Hospital, Huddinge, Sweden and *Department of Human Physiology, University of Modena, Modena, Italy

Abstract. One important neuroendocrine action of nicotine in the male rat is an increase in the secretion of corticosterone which is seen upon acute and acute intermittent exposure to nicotine. Tolerance develops to this action of nicotine upon chronic exposure, and in the withdrawal phase serum corticosterone levels are substantially reduced. In contrast, no significant increases of serum corticosterone levels were observed upon acute intermittent treatment with nicotine in the dioestrous rat. Available evidence indicates that corticosterone can modulate dopamine transmission in the basal ganglia via glucocorticoid receptors within the nucleus accumbens and neostriatum, and via glucocorticoid receptor immunoreactivity in nigrostriatal and mesolimbic dopamine pathways. Through concerted pre- and postsynaptic actions glucocorticoids may decrease dopamine transmission, especially that mediated by D2 receptors in these regions. In view of the hypothesis that the mesolimbic dopamine pathways mediate the euphoric effects of nicotine, the secretion of corticosterone induced by nicotine in the smoking male may substantially influence the mood elevating activity of nicotine. Thus, individual smoking habits may depend on the ability of nicotine to induce corticosterone secretion, which obviously would also vary with the degree of stress. The glucocorticoids may in a similar way influence the arousal action of nicotine because of the high number of glucocorticoid receptors present both in noradrenaline cell bodies of the locus ceruleus and within the entire cerebral cortex.

1990 The biology of nicotine dependence. Wiley, Chichester (Ciba Foundation Symposium 152) p 113–130

The neuroendocrine actions of nicotine are complex and highly dependent on the mode of administration—acute, acute intermittent or chronic (see Fuxe et al 1987a, 1989a,c). In this paper, we summarize the neuroendocrine actions of nicotine in adults and the effects of pre- and/or postnatal treatment of nicotine on the development of neuroendocrine function (Jansson et al 1989, 1990a). We focus on the effects of nicotine on adrenocorticotropic hormone (ACTH) and corticosterone secretion, since the mesolimbic dopamine (DA) pathways which mediate the euphoric actions of nicotine (see Andersson et al 1981a,b, Singer et al 1982, Clarke et al 1988, DiChiara & Imperato 1988) appear to be regulated by glucocorticoids (Fuxe et al 1985, Härfstrand et al 1986, von Euler et al 1989, Zoli et al 1990, Tanganelli et al 1990). It has also recently been demonstrated that the adrenocortical hormones control nicotine sensitivity in mice (Pauly et al 1988). Adrenalectomy increased nicotine sensitivity as measured in biological tests, although the brain nicotinic cholinergic receptors were not altered nor was nicotine metabolism.

Neuroendocrine actions of nicotine in adult rats

The initial effects of nicotine in the adult male rat are a marked hypersecretion of ACTH, vasopressin, β-endorphin, prolactin and luteinizing hormone (LH), associated with a delayed increase of serum corticosterone levels due to the very rapid increase in the ACTH secretion (Table 1) (for review, see Fuxe et al 1987a, 1989a,b). Acute intermittent treatment with nicotine (30 minute intervals) or intermittent exposure to cigarette smoke leads to inhibitory effects on prolactin, LH and thyroid stimulating hormone (TSH) secretion. However, the hypersecretion of corticosterone is maintained after this type of intermittent treatment with nicotine in the male rat (Table 2). Rapid desensitization of the acute stimulatory effects of nicotine on rat plasma ACTH takes place on acute intermittent treatment of high frequency (Sharp & Bayer 1986). This also occurs on chronic exposure to nicotine or to cigarette smoke (Table 2), whereas the inhibitory effects on LH and prolactin secretion are maintained (Balfour et al 1975, Balfour & Morrison 1975, Cam & Bassett 1979, Andersson et al 1983, 1985b, Fuxe et al 1987a, 1989a,b).

Nicotine may release ACTH and thus increase serum corticosterone levels in the rat, not only by activation of central nicotinic receptors that control corticotropin releasing factor neuronal pathways, but also via release of catecholamines from the adrenal medulla, which can release ACTH from the pituitary gland via activation of β-adrenergic receptors (Reisine et al 1984). It is also possible that nicotine acts additively with ACTH to stimulate adrenal steroidogenesis (see Rubin & Warner 1975, Balfour et al 1975).

There are sex-specific differences in the nicotine-induced changes in ACTH and corticosterone secretion. Acute intermittent exposure to cigarette smoke in the male rat increases corticosterone secretion (Andersson et al 1985a), while exposure to cigarette smoke in the dioestrous rat does not lead to any significant alterations in ACTH and corticosterone secretion (Table 2) (Andersson et al 1988a). Thus, gonadal steroids may regulate the sensitivity of cholinergic nicotinic receptors or the networks controlling secretion of corticotropin releasing factor.

Another factor of importance for the effect of nicotine on corticosterone secretion is the type of exposure to nicotine. Andersson et al (1987) showed that

TABLE 1 Effects of nicotine on plasma levels of pituitary hormones and on homeostatic and behavioural responses

Pituitary hormones	Change in plasma levels after nicotine	Homeostatic responses affected[a]	Behavioural responses affected[a]	Development of tolerance[b]
Adrenocorticotrophic hormone	↑	Control of catabolism (GC) Immune responses (GC)	Fear-motivated behaviour (activated by ACTH; inhibited by GC)	Partial
β-Endorphin	↑	?	Reinforcement Pain threshold	Partial
Growth hormone	↑ (man) ↓ (rat)	Control of anabolism Immune responses	?	?
Luteinizing hormone	↑, ↓ acute	?	Sexual behaviour	Partial ↑ No ↓
Follicle stimulating hormone	–, ↓	?	?	No
Prolactin	↑, ↓ acute	Control of extracellular fluid Immune responses	Sexual and parental behaviour	Partial ↑ No ↓
Thyroid stimulating hormone	↓	Control of energy metabolism, anabolism	?	Yes
Vasopressin	↑	Control of extracellular fluid, arterial blood pressure, immune responses	Cognitive behaviour	No

ACTH, adrenocorticotropic hormone; GC, glucocorticoid hormones; ↑, increased; ↓ decreased; ?, unknown.
[a]Possibly mediated by changes in secretion of pituitary hormones. These responses are biphasic, an early increase being followed by a later decrease in activity.
[b]Partial refers to the acute early increase; No refers to the late decrease.

TABLE 2   Effects of nicotine and exposure to cigarette smoke on the pituitary-adrenal axis and regional utilization of catecholamine

Nicotine treatment	ACTH	Corticosterone	Median eminence dopamine	PA noradrenaline
Single dose (male)	↑	↑ (delayed)	—	↑
Acute intermittent (male)	↑	↑	↑	↑
Chronic exposure to cigarette smoke (male)	—	—	↑	—
Acute continuous exposure to cigarette smoke (male)	↑	—	—	↑
Acute intermittent exposure to cigarette smoke (female)	—	—	↑	↑

↑, increase; —, no change; ACTH, adrenocorticotropic hormone; PA, paraventricular hypothalamic nucleus. Summary of results obtained from Andersson et al (1983, 1985a,b, 1987, 1988a), Fuxe et al (1989a).

acute continuous exposure of male rats to cigarette smoke does not lead to any changes in serum ACTH and corticosterone levels (Table 2).

Of substantial interest are the findings that by 48 hours after withdrawal from chronic exposure to cigarette smoke there is a highly significant lowering of corticosterone serum levels in spite of maintained blood levels of ACTH. This is no longer seen after 72 hours (Table 3) (Andersson et al 1989). These types of endocrine changes may lead to alterations in fear-motivated behaviour and contribute to the behavioural withdrawal reactions, since glucocorticoids suppress fear-motivated behaviours, while ACTH enhances them (DeWied 1980, Bohus et al 1982). Thus, the endocrine disturbance observed after cessation of exposure to nicotine could facilitate fear-motivated behaviour, which may contribute to the withdrawal symptoms. One important site of interaction of ACTH peptides and glucocorticoids is the locus ceruleus, which contains glucocorticoid receptor (GR)-immunoreactive noradrenaline (NA) cell bodies (Fuxe et al 1985) and which can be modulated by ACTH (Markey & Sze 1984).

Studies in humans have demonstrated significant dose-related increases in serum cortisol levels on smoking of high nicotine cigarettes (see Pomerleau & Rosecrans 1989, Seyler et al 1984). However, Seyler et al (1984) found increases of ACTH secretion only in smokers showing nausea, while Novac & Allen-Rowlands (1985) observed increases of ACTH, cortisol and β-endorphin also in the absence of nausea. Thus, activation of the pituitary–adrenal axis by nicotine in humans may not be caused by the induction of nausea by nicotine but be related to an effect on central nicotinic cholinergic receptors in the brain. Increases of corticosterone secretion may be an important factor in the development of nicotine dependence and/or nicotine withdrawal reactions in view of the widespread presence of GR immunoreactivity in DA pathways and

TABLE 3 **Effects of withdrawal from exposure to cigarette smoke on neuroendocrine function**

Time after withdrawal	Follicle stimulating hormone	Adreno-corticotropic hormone	Corticosterone	Prolactin
48 hours	↓	—	↓	↓
72 hours	—	—	—	↓
7 days	—	—	—	—

↓, decrease; —, no change. Summary of results obtained from Andersson et al (1989).

NA pathways and their target areas, such as the nucleus accumbens and the cerebral cortex (Härfstrand et al 1986, Fuxe et al 1987b) (see below and Figs. 1 and 2).

Neuroendocrine actions of nicotine after pre- and/or postnatal treatment in the male and female rat

We have studied whether combined chronic pre- and postnatal exposure to high concentrations of nicotine in the drinking water can lead to long-lasting changes in discrete catecholamine nerve terminal systems and in neuroendocrine function in male and female rats (Jansson et al 1989). The concentration of nicotine hydrogen (+)tartrate in the drinking water was 160 mg/l, corresponding to a dose of 12 mg nicotine free base per kg per day. The treatment was maintained for the entire prenatal period and three weeks after birth. Analysis of catecholamines and of neuroendocrine function was performed one week after withdrawal from the nicotine treatment and at six months of age. Serum corticosterone levels were not influenced by this pre- and postnatal nicotine treatment. The major alteration was found in prolactin secretion (Table 4). In the female but not in the male rat a marked reduction of serum prolactin levels was observed after one week of withdrawal. Control levels were restored in adults. The pre- and postnatal nicotine treatment resulted in a marked activation of the tuberoinfundibular DA neurons of the median eminence of the female rat, which was maintained in adults, although serum prolactin levels had returned to normal (Table 4) (Jansson et al 1989). The permanent activation of the tuberinfundibular DA neurons in the female rat may have important functional consequences for the regulation of LH, prolactin and TSH secretion in view of the inhibition of the release of LH releasing hormone, prolactin and thyrotropin releasing hormone (see Fuxe et al 1989a,b). The pre- and postnatal treatment with nicotine did not significantly reduce the prolactin serum levels in the male rat at seven days after cessation of treatment, suggesting that the inhibitory effects on prolactin secretion are sex specific. The activation of the tuberoinfundibular DA neurons at this time in male rats was much less than in the female (Table 4).

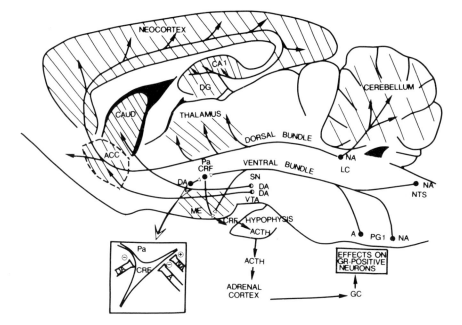

FIG. 1. Illustration of distribution of glucocorticoid receptors in relation to the mesolimbic dopamine neurons, the non-locus ceruleus and locus ceruleus noradrenaline neurons and the corticotropin releasing factor pathways to the median eminence. A, adrenaline; ACC, nucleus accumbens; ACTH, adrenocorticotropic hormone; CAUD, nucleus caudatus; CRF, corticotropin releasing factor; DA, dopamine; DG, dentate gyrus; GC, glucocorticoid hormones; GR, glucocorticoid receptor; LC, locus ceruleus; ME, median eminence; NA, noradrenaline; NTS, nucleus tractus solitarius; Pa, paraventricular hypothalamic nucleus; PG1, paragigantocellular reticular nucleus; SN, substantia nigra; VTA, ventral tegmental area. ▨ GR-rich areas. GR/transmitter coexistence: ●, 100%; ◑, 50%; ○, 0%.

We also evaluated the effects of combined pre- and postnatal nicotine exposure on DA levels and utilization in various forebrain DA nerve terminal systems in the postnatal and adult male rat. There was a selective increase in DA levels and utilization in the anterior but not in the posterior part of the nucleus accumbens seven days after cessation of treatment (Table 4) (Jansson et al 1990b). No effects were observed on DA nerve terminals in the nucleus caudatus putamen and tuberculum olfactorium. In seven month old male rats these effects were no longer significant, but a trend for increased DA utilization within the anterior nucleus accumbens was still present.

This long-term activation of DA synthesis and release in nerve terminals of the anterior nucleus accumbens may contribute to the increased spontaneous locomotion observed in adult rodents after prenatal nicotine exposure. Pre- and postnatal nicotine treatment may, therefore, selectively disrupt the mechanisms

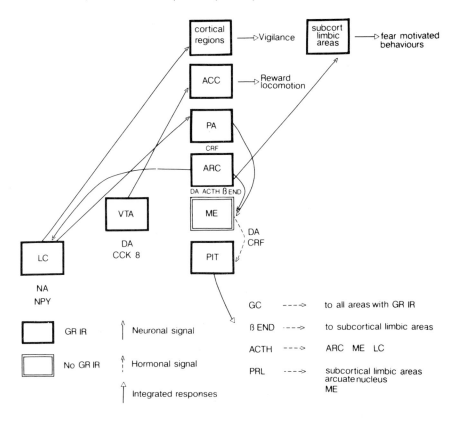

FIG. 2. Summary scheme of the catecholamine pathways and hormonal signals involved in the control of arousal, fear-regulated behaviours and mood, focusing on the role of mesolimbic dopamine pathways and the locus ceruleus noradrenaline system. ACC, nucleus accumbens; ACTH, adrenocorticotropic hormone; ARC, arcuate nucleus; β-end, β-endorphin; CRF, corticotropin releasing factor; DA, dopamine; GC, glucocorticoid hormone; GR IR, glucocorticoid immunoreactivity; LC, locus ceruleus; ME, median eminence; PA, paraventricular hypothalamic nucleus; PIT, pituitary gland; PRL, prolactin; VTA, ventral tegmental area.

that regulate cellular replication and/or differentiation in regions controlling the meso-accumbens DA pathways. Further work will be performed to evaluate the neurochemical mechanisms underlying the possible permanent activation of the DA nerve terminal networks of the anterior nucleus accumbens and those within the median eminence (see Slotkin et al 1987).

It should be pointed out that the withdrawal reaction in the hypothalamic catecholamine nerve terminal systems is observed only 48 and 72 hours after the last exposure (Andersson et al 1989). Therefore, it is possible that the activation of the accumbens DA nerve terminals seen one week after cessation

TABLE 4   Long-term effects of pre- and postnatal exposure to nicotine on hypothalamic catecholamine utilization and hypophyseal hormone secretion

Time after treatment	Catecholamine utilization			Hormone levels		
	ME	ACC	PA	LH	PRL	CORT
7 days						
Female	↑	NT	—	—	↓	—
Male	(↑)	↑	—	—	—	—
Adulthood						
Female	↑	NT	—	—	—	—
Male	(↑)	(↑)	↑NA	↑	—	—

↑, increase; ↓, decrease; —, no change; NT, not tested; ACC, nucleus accumbens; CORT, corticosterone; LH, luteinizing hormone; ME, median eminence; NA, noradrenaline; PA, paraventricular hypothalamic nucleus; PRL, prolactin. Summary of results obtained from Jansson et al (1989, 1990b).

of the postnatal exposure to nicotine is a long-term action related to the teratological effects of nicotine (Slotkin et al 1987). These results are very interesting in view of the fact that the accumbens DA nerve terminals probably play an important role in reward mechanisms, as pointed out above. DA in the nucleus accumbens also induces locomotor behaviour. A long-term activation of the accumbens DA nerve terminals after prenatal nicotine exposure would support the notion that smoking during pregnancy is one cause of the hyperkinetic syndrome in new-born babies.

We have also evaluated the effects of postnatal exposure to cigarette smoke on neuroendocrine function in the male rat (Table 5) (Jansson et al 1990a). Marked but temporary increases in LH secretion occur 24 hours after postnatal exposure to cigarette smoke, while increases in prolactin and corticosterone secretion develop only in adult life, when maturation of the brain and the anterior pituitary gland is complete (Table 5). Thus, exposure to cigarette smoke, which produces no alterations in catecholamine function in adults, in postnatal

TABLE 5   Effects of daily postnatal exposure to cigarette smoke for three weeks on hypothalamic utilization of catecholamine and hypophyseal hormone levels

Time after treatment	Catecholamine utilization			Hormone levels		
	MPZ	PA	LPZ	PRL	LH	CORT
24 hours	↑	↓	—	—	↑	—
7 days	—	—	—	—	—	—
Adulthood	—	—	—	↑	—	↑

↑, increase; ↓, decrease; —, no change; NT, not tested; CORT, corticosterone; LH, luteinizing hormone; LPZ, lateral palisade zone; MPZ, medial palisade zone; PA, paraventricular hypothalamic nucleus; PRL, prolactin. Summary of results obtained from Jansson et al (1990a).

rats leads to alterations within the endocrine system. This may have consequences for hormonally regulated behaviours and stress responses, especially in view of the elevations of serum corticosterone levels in adulthood (Jansson et al 1990a). These increases in serum corticosterone levels may lead to alterations in GR activity in the central nervous system, which may lead to changes, for example, in DA and nicotinic receptor-mediated responses.

Studies on glucocorticoid receptor-immunoreactive neurons in relation to the mesolimbic and nigrostriatal dopamine pathways

Nuclear GR immunoreactivity has been demonstrated within the nigral DA cell bodies and DA cell bodies of the ventral tegmental area, as well as within the neostriatum and the nucleus accumbens (Fig. 1), where many of the nigrostriatal and mesolimbic DA pathways terminate (Fuxe et al 1985, 1987a, Härfstrand et al 1986, Zoli et al 1990). Fifty percent of the nigral DA cells and the ventral tegmental DA cells contain moderate GR immunoreactivity; in the interfascicular nucleus and in the linear caudal nucleus of the ventral tegmental area a strong GR immunoreactivity is observed (Härfstrand et al 1986). Ninety percent of the entire striatal and accumbens neuronal population in the rat contain nuclear GR immunoreactivity of weak to moderate intensity. Thus, it is likely that the D1 and D2 receptors in these regions are located on GR immunoreactive nerve cells. However, the large striatal choline acetylase-immunoreactive interneurons and the striatal neuropeptide Y-immunoreactive interneurons were shown to lack GR (Zoli et al 1990). The absence of GR in these striatal neuronal populations may explain their resistance to metabolic and toxic injuries (see Sapolsky 1985). The findings from the nucleus accumbens and neostriatum indicate that the entire basic organization of the basal ganglia in the forebrain is under glucocorticoid control. Thus, the glucocorticoids could represent a way to alter the functional states of these regions, so that the animal can respond to stressful situations. Finally, the GR-immunoreactive nerve cells form clusters in the dorsal striatum and in the nucleus accumbens. The islands most frequently found consisted of three to ten nerve cells, in both regions. However, the tyrosine hydroxylase, enkephalin and DARPP-32 islands and striae of the dorsal striatum (Agnati et al 1988) are much larger and less uniformly distributed than the GR islands demonstrated in the study of Zoli et al (1990). It will be of interest to evaluate the relationships between these two types of neuronal compartments within the dorsal striatum and the nucleus accumbens.

In conclusion, GR may influence the mesolimbic and nigrostriatal DA pathways both at the cell body–dendritic level and at the postsynaptic level within the nucleus accumbens and neostriatum.

Effects of the pituitary-adrenal axis on dopamine transmission in the basal ganglia

We have used intrastriatal microdialysis to investigate whether corticosterone suppression by adrenalectomy affects DA release and its regulation by apomorphine and cholecystokinin-8 (CCK-8) and whether replacement treatment with corticosterone counteracts these effects. The apomorphine-induced reduction in DA release was attenuated one week after adrenalectomy. This action was partially counteracted by corticosterone replacement treatment (5 mg/kg, twice daily for seven days) (Tanganelli et al 1990). These results suggest that GR have a role in maintaining the sensitivity of the D2 autoreceptors, and thereby reduce DA neurotransmission.

Thus, the increase in serum corticosterone levels that follows acute single intermittent treatment with nicotine may increase the sensitivity of the D2 autoreceptors and thus dampen the nicotine-induced release. It is possible that corticosterone acts via GR in the nigral DA cells, controlling *inter alia* the synthesis of G proteins involved in the regulation of DA autoreceptors (Tanganelli et al 1990).

CCK-8 administered via the microdialysis probe was one hundredfold more effective in increasing DA release in the neostriatum after adrenalectomy. This increase in potency of CCK-8 was fully counteracted by replacement treatment with corticosterone. These findings suggest that corticosterone can regulate the function of striatal CCK-8 receptors, at least those controlling DA release, leading to reduction of striatal DA transmission.

The reduction of the D2 autoreceptor function after adrenalectomy may be caused by a reduction in the affinity of these receptors, since adrenalectomy increases the K_D of the D2 agonist binding sites without affecting the B_{max} (von Euler et al 1989). This increase in the K_D was fully counteracted by replacement treatment with corticosterone (5 mg/kg, twice daily for one week, last injection two hours before killing). However, adrenalectomy does not alter the binding characteristics of D2 antagonist binding sites (Faunt & Crocker 1988). Although adrenalectomy reduces the affinity of the D2 receptors, it potentiates D2-regulated behaviours, an effect which is counteracted by corticosterone treatment (Faunt & Crocker 1989). These results indicate that for the postsynaptic D2 receptors the reduced affinity may reflect an increase in the coupling to signal-transducing proteins, such as the G protein. Since both these effects of adrenalectomy on D2 receptor function are reversed by corticosterone treatment, it is possible that corticosterone, via a combined pre- and postsynaptic action on the ascending DA pathways to the neostriatum and nucleus accumbens, reduces DA transmission, especially that mediated by D2 receptors. Thus, glucocorticoids seem capable of producing concerted responses in the nigrostriatal and mesolimbic DA systems, allowing a fine tuning of DA neurotransmission. Such an action may be brought about by a differential regulation of the expression of D2 receptor-coupled G_i proteins (Kuno et al 1983, Saito et al 1989) or of the phosphorylation state of these G_i proteins or of the D2 receptor itself (von Euler et al 1989).

Glucocorticoids and the action of nicotine

The available evidence indicates that the euphoric actions of nicotine may be mediated via increased DA release, leading to an increase of DA neurotransmission within the nucleus accumbens, especially the anterior part (Table 6) which contains a diffuse DA fluorescence because of densely packed DA terminals. From the observations described above, that glucocorticoids reduce DA neurotransmission, at least that related to activation of D2 receptors, it is likely that glucocorticoids reduce the euphoric actions of nicotine. Thus, in conditions of stress the euphoric actions of nicotine may be reduced by the hypersecretion of glucocorticoids. It cannot be excluded that mineralocorticoids are also involved, but the presence of mineralocorticoid receptors has not been demonstrated within the DA neurons or within the nucleus accumbens (DeKloet et al 1987).

In support of these results, it has been shown that adrenocortical hormones can regulate nicotine sensitivity in the mouse, as measured in physiological and behavioural tests. Corticosterone treatment counteracted the effects of adrenalectomy (Pauly et al 1988). Also, corticosterone treatment of intact animals reduced the sensitivity to nicotine in various tests. However, the number of nicotinic cholinergic receptors in brain was unaltered, as was nicotine metabolism. It is therefore suggested that the ability of glucocorticoids to reduce nicotine sensitivity in rodents may be related, at least in part, to a suppression

TABLE 6 Effects of nicotine and exposure to cigarette smoke on dopamine utilization in the nucleus accumbens and on corticosterone secretion

Treatment	Dopamine utilization in nucleus accumbens neurons		Corticosterone secretion
	dotted CCK	diffuse CCK	
Single dose of nicotine	—	↑	↑
Intraventricular (1 h) or intravenous infusion (1 h) of nicotine	↑ ↑	↑ ↑	↑ ↑
Acute intermittent exposure to cigarette smoke	—	↑	↑
Chronic treatment with nicotine (via minipumps)	—	—	—

↑, increase; —, no change; CCK, cholecystokinin. Summary of results obtained from Andersson et al (1981a,b), Fuxe et al (1987a, 1989b).

of DA neurotransmission, especially that mediated by D2 receptors, within the mesotelencephalic DA pathways. Recently, however, we have observed that after a one week treatment with corticosterone (2×5 mg/kg, i.p.) the IC_{50} value of ($\pm$)nicotine to displace N-[^{3}H]methylcarbamylcholine (Aranjo et al 1989) from its binding sites in limbic membranes (nucleus accumbens and tuberculum olfactorium) is significantly increased. These results suggest that corticosterone reduces the affinity of high affinity nicotinic cholinergic receptors present in the subcortical limbic forebrain. Thus, glucocorticoids may dampen the intensity of the euphoric effect of nicotine via effects both on DA neurotransmission and on nicotinic cholinergic receptors. Glucocorticoids may in this way participate in the regulation of nicotine dependence, as well as in the regulation of withdrawal reactions to nicotine.

Acknowledgements

This work has been supported by a grant from Svenska Tobaks AB, Stockholm, Sweden.

References

Agnati LF, Fuxe K, Zoli M et al 1988 Morphometrical evidence for a complex organization of tyrosine hydroxylase-, enkephalin- and DARPP-32-like immunoreactive patches and their codistribution at three rostrocaudal levels in the rat neostriatum. Neuroscience 27:785–797

Andersson K, Fuxe K, Agnati LF 1981a Effects of single injections of nicotine on the ascending dopamine pathways in the rat. Acta Physiol Scand 112:345–347

Andersson K, Fuxe K, Agnati LF, Eneroth P 1981b Effects of acute central and peripheral administration of nicotine on ascending dopamine pathways in the male rat brain. Evidence for nicotine induced increases of dopamine turnover in various telencephalic dopamine nerve terminal systems. Med Biol (Helsinki) 59:170–176

Andersson K, Siegel R, Fuxe K, Eneroth P 1983 Intravenous injections of nicotine induced very rapid and discrete reduction of hypothalamic catecholamine levels associated with increases of ACTH, vasopressin and prolactin secretion. Acta Physiol Scand 118:35–40

Andersson K, Fuxe K, Eneroth P, Mascagni F, Agnati LF 1985a Effects of acute intermittent exposure to cigarette smoke on catecholamine levels and turnover in various types of hypothalamic DA and NA nerve terminal systems as well as on the secretion of adenohypophyseal hormones and corticosterone. Acta Physiol Scand 124:277–285

Andersson K, Eneroth P, Fuxe K, Mascagni F, Agnati LF 1985b Effects of chronic exposure to cigarette smoke on amine levels and turnover in various hypothalamic catecholamine nerve terminal systems and on the secretion of pituitary hormones in the male rat. Neuroendocrinology 41:462–466

Andersson K, Fuxe K, Eneroth P, Agnati LF, Härfstrand A 1987 Effects of acute continuous exposure of the rat to cigarette smoke on amine levels and utilization in discrete hypothalamic catecholamine nerve terminal systems and on neuroendocrine function. Arch Pharmacol 335:521–528

Andersson K, Eneroth P, Fuxe K, Härfstrand A 1988a Effects of acute intermittent exposure to cigarette smoke on hypothalamic and pre-optic catecholamine nerve terminal systems and on neuroendocrine function in the diestrous rat. Arch Pharmacol 337:131–139

Andersson K, Fuxe K, Eneroth P, Härfstrand A, Agnati LF 1988b Involvement of D1 dopamine receptors in the nicotine-induced noradrenaline release from hypothalamic and preoptic noradrenaline nerve terminal systems. Neurochem Int 13:159–163

Andersson K, Fuxe K, Eneroth P, Jansson A, Härfstrand A 1989 Effects of withdrawal from chronic exposure to cigarette smoke on hypothalamic and preoptic catecholamine nerve terminal systems and on the secretion of pituitary hormones in the male rat. Arch Pharmacol 339:387–396

Aranjo DM, Lapchak PA, Collier B, Quirion R 1989 N-(^{3}H)methylcarbamylcholine binding sites in the rat and human brain: relationship to functional nicotinic autoreceptors and alterations in Alzheimer's disease. In: Nordberg A, Fuxe K, Holmstedt B, Sundvall A (eds) Progress in Brain Research 79:345–352

Balfour DJK, Morrison CF 1975 A possible role for the pituitary-adrenal system in the effects of nicotine on avoidance behaviour. Pharmacol Biochem Behav 3:349–354

Balfour DJ, Khullar AK, Longden A 1975 Effects of nicotine on plasma corticosterone and brain amines in stressed and unstressed rats. Pharmacol Biochem Behav 3:179–184

Bohus B, DeKloet ER, Veldhuis HD 1982 Adrenal steroids and behavioral adaptation: relationship to brain corticoid receptors. In: Ganten D, Pfaff D (eds) Current topics in neuroendocrinology. Springer-Verlag, Heidelberg, p 107–148

Cam TR, Bassett JR 1979 The action of nicotine on the pituitary-adrenal cortical axis. Arch Int Pharmacodyn Ther 237:49–66

Clarke PB, Fu DS, Jakubovic A, Fibiger HC 1988 Evidence that mesolimbic dopaminergic activation underlies the locomotor stimulant action of nicotine in rats. J Pharmacol Exp Ther 246:701–708

DeKloet ER, Ratka A, Reul JMHM, Sutanto W, Van Eekelen JAM 1987 Corticosteroid receptor types in brain: regulation and putative function. Ann NY Acad Sci 512:351–361

DeWied D 1980 Peptides and adaptive behaviour. In: DeWied D, Van Keep PA (eds) Hormones and the brain. MTP Press, Lancaster, p 103–113

DiChiara G, Imperato A 1988 Drugs abused by humans preferentially increase synaptic dopamine concentrations in the mesolimbic system of freely moving rats. Proc Natl Acad Sci USA 85:5274–5278

Faunt JE, Crocker AD 1988 Adrenocortical hormone status affects responses to dopamine receptor agonists. Eur J Pharmacol 152:255–261

Faunt JE, Crocker AD 1989 Effects of adrenalectomy on responses mediated by dopamine D1 and D2 receptors. Eur J Pharmacol 162:237–244

Fuxe K, Wikström AC, Okret S et al 1985 Mapping of glucocorticoid receptor immunoreactive neurons in the rat tel- and diencephalon using a monoclonal antibody against rat liver glucocorticoid receptor. Endocrinology 177:1803–1812

Fuxe K, Andersson K, Eneroth P, Härfstrand A, Nordberg A, Agnati LF 1987a Effects of nicotine and exposure to cigarette smoke on discrete dopamine and noradrenaline nerve terminal systems of the telencephalon and diencephalon of the rat: relationship to reward mechanisms and neuroendocrine functions and distribution of nicotinic binding sites in brain. In: Martin WR et al (eds) Tobacco smoking and nicotine. Plenum, New York, p 225–262

Fuxe K, Cintra A, Härfstrand A et al 1987b Central glucocorticoid receptor immunoreactive neurons: new insights into the endocrine regulation of the brain. Ann NY Acad Sci 512:362–393

Fuxe K, Andersson K, Eneroth P et al 1989a Neurochemical mechanisms underlying the neuroendocrine actions of nicotine: focus on the plasticity of central cholinergic nicotinic receptors. In: Nordberg A et al (eds) Progress in Brain Research 79:197–207

Fuxe K, Janson AM, Jansson A, Andersson K, Eneroth P, Agnati LF 1989b Chronic nicotine treatment increases dopamine levels and reduces dopamine utilization in substantia nigra and in surviving forebrain dopamine nerve terminal systems after a partial di-mesencephalic hemitransection. Arch Pharmacol, in press

Fuxe K, Andersson K, Eneroth P, Härfstrand A, Agnati LF 1989c Neuroendocrine actions of nicotine and of exposure to cigarette smoke: medical implications. Psychoneuroendocrinology 14:19–41

Härfstrand A, Fuxe K, Cintra A et al 1986 Demonstration of glucocorticoid receptor immunoreactivity in monoamine neurons of the rat brain. Proc Natl Acad Sci USA 83:9779–9783

Jansson A, Andersson K, Fuxe K, Bjelke B, Eneroth P 1989 Effects of combined pre- and postnatal treatment with nicotine on hypothalamic catecholamine nerve terminal systems and neuroendocrine function in the four week old and adult male and female diestrous rat. J Neuroendocrinol 1:455–464

Jansson A, Andersson K, Bjelke B, Eneroth P, Fuxe K 1990a Effects of postnatal exposure to cigarette smoke on hypothalamic catecholamine nerve terminal systems and on neuroendocrine function in the postnatal and adult male rat. Evidence for long-term modulation of anterior pituitary function. Acta Physiol Scand, in press

Jansson A, Fuxe K, Andersson K, Agnati LF, Eneroth P 1990b Effects of combined prenatal and postnatal nicotine exposure on dopamine levels and utilization in various forebrain dopamine nerve terminal systems in the postnatal and adult female rat. Selective action on a subset of accumbens dopamine nerve terminals. Acta Physiol Scand, submitted

Kuno T, Shirakawa O, Tanaka C 1983 Selective decrease in the affinity of D2 dopamine receptor for agonist induced by islet-activating protein, pertussis toxin, associated with ADP-ribosylation of the specific membrane protein of bovine striatum. Biochem Biophys Res Comm 115:325–330

Markey KA, Sze PY 1984 Influence of ACTH on tyrosine hydroxylase activity in the locus coeruleus of mouse brain. Neuroendocrinology 38:269–275

Novack DH, Allen-Rowlands CF 1985 Pituitary-adrenal response to cigarette smoking (abstract). Psychosom Med 47:78

Pauly JR, Ullman EA, Collins AC 1988 Adrenocortical hormone regulation of nicotine sensitivity in mice. Physiol Behav 44:109–116

Pomerleau 'OF, Rosecrans J 1989 Neuroregulatory effects of nicotine. Psychoneuroendocrinology 14:1–17

Reisine TD, Mezey E, Palkovits M, Heisler S, Axelrod J 1984 Beta-adrenergic control of adrenocorticotropic hormone release from the anterior pituitary. In: Usdin E et al (eds) Catecholamines: neuropharmacology and central nervous system theoretical aspects. Alan R Liss, New York, p 419–423

Rubin RP, Warner W 1975 Nicotine-induced stimulation of steroidogenesis in adrenocortical cells of the cat. Br J Pharmacol 53:357–362

Saito N, Guitart X, Hayward M, Tallman JF, Duman RS, Nestler EJ 1989 Corticosterone differentially regulates the expression of $G_{s\alpha}$ and $G_{i\alpha}$ messenger RNA and protein in rat cerebral cortex. Proc Natl Acad Sci USA 86:3906–3910

Sapolsky RM 1985 A mechanism for glucocorticoid toxicity in the hippocampus: increased neuronal vulnerability to metabolic insults. J Neurosci 5:1228–1232

Seyler LE, Fertig JB, Pomerleau OF, Hunt D, Parker K 1984 The effects of smoking on ACTH and cortisol secretion. Life Sci 34:57–65

Singer G, Wallace M, Hall R 1982 Effects of dopaminergic nucleus accumbens lesions on the acquisition of schedule induced self injection of nicotine in the rat. Pharmacol Biochem Behav 17:579–581

Sharp BM, Beyer HS 1986 Rapid desensitization of the acute stimulatory effects of nicotine on rat plasma adrenocorticotropin and prolactin. J Pharmacol Exp Ther 238:486–491

Slotkin TA, Orband-Miller K, Queen KL, Whitmore WL, Seidler F 1987 Effects of prenatal nicotine exposure on biochemical development of rat brain regions: maternal drug infusions via osmotic minipumps. J Pharmacol Exp Ther 240:602–611

Tanganelli S, Fuxe K, von Euler G, Eneroth P, Agnati LF, Ungerstedt A 1990 Changes in pituitary-adrenal activity affect the apomorphine- and cholecystokinin-8-induced changes in striatal dopamine release using microdialysis. J Neural Trans, in press

von Euler G, Fuxe K, Tanganelli S, Finnman UB, Eneroth P 1989 Changes in pituitary-adrenal activity affect the binding properties of striatal dopamine D2 receptors but not their modulation by neurotensin and cholecystokinin-8. Neurochem Int, in press

Zoli M, Cintra A, Zini I et al 1990 Nerve cell clusters in dorsal striatum and nucleus accumbens of the male rat demonstrated by glucocorticoid receptor immunoreactivity. J Chem Neuroanatomy, in press

DISCUSSION

Pomerleau: You have emphasized the role of the GR, but corticosterone has relatively little affinity for that receptor. It acts preferentially at the mineralocorticoid type 1 receptor.

Fuxe: At low doses, corticosterone does act preferentially at the mineralocorticoid receptors. But these receptors have a restricted distribution within the brain; they are predominantly located in the hippocampus and in the septal region. There is no doubt that the major impact of corticosterone will be in relation to stress. Whether or not an individual is under stress when they smoke will modulate the response to nicotine.

Iversen: Could you explain how rats smoke!

Fuxe: They are exposed to smoke in special chambers for different amounts of time: one cigarette takes about 10 minutes.

Iversen: What plasma level of nicotine does smoke from one cigarette in such a chamber generate?

Fuxe: Intermittent exposure to two cigarettes gives 40–80 ng per ml. In a human smoker the peak concentration of nicotine in the plasma would be 40–50 ng/ml.

Heinemann: What about the carbon monoxide levels?

Fuxe: We controlled for that by using filter cigarettes to remove particulate matter from the smoke.

Rose: It's not enough to filter out particulates, because nicotine is one of the most irritating things in cigarette smoke. As an anecdote, I as a non-smoker can inhale smoke from a cigarette from which nicotine has been extracted but everything else is there and not cough at all, but if I puff on a cigarette that contains nicotine, I find it very irritating. Laboratory studies with smokers also show that nicotine is a key irritant in smoke (Herskovic et al 1986, Rose et al 1989).

It is very difficult to keep irritation constant and manipulate the amount of nicotine in that paradigm.

Fuxe: The only thing I can say is that we have a good correlation between our results obtained with nicotine exposure and those obtained with exposure to cigarette smoke. I believe that these data on exposure to cigarette smoke are relevant.

Grunberg: Dr Fuxe, you mentioned sex-specific differences in the responses of the rats to nicotine. It was not clear whether those were shifts of dose–response curves or absolute differences between the sexes.

Fuxe: We haven't done those dose–response curves properly for nicotine in the dioestrous rat. The exposure to cigarette smoke from one, two or four cigarettes led to dose-related increases in nicotine in the serum. There was no effect on the corticosterone level in the serum in the dioestrous rat. It may be just a shift in the dose–response curve, perhaps due to modulation by oestrogen or progesterone.

Grunberg: I think it is very important. We have found sex-specific differences in the effects of nicotine on body weight and eating behaviour (Grunberg et al 1986, 1987). We expected only a shift in the dose–response curve, but it's more than that. Nicotine had greater effects on the eating behaviour and body weight of females. Have you corrected statistically for the size of the animal? Females are smaller on the average at the same age, by 20–30%.

Fuxe: The difference in body weight was not significant.

Grunberg: It is also important to know the concentrations of nicotine in the blood.

Fuxe: The blood levels of nicotine were in the same range in the male and female rats, i.e. 40–80 ng/ml after exposure to two cigarettes. Again, I would like to emphasize the marked difference in the effects of nicotine on serum concentrations of TSH and ACTH in the dioestrous and male rats (Andersson et al 1988). There does seem to be a true sex difference.

Grunberg: When we looked at nicotine administration, we expected just a shift in dose–response curves that was due to the size of the animal, but we actually see sex-specific behavioural differences. That's why I am so interested in your results.

Fuxe: If these sex-specific differences in endocrine responses to nicotine are also true for humans, in conditions of stress there should be marked differences in the effects of nicotine in males and females on brain activity, since adrenocorticoids modulate neurotransmission.

Grunberg: That's completely consistent with our data.

Collins: In our laboratory, we find that there are sex differences in nicotine-induced corticosterone release, but they are quantitative, the dose–response curves are different—the males are more sensitive to nicotine.

Svensson: What happens to steroid concentrations in the plasma during withdrawal from other drugs? Is this a general phenomenon?

Fuxe: I don't know what happens after withdrawal from heroin or cocaine. That would be interesting to study.

Svensson: Do you think that steroid treatment might be an interesting thing to try to help people give up smoking?

West: There was an uncontrolled trial reported by Bourne (1985) of ACTH treatments for cigarette smokers with supposedly a high level of success, but with no follow-up or validation of claims of abstinence. However, from my understanding of the literature I felt that the trial was misconceived. In humans, ACTH mediates an increase in cortisol levels only in 'oversmoking', in a situation where there are all sorts of other things going on—stress and nausea and so on. When a smoker smokes a cigarette in the normal way, there may be increases in cortisol in the plasma but this is probably not mediated by ACTH.

Fuxe: What is the mechanism?

West: Nicotine is probably acting directly on the adrenal gland.

Clarke: In relation to that, I feel that you are using very high doses of nicotine in your rats. I think the cigarettes are in the right range, but you use 2 mg/per/kg i.p. of nicotine. When I give that to a rat the rat convulses, it stops breathing for about a minute. You gave that dose four times within a few hours.

Fuxe: We have dose–response curves for everything and we have done so much work on this. I only showed the high doses, because I wanted to demonstrate clearly the biphasic endocrine effects: from the initial hormone release to a delayed hormone response where the inhibitory effects of nicotine on hormone secretion dominate. When we give high doses, we know we get other effects as well, but the important aspect is the dose–response relationship.

Collins: Concerning the doses of nicotine and tobacco that are necessary to elicit an increase in ACTH or cortisol release in a smoker, it is important to remember that those studies are probably done in people who are very tolerant to those releases. Kjell Fuxe's data and some data that we have are consistent with the argument that chronic exposure to nicotine or smoke elicits tolerance to nicotine-induced release of cortisol and ACTH.

Kellar: Do you expect to find nicotinic receptors on the dopamine neurons in the hypothalamus? These neurons are structurally and probably functionally different from those in the forebrain. Is there any evidence that there are nicotinic receptors on these neurons?

Fuxe: The data would be compatible with such an assumption, because nicotine increases dopamine turnover in the tuberolafundibular dopaminergic neurons, but the effects could be indirect. It is possible to show this now that we have antibodies against the cholinergic nicotinic receptors.

Kellar: Could nicotine release steroids from the adrenal without releasing ACTH?

Pomerleau: There was such an experiment done *in vitro* by Rubin & Warner (1975). I don't think it was followed up, but there was a direct release using isolated cat adrenocortical cells.

Collins: Those cells do have receptors that bind bungarotoxin. L.L. Miner in Pittsburgh has shown that.

Russell: I was very interested in the slightly different responses you obtained according to the maturity of the animal. Cigarette smoking is a habit that seems to be established at the time of puberty. There is evidence that smoking something like three or four cigarettes at that time gives a 90% probability that that person will become a regular smoker. People who take up smoking after the age of 20 tend not to get quite so hooked, and it is uncommon to take it up at that stage of life. I know there are other explanations, but if you consider that puberty is the time when hormones and other adjustments are in turmoil, these effects of nicotine might have special piquancy and significance. There might be something in these hormonal changes and what nicotine does at that time which make puberty a specially sensitive period for developing dependence. Could you speculate on that in any way?

Fuxe: It's a very important issue. That was one of the reasons for studying the effects of exposure to nicotine or cigarette smoke before and after birth. We were fascinated by the highly selective action of nicotine within the anterior part of the nucleus accumbens. We believe that dopamine release in this area is associated with reward. Even one week after cessation of nicotine administration or exposure to smoke, there was a maintained activation of dopamine utilization in the accumbens.

We can speculate that perhaps this high responsivity and selectivity for activation of dopaminergic mechanisms in the accumbens might contribute to the feeling of well being that people get when smoking cigarettes, and this might contribute to the development of dependence in young smokers.

References

Andersson K, Eneroth P, Fuxe K, Harfstrand A 1988 Effects of acute intermittent exposure to cigarette smoke on hypothalamic and pre-optic catecholamine nerve terminal systems and on neuroendocrine function in the diestrous rat. Arch Pharmacol 337:131–139

Bourne S 1985 Treatment of cigarette smoking with short term high dosage corticotropin therapy: preliminary communication. J R Soc Med 78:649–650

Grunberg NE, Bowen DJ, Winders SE 1986 Effects of nicotine on body weight and food consumption in female rats. Psychopharmacology 90:101–105

Grunberg NE, Winders SE, Popp KA 1987 Sex differences in nicotine's effects on consummatory behavior and body weight in rats. Psychopharmacology 91:221–225

Herskovic JE, Rose JE, Jarvik ME 1986 Cigarette desirability and nicotine preference in smokers. Pharmacol Biochem Behav 24:171–175

Rose JE, Sampson A, Levin ED, Henningfield JE 1989 Mecamylamine increases nicotine preference and attenuates nicotine discrimination. Pharmacol Biochem Behav 32:933–938

Rubin RP, Warner W 1975 Nicotine induced stimulation of steroidogenesis in adrenocortical cells in the cat. Br J Pharmacol 53:357–362

Effects of nicotine
on cerebral metabolism

Edythe D. London

Neuropharmacology Laboratory, Neuroscience Branch, Addiction Research Center, National Institute on Drug Abuse, P.O. Box 5180, Baltimore, MD 21224, USA

Abstract. Interest in identifying brain areas mediating the behavioural effects of nicotine led to autoradiographic studies on the distribution of cerebral metabolic responses to nicotine. The 2-deoxy-D-[1-^{14}C]glucose method was used to map and quantitate nicotine's effects in the rat brain. The method allows simultaneous measurement of the regional cerebral metabolic rate(s) for glucose (rCMRglc), an index of functional activity, throughout the central nervous system. It provides information about sites of initial drug interactions, and of secondary effects propagated via afferents to remote areas.

In rats given acute systemic (−)nicotine, stimulation occurs in brain areas which contain specific binding sites for [^{3}H]nicotine, indicating that the sites are true receptors, linked to functional activity. Doses of nicotine that are discriminated by rats and that produce behavioural and physiological effects stimulate rCMRglc. The stimulation is transient and is antagonized by mecamylamine. Affected areas include limbic structures, components of the visual system, brainstem nuclei important in cardiovascular reflexes, and areas involved in motor function. The distribution of nicotine's *in vivo* effects on rCMRglc implicates various brain regions in the behavioural and physiological effects of nicotine. Future studies employing positron emission tomography will assess relations between nicotine's effects on mood and rCMRglc in man.

1990 The biology of nicotine dependence. Wiley, Chichester (Ciba Foundation Symposium 152) p 131–146

Nicotine receptors

Nicotine produces a host of behavioural effects. The drug can act as a reinforcer and is self administered (Henningfield 1984). It also facilitates memory, increases locomotor activity, acts as an antinociceptive agent, reduces irritability and suppresses appetite (Aceto & Martin 1982, Larson & Silvette 1971). Interest in identifying sites in the brain that might contribute to these effects has inspired studies to map the distribution of receptors for nicotine (Clarke et al 1984, London et al 1985b). In these studies [^{3}H]nicotine has been used to label binding sites, which can be visualized by light microscopic autoradiography.

High densities of specific sites are seen in the interpeduncular nucleus and medial habenula of the limbic system. Dense labelling also is seen in thalamic nuclei, components of the visual system, and the cerebral cortex. Marked similarities in the binding patterns of [^{3}H]nicotine and [^{3}H]acetylcholine support the view that nicotine binds to cholinergic nicotinic receptors in the brain (Clarke et al 1984).

Because of interest in visualizing and quantitating nicotinic binding in the living human brain by positron emission tomography, we also studied the *in vivo* labelling of nicotinic sites after the intravenous injection of [^{3}H]nicotine in mice (Broussolle et al 1989). Entry of the radiotracer into the brain was almost instantaneous. A plateau was reached 5–7.5 minutes after injection, when about 30% of the injected radioactivity was in the brain. Brain radioactivity declined rapidly; only 10–20% of the maximum tissue radioactivity remained after 30 minutes. Pretreatment with 5 mg/kg unlabelled (–)nicotine reduced brain radioactivity at all times, except at one minute after injection. Using the difference between radioactivity measured in animals with and without unlabelled nicotine pretreatment as an estimate of non-specific binding, estimated specific binding of the radiotracer reached a maximum after five minutes. The greater level of radioactivity at one minute in animals pretreated with 5 mg/kg nicotine probably reflected stimulation of cerebral blood flow, which would increase the concentration of radiotracer in the brain available for binding at this early time. Pharmacological studies of binding demonstrated that, as in *in vitro* studies, agonists of the nicotinic receptor were generally better inhibitors of [^{3}H]nicotine binding than were antagonists.

Light microscopic autoradiography demonstrated that total binding was markedly heterogeneous, with the densest labelling in thalamus, particularly in anterior nuclei (Fig. 1). High levels of radioactivity also occurred in the cerebral cortex and, to a lesser extent, the dentate gyrus, subicular regions, medial geniculate body and caudate/putamen. Binding was inhibited by pretreatment with unlabelled nicotine. However, radioactivity representing non-specific binding was not homogeneous, probably because the dose of unlabelled nicotine was inadequate to saturate specific binding sites. Studies on *in vivo* nicotine binding have been extended with the use of [^{11}C]nicotine, a positron-emitting tracer that can be used in conjunction with positron emission tomography. Nicotine receptors have been visualized non-invasively with [^{11}C]nicotine in the monkey and human brain (Nybäck et al 1989). However, full quantitation of specific receptor densities and affinities using [^{11}C]nicotine has not yet been reported.

Metabolic mapping with deoxyglucose

In addition to studies of receptor binding, metabolic mapping by the deoxyglucose technique can be used to visualize and quantitate the actions of

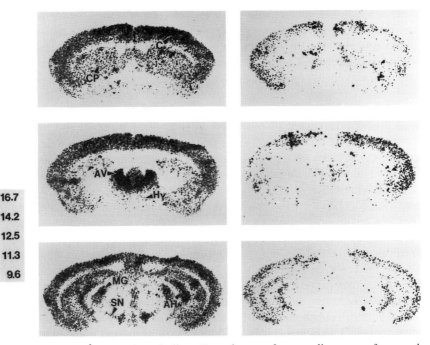

FIG. 1. *In vivo* [³H]nicotine binding. Transforms of autoradiograms of coronal sections from four anteroposterior levels of mouse brain. Mice were given 10 μCi of the [³H]nicotine, i.v., five minutes before sacrifice. Micrographs on the left (total binding) are from a mouse pretreated with unlabelled (−)nicotine to inhibit specific binding. Nicotine binding is indicated on the grey scale in fmol/mg tissue. Images appear wider than the actual autoradiograms owing to an influence of the aspect ratio of the display monitor. AH, Ammons horn of the hippocampus; AV, anteroventral nucleus, thalamus; C, cortex; CP, caudate/putamen; HY, hypothalamus; MG, medial geniculate body; SN, substantia nigra pars compacta. (Data from Broussolle et al 1989.)

various abused drugs, including nicotine, in the brain of an intact animal or human subject (McCulloch 1982, London et al 1986, London 1989). In animals, 2-deoxy-D-[1-¹⁴C]glucose (DG) is used as a radiotracer to determine regional rates of glucose utilization throughout the central nervous system (Sokoloff et al 1977). Rates of glucose utilization in individual neuroanatomical areas are determined from autoradiographic measures of tissue radioactivity, the time course of the radiotracer in arterial plasma, and the arterial glucose concentration. The method has been adapted for human studies with the use of 2-deoxy-2-[¹⁸F]fluoro-D-glucose and positron emission tomography (Phelps et al 1979). As glucose is the major substrate for oxidative metabolism in the adult brain, rates of glucose utilization provide an index of local brain function (Sokoloff et al 1977).

Several studies have focused on the effects of acute, systemic nicotine treatment on regional glucose utilization in the brain (Grunwald et al 1987, London et al 1988a,b). The general finding from these studies is that nicotine stimulates glucose utilization. The effects are localized primarily to brain areas that contain specific binding sites for [^{3}H]nicotine (see Table 1). Subcutaneous injection of nicotine produces increases of 100% or more over control in the medial habenula, fasciculus retroflexus, superior colliculus and median eminence (see Fig. 2). Increases of 50–100% over control occur in the cerebellum, interpeduncular nucleus, and some thalamic nuclei. Increases of 20–50% are seen in the reticular nucleus of the medulla, paramedian lobule, subicular areas, various brainstem nuclei, and areas of the midbrain. The correlation of nicotine-induced stimulation of glucose utilization with the presence of specific binding sites for [^{3}H]nicotine indicates that the binding sites are true receptors that are coupled to energy metabolism.

There are some discrepancies between the densities of binding sites for [^{3}H]nicotine and the effects of nicotine on glucose utilization (London et al 1988a). Some brain regions, such as the caudate/putamen and parts of the neocortex, show moderate levels of binding (London et al 1985b) but no effects of systemic nicotine on glucose utilization. This discordance may reflect the dilution of effects on nicotine-responsive cells in regions with heterogenous cell populations. Furthermore, brain regions, such as the red nucleus and median eminence, which lack [^{3}H]nicotine binding sites but show nicotine-induced

TABLE 1   Nicotine binding and effects on glucose utilization in selected regions of the rat brain

Brain region	Binding site density[a]	LCGU activation[b]
Caudate/putamen	+	−
Thalamus, ventral posterior nucleus	+ +	−
Lateral geniculate body, dorsal nucleus	+	+
Superior colliculus	+ +	+ +
Interpeduncular nucleus	+ + +	+ +
Medial habenula	+ + +	+ + +
Hippocampus, CA$_1$	−	−
Subiculum	+	−
Periaqueductal grey matter	−	−

[a]Specific binding of 50 nM [^{3}H]($\pm$)nicotine was determined autoradiographically in 10 µm slide-mounted brain sections. Data are from London et al (1985a,b). Specific binding: −, 1 fmol/mg tissue; +, 1–9 fmol/mg; + +, 10–19 fmol/mg; + + +, >20 fmol/mg. [b]Local cerebral glucose utilization was determined as described previously (Sokoloff et al 1977) two minutes after the subcutaneous injection of 0.9% NaCl (control) or 1 mg/kg (−)nicotine (free base). −, no significant difference from control; +, increase of 20–49%; + +, 50–99%; + + +, 100%.

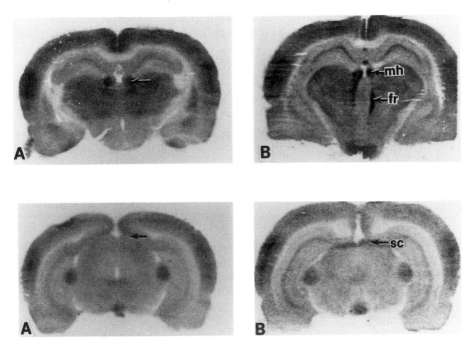

FIG. 2. Effect of subcutaneous (−)nicotine on autoradiographic grain densities, representing glucose utilization in the rat brain. These are photographs of X-ray film exposed to 20 μm brain sections from a control rat (A) given 0.9% NaCl (1 ml/kg), and another rat (B) given nicotine (1 mg/kg, two minutes before [^{14}C]DG). Note the increased density in the medial habenula (mh), fasciculus retroflexus (fr), and superior colliculus (sc) after nicotine treatment.

stimulation of glucose utilization, may reflect propagation of nicotine's effects from receptor-rich areas to remote regions.

Components of the visual system are primary targets for nicotine-induced stimulation of glucose utilization, suggesting a role of the nicotinic cholinergic system and an effect of nicotine on the processing of visual information or visual-motor function. The visual cortex, nucleus of the optic tract, lateral geniculate bodies and superior colliculus all show significant densities of nicotinic binding sites, as labelled with [^{125}I]α-bungarotoxin (Oswald & Freeman 1981) and [^{3}H]nicotine (London et al 1985b). Nicotinic receptors also have been localized to the inner plexiform layer of the retina (Schwartz & Bok 1979). It was of interest to determine whether the effects of nicotine throughout the rat visual system were due primarily to direct interactions of the drug with nicotinic receptors or if they reflected actions in the retina.

Rats were enucleated unilaterally before treatment with nicotine and DG. Enucleation completely abolished the stimulatory action of nicotine throughout visual pathways in the contralateral side of the brain, suggesting that direct effects of nicotine in the retina are necessary for this general stimulation of glucose utilization. Similarly, enhancement of glucose utilization in the superior colliculus by cholinomimetic drugs was blocked by intraocular injection of kainic acid, a neurotoxin which depleted chemical markers for cholinergic neurons (Gomez-Ramos et al 1982). These findings demonstrate that retinal input is necessary for the action of nicotine and other cholinomimetics on glucose utilization throughout visual pathways. The retinal involvement derives from the presence of nicotinic receptors presynaptically on retinal afferents, which are no longer active despite the persistence of nicotinic receptors in the acutely enucleated rat.

Effects of nicotine on behaviour and on glucose utilization throughout the brain are blocked by mecamylamine, a ganglionic blocking drug which enters the brain readily (London et al 1985a, London et al 1988a,b). However, they are unaffected by prior treatment with hexamethonium, a quaternary ganglionic blocking drug. Therefore, these effects are specific pharmacological and central effects of nicotine.

As nicotine is used chronically, more recent studies have focused on chronic effects of nicotine on cerebral glucose utilization (Grunwald et al 1988, London et al 1990c). In one of these studies (London et al 1990c), either $(-)$nicotine or saline was injected subcutaneously twice daily for 10 days and once in the morning on the eleventh day. On the following afternoon, rats received either nicotine challenge (0.3 mg/kg) or saline subcutaneously two minutes before DG. As seen in other studies (London et al 1985a, 1988a,b, Grunwald et al 1987), drug-naïve rats showed regional increases in glucose utilization in response to the nicotine challenge. Of forty-five regions sampled, only the superior colliculus and lateral geniculate body showed effects of chronic nicotine (Fig. 3). Glucose utilization of the superior colliculus in the basal state, as well as after nicotine challenge, was reduced compared with that in drug-naïve rats. The lateral geniculate body showed complete tolerance to nicotine challenge; no region showed sensitization. Since the chronic nicotine treatment regimen used previously increased the densities of nicotinic receptors in several brain regions (Schwartz & Kellar 1985), it appeared that cerebral metabolic responses to nicotine depend on factors other than the densities of nicotinic receptors.

Another study was concerned with the effects of chronic nicotine infusion on cerebral glucose utilization (Grunwald et al 1988). Several brain regions which previously showed enhanced glucose utilization in response to acute nicotine also showed stimulation in response to the chronic infusion. In contrast to the findings with repeated injections of nicotine (London et al 1990c), infusion produced a stimulation rather than tolerance in the lateral geniculate body.

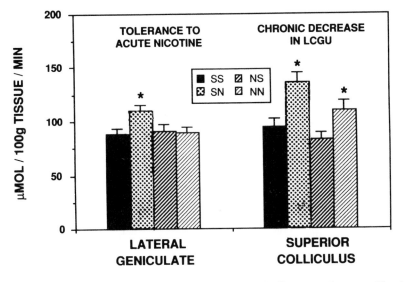

FIG. 3.   Effects of chronic nicotine and acute nicotine challenge on glucose utilization in the lateral geniculate body and superior colliculus. *Indicates the group was significantly different from its respective control ($P < 0.05$). The treatments are abbreviated as follows: SS, chronic saline (0.9% NaCl, 1 ml/kg, twice daily for 10 days), acute saline; SN, chronic saline, acute nicotine (0.3 mg/kg as the base); NS, chronic nicotine (1 mg/kg), acute saline; NN, chronic nicotine, acute nicotine. Chronic nicotine induced tolerance to the effect of acute nicotine challenge on glucose utilization in the lateral geniculate body. Chronic nicotine reduced basal glucose utilization in the superior colliculus. LCGU, local cerebral glucose utilization.

However, in the rats which received the chronic infusion, the plasma concentrations of nicotine (mean = 77 ng/ml) were close to levels produced by acute challenge in the other study (London et al 1990c). Therefore, some of the stimulatory effects of the chronic infusion may not have been due to a chronic effect. Nonetheless, the stimulation in the lateral geniculate body indicated that complete tolerance was not produced in this region by the chronic infusion. These findings suggest that the treatment regimen is an important factor in determining the effects of chronic nicotine administration.

Future direction

A future direction for work on mapping the metabolic response to nicotine is its extension to human studies using positron emission tomography. This technique does not offer the fine anatomical resolution achievable in *ex vivo* autoradiographic studies in animals. However, it allows simultaneous non-invasive measurement of biochemical processes in the brain and measurements of drug effects on mood and feeling state. Studies in human volunteers have demonstrated that euphorigenic treatment with morphine or cocaine reduces cortical glucose utilization, suggesting that a reduction of cortical activity may be a common mechanism of drug-induced euphoria (London et al 1990a,b). If this hypothesis is correct, euphorigenic doses of nicotine also would reduce cortical glucose utilization in humans.

It is now known that nicotinic receptors are localized to neurons of the mesolimbic dopamine system, which has been implicated in the reinforcing properties of many abused drugs (Clarke 1990). Therefore, the reinforcing, and possibly the euphoriant, properties of nicotine and other drugs of abuse might act through a circuit that involves the mesolimbic dopamine system, which originates in the ventral tegmentum and projects to the nucleus accumbens. According to a model proposed by Swerdlow & Koob (1987), nicotine or cocaine could increase dopaminergic inhibition in the nucleus accumbens, thereby disinhibiting neurons in the ventral pallidum, which inhibit neurons in the dorsal medial thalamic nucleus. Therefore, thalamic stimulation of the limbic cortex would be reduced. Interactions of opioids in the ventral tegmental area could produce the same effect through afferents to the nucleus accumbens. Current positron emission tomography instruments lack the spatial resolution to visualize the ventral tegmental area or nucleus accumbens. However, they can be used to image brain regions, such as the limbic cortex, into which these areas project and which may play a fundamental role in drug-induced reward.

Conclusions

Specific binding of [³H] nicotine has been demonstrated in the rat brain, with high densities in limbic areas, components of the visual system, thalamic nuclei and the cerebral cortex. Studies in mice have demonstrated that nicotinic receptors can be visualized and quantitated using radiolabelled nicotine *in vivo*, indicating that such quantitative studies might ultimately be performed non-invasively in humans using positron emission tomography.

Metabolic mapping with DG has been used in rats to delineate the distribution of the *in vivo* metabolic effects of nicotine in the brain. These studies have demonstrated that acute nicotine stimulates cerebral metabolism primarily in regions that show high densities of nicotinic receptors. Therefore, the binding sites identified with radiolabelled nicotine appear to be true receptors that are coupled to functional activity. When nicotine is given chronically, by intermittent injection, the effect is a reduction of basal metabolic activity in the superior colliculus, and the production of tolerance in the lateral geniculate body. These findings suggest an effect of chronic nicotine on visual processing or visual-motor function.

A new frontier for metabolic mapping studies with nicotine is the extension of this work to include studies in human volunteers. The use of positron emission tomography offers the promise of relating nicotine's effects on mood to specific metabolic effects in the human brain.

Acknowledgements

Supported in part by a grant from the Council for Tobacco Research, USA, Inc.

References

Aceto MD, Martin BM 1982 Central actions of nicotine. Med Res Rev 2:43–62

Broussolle EP, Wong DF, Fanelli RJ, London ED 1989 In vivo specific binding of [^{3}H]l-nicotine in the mouse brain. Life Sci 44:1123–1132

Clarke PBS 1990 Mesolimbic dopamine activation—the key to nicotine reinforcement? In: The biology of nicotine dependence. Wiley, Chichester (Ciba Found Symp 152) p 153–168

Clarke PBS, Pert CB, Pert A 1984 Autoradiographic distribution of nicotine receptors in rat brain. Brain Res 323:390–395

Gomez-Ramos PS, Nelson S, Walter D, Cross R, Samson FE 1982 Kainic acid alters cholinergic responses in the rat retina: a 2-deoxyglucose study. J Neurosci Res 7:297–303

Grunwald F, Schrock H, Kuschinsky W 1987 The effect of an acute nicotine infusion on the local cerebral glucose utilization of the awake rat. Brain Res 400:232–238

Grunwald F, Schrock H, Theilen H, Biber A, Kuschinsky W 1988 Local cerebral glucose utilization of the awake rat during chronic administration of nicotine. Brain Res 456:350–356

Henningfield JE 1984 Behavioral pharmacology of cigarette smoking. In: Thompson T et al (eds) Advances in behavioral pharmacology. Academic Press, New York, vol 4:131–210

Larson PS, Silvette H 1971 Tobacco: experimental and clinical studies, Suppl II. Williams & Wilkins, Baltimore

London ED 1989 The effects of drug abuse on glucose metabolism. J Neuropsychiatry 1:S30–S36

London ED, Connolly RJ, Szikszay M, Wamsley JK 1985a Distribution of cerebral metabolic effects of nicotine in the rat. Eur J Pharmacol 110:391–392

London ED, Waller SB, Wamsley JK 1985b Autoradiographic localization of [^{3}H]nicotine binding sites in the rat brain. Neurosci Lett 53:179–184

London ED, Szikszay M, Dam M 1986 Metabolic mapping of the cerebral effects of abused drugs In: Harris LS (ed) Problems of drug dependence, (Proceedings of 47th Annual Scientific Meeting, The Committee of Problems of Drug Dependence, Inc. NIDA Research Monograph 67) Washington, DC, p 26–35

London ED, Connolly RJ, Szikszay M, Wamsley JK, Dam M 1988a Effects of nicotine on local cerebral glucose utilization in the rat. J Neurosci 8:3920–3928

London ED, Dam M, Fanelli RJ 1988b Nicotine enhances cerebral glucose utilization in central components of the rat visual system. Brain Res 20:381–385

London ED, Broussolle EPM, Links JM et al 1990a Morphine-induced metabolic changes in human brain: studies with positron emission tomography and [fluorine 18]fluorodeoxyglucose. Arch Gen Psychiatry 47:73–81

London ED, Cascella NG, Wong DF et al 1990b Cocaine-induced reduction of glucose utilization in human brain. A study using positron emission tomography and [fluorine 18]fluorodeoxyglucose. Arch Gen Psychiatry, in press

London ED, Fanelli RJ, Kimes AS, Moses RL 1990c Effects of chronic nicotine on cerebral glucose utilization in the rat. Brain Res, in press

McCullough J 1982 Mapping functional alterations in the CNS with [^{14}C]deoxyglucose. In: Iversen LL et al (eds) Handbook of psychopharmacology. Plenum, New York, vol 15:321–410

Nybäck H, Nordberg A, Langström B et al 1989 Attempts to visualize nicotinic receptors in the brain of monkey and man by positron emission tomography. In: Nordberg A et al (eds) Progress in brain research. Elsevier Science Publishers, Amsterdam, vol 79:313–319

Oswald RE, Freeman JA 1981 Alpha-bungarotoxin binding and central nervous system nicotinic acetylcholine receptors. Neuroscience 6:1–14

Phelps ME, Huang SC, Hoffman EJ, Selin C, Sokoloff L, Kuhl DE 1979 Tomographic measurement of local cerebral glucose metabolic rate in humans with (18F)2-fluoro-2-deoxy-D-glucose: validation of method. Ann Neurol 6:371–388

Schwartz IR, Bok D 1979 Electron microscopic localization of [^{125}I]α-bungarotoxin binding sites in the outer plexiform layer of the goldfish retina. J Neurocytol 8:53–66

Schwartz RD, Kellar KJ 1985 In vivo regulation of [^{3}H]acetylcholine recognition sites in brain by nicotinic cholinergic drugs. J Neurochem 45:427–433

Sokoloff L, Reivich M, Kennedy C et al 1977 The [^{14}C]deoxyglucose method for the measurement of local cerebral glucose utilization: theory, procedure, and normal values in the conscious and anesthetized albino rat. J Neurochem 28:897–916

Swerdlow NR, Koob GF 1987 Dopamine, schizophrenia, mania, and depression: toward a unified hypothesis of cortico-striato-pallido-thalamic function. Behav Brain Sci 10:197–245

DISCUSSION

Gray: The large areas of stimulation that you showed are areas of the brain concerned with cognition. We shouldn't forget the cognitive effects of nicotine, which are very well established.

Concerning the interpretation of 2-deoxyglucose pictures, I thought that the 2-deoxyglucose technique detects activity in the terminals that arrive in a particular region rather than in the cell bodies that are fired in a particular region. Presumably, you are seeing nicotine acting presynaptically to activate the terminals.

London: In about 1979 everybody believed that the 2-deoxyglucose procedure visualized activity in terminals more than in other neuronal elements. This view reflected the fact that the surface:volume ratio is greater in terminals. However, we found that, in some systems, glucose utilization in the entire neuron—cell bodies, fibre pathways and terminals—is affected (Dam & London 1984, London et al 1988). When entire neurons are seen to be activated, it generally involves a brain region that has a metabolic increase of 40% or more.

Nicotine is a unique drug with the deoxyglucose procedure. We have mapped metabolic responses to drugs of many different classes, and nicotine is the only one that shows good correspondence between the distribution of specific binding sites for the drug and stimulation or inhibition of metabolic response.

Gray: Could the reason be that, if the nicotinic receptors are largely presynaptic, you are looking at switched on terminal activity?

London: That's right. The nicotinic system could differ from other systems in metabolic mapping because of the preponderance of receptors localized to presynaptic terminals.

Awad: I would like to compare your data with Dr Stolerman's results from behavioural studies on nicotinic receptor heterogeneity. Have you used other nicotinic agonists?

London: No, but I think our results are consistent with heterogeneity of nicotinic receptors. The metabolic responses to nicotine of various brain regions are different. For example, when rats are treated chronically with nicotine, some brain regions show tolerance to nicotine challenge, whereas others do not (London et al 1990a).

Stolerman: Evidence is certainly growing that different behavioural effects of nicotine are mediated through different brain areas. That is true for the three effects that I talked about. Because it's possible to dissociate the ability of other nicotinic agonists to produce those behavioural effects, it would be of great interest to see what would happen with some of these other agonists in the assay of metabolic activity in the brain.

Collins: Ron Freund, an electrophysiologist, has evidence that under certain circumstances nicotine will decrease the activity of GABAergic systems (Freund et al 1988). Inhibiting an inhibitor such as GABA might explain how you could see metabolic activation as well as behavioural inhibition in the type of experiments that you are doing.

Svensson: I wonder about the significance of the reduction in cortical activity you describe. Morphine and cocaine gave similar results in your study (London et al 1990b,c). You saw a reduction in cortical activity, and you think this is correlated with disinhibition of lower pleasure centres. With nicotine, cognitive functions do not seem to be impaired.

London: Nor are they necessarily impaired with high doses of cocaine.

Svensson: With morphine, however, this is clearly a problem. The clouding of consciousness is one of the classical effects of morphine. And we do think with our cortex, not with our brainstem pleasure centres.

London: It is a problem that needs to be addressed. All of these drugs produce effects other than euphoria. We have begun to approach this issue by doing multiple correlational studies, relating the metabolic findings for different brain regions to various functional effects.

Fuxe: We should remember the potential euphoric action of arousal itself. What happened in the locus ceruleus and the thalamus in response to nicotine?

London: Glucose metabolism in the thalamus, but not in the locus ceruleus, was stimulated.

Fuxe: Perhaps the euphoria of the nicotine is potentiated because there is arousal at the same time. What do you think?

London: The autoradiograms I showed were obtained with acute nicotine administration in rats. We don't really know that they like nicotine at all! The euphoria would have to be measured in a different paradigm, perhaps in people that have chronically self-administered nicotine because they enjoy it. It is difficult to make generalizations. Metabolic responses to acute drug treatments in naive rats don't resemble the responses to similar treatments in experienced human substance users.

Clarke: Several people have reported that presumed channel blocking drugs, such as mecamylamine, do not inhibit high affinity [³H]nicotine binding.

London: They do inhibit binding at ACh recognition sites. However, at least with mecamylamine, inhibition occurs only at high concentrations, at which the drug acts as a non-competitive antagonist (Takayama et al 1989).

Clarke: We have all been thinking of high affinity binding as a result of desensitization, but maybe that's not the case. Mecamylamine is presumably blocking activation of the receptor; is it blocking the desensitization?

Schwartz: In the nicotinic receptor, mecamylamine can promote desensitization in certain paradigms.

Colquhoun: It's often not easy to distinguish between slow channel block and desensitization.

Heinemann: Did any areas of the brain show depressed metabolic activity?

London: No.

Heinemann: So there is no evidence that nicotine acts as an antagonist in the brain?

London: No, not from the 2-deoxyglucose studies.

Kellar: I would have expected to see some decreases for two reasons. Firstly, if the cholinergic system was tonically active. Secondly, the timing of this technique is that you inject the drug, then you take a cut through a 45 minute window. I don't know where the peak is. Are some of the effects that you see peak effects in some areas and perhaps effects that are either before or after maximum in other areas?

London: According to the Sokoloff procedure, we inject the radiotracer and collect samples to obtain the integrated specific activity of the radiotracer in the arterial plasma over 45 minutes. However, most of the incorporation of the radiotracer in the rat takes place within the first ten minutes after the radioisotope is injected. Between 10 and 45 minutes, the precursor (2-deoxyglucose) is cleared from the arterial plasma and the brain. The autoradiograms show radioactivity that is due, primarily, to the phosphorylated radiotracer. The mathematical model is such that errors in rate constants for the transport and phosphorylation of the radiotracer diminish with time. At 45 minutes, these constants are exponentials that approach zero. Thus, the procedure measures brain responses during the first 10 minutes after radiotracer injection.

Kellar: Have you looked at deoxyglucose responses at various times relative to nicotine administration?

London: Yes, we noted that the effect on cerebral glucose utilization was greatest and roughly comparable when nicotine was given either two minutes before or two minutes after the radiotracer. However, most brain regions showed no response when nicotine was given 15 minutes or more before the 2-deoxyglucose. Exceptions were the medial habenula, which had a persistent metabolic effect 15 minutes after nicotine injection, and the superior colliculus, which showed stimulation for up to two hours after nicotine treatment (London et al 1988).

Collins: To address a comment Paul Clarke made, I would like to remind you of the results of our mecamylamine experiments. The up-regulation of nicotine binding seen in animals treated chronically with mecamylamine suggests that you can increase the numbers of nicotinic receptors, if you just block the existing receptors. But when we infused mecamylamine and nicotine together we got additivity or even synergy. This suggests that mecamylamine does not block the desensitization process, if that is what is involved in the up-regulation.

Clarke: I would be interested to know whether mecamylamine affects B_{max} or K_d of [^{3}H]nicotine binding. I have tried chlorisondamine, which is a long term nicotinic blocker that will block the central effects of nicotine for weeks. I saw no increase in B_{max} for [^{3}H]nicotine binding.

Collins: We have done the same experiment and get exactly the same result—chlorisondamine treatment does not result in any change in B_{max} or K_d. Chronic mecamylamine infusion results in an increase in B_{max} but no change in the K_d.

Clarke: There is at least one paper showing that mecamylamine blocks N-methyl-D-aspartate (NMDA) receptors, so it's interesting that mecamylamine doesn't seem to affect glucose uptake.

Heinemann: I think that mecamylamine is a glutamate blocker.

London: It may be an antagonist at the level of cationic channels associated with some glutamate receptors. We found that mecamylamine inhibits the binding of radioligands that label the channel coupled to NMDA-preferring glutamate receptors (M. D. Majewska, H. Takayama, E. D. London, unpublished findings).

Changeux: When you take these pictures, you see clearly an effect on the steady-state level of electrical activity. But this is derived from averaging the signals from many nerve cells and fibres. It may not reflect other kinds of electrical activity, which might be physiologically more significant, but concern only a small number of fibres which would not contribute much to the average measurement. Can you correlate electrical recordings with your results on brain metabolism?

London: It might be worthwhile to test such a correlation. However, a negative result would not be conclusive. The 2-deoxyglucose technique averages both over time and over heterogeneous populations of cells within brain regions. Therefore, there is a dilution of activity in individual cells that express the appropriate receptors by metabolism in irrelevant neurons.

Changeux: Some receptors do not seem to desensitize, for example, some glutamate receptors do not. Peter Seeburg has found that some combinations of GABA receptor subunits form a receptor that does not desensitize (personal communication). On the other hand, other combinations of subunits do desensitize. Could there be some combination of subunits of the ACh receptor of the brain that form a receptor which does not desensitize? I don't think anybody has found a nicotinic receptor which does not desensitize, but why not?

London: To answer this question, it may be useful to look at the subunit composition of nicotinic receptors in different brain regions. Is the subunit composition in the visual system, which shows a prolonged response to nicotine, different from the composition in thalamic nuclei, which show transient responses?

Heinemann: The major nicotinic receptor type is $\alpha4\beta2$, which is found everywhere throughout the brain, so this is not very helpful.

Kellar: In the peripheral receptor, phosphorylation is mostly on the δ and γ subunits. In a receptor that doesn't contain those subunits, where would you think the desensitization might occur?

Changeux: There are two questions: the role of particular subunits in desensitization, and the role of phosphorylation in desensitization. Sumikura and Miledi have shown a differential role of the γ subunit in desensitization by making chimaeric receptor molecules with *Torpedo* receptors.

The role of phosphorylation is debatable. It does not seem to be required for desensitization. But, several groups have published that phosphorylation accelerates desensitization of *Torpedo* and mammalian receptors. The phosphorylated subunits are the γ and δ subunits. We have shown that calcitonin gene related peptide (CGRP), a neuropeptide present in spinal and motoneurons, both increases levels of cAMP and enhances desensitization in a mouse muscle cell line.

The question is whether or not some particular amino acids are the target of phosphorylation and control desensitization. These amino acids could be substrates for protein kinases A and C. Site-directed mutagenesis might have to be used to prove that these amino acids are involved in the regulation of desensitization.

Kellar: γ and δ subunits may be involved in regulating desensitization but we don't think they are present in the brain receptor.

Heinemann: We get very nice desensitization in *Xenopus* oocytes that express only α and β subunits. Concerning the phosphorylation, there are many potential phosphorylation sites in all the neuronal receptor subunits. We have mutated some sites that could be targets for cAMP-dependent kinase and we still see desensitization. We are looking at a very slow form of desensitization, so phosphorylation could be affecting a fast form.

Benowitz: It bothers me that you give extremely high doses of nicotine that blast the brains of these rats. Rodents eliminate nicotine very quickly, so with your dosing regimen there is a very high but brief exposure to nicotine then it's gone. If you are interested in simulating exposure to nicotine in human tobacco users, it is the wrong paradigm. It will be hard to interpret these data in terms of the pharmacology of nicotine in humans.

London: The value of these data is that they indicate differences in responsivity of different parts of the brain. These differences are not necessarily relevant to chronic human nicotine consumption; however, they indicate that certain nicotinic receptors differ from others.

Heinemann: The interesting finding is that the areas in which Eydie London sees large changes in metabolic activity are the same as those where we see large amounts of mRNA that codes for functional nicotinic receptors. That's a nice correlation. To go beyond that to differences in different cell types is too big a jump, because you have to think of the neuronal network. The different responses, I think, are pretty likely to be due to the specific networks.

Benowitz: Why is there so much metabolic activity in the visual system?

London: There is an abundance of nicotinic receptors in the retina and throughout central visual pathways.

Benowitz: Why is that so?

London: ACh apparently is an important neurotransmitter in visual systems.

Iversen: One of the highest densities of nicotinic binding sites is in the colliculus. These, we presume from the lesion studies, are located on fibres that come straight from the retina. Unfortunately, it is not known what transmitter those fibres secrete, so the nicotinic receptors control the release of something, but we don't know what that something is.

Collins: I would like to make a comment about Eydie London's very provocative finding that the 2-deoxyglucose studies indicate no attenuation of response in the colliculus over time. The colliculus is a brain region that has a relatively high number of α-bungarotoxin (α-Bgt) binding sites. It is also one of the three brain regions where the Bgt binding site changes when we treat chronically with nicotine. Does that mean that in this particular region we are not talking about a vestigial organ and the Bgt binding site is functional?

Along those lines, in our hands the Bgt binding site is a low affinity binding site. The work of Jean-Pierre Changeux and other people who have studied desensitization in the *Torpedo* nicotinic receptor indicates that the desensitization process is concentration dependent. So if you have a relatively low concentration of nicotine for the receptor involved, it may be that over a time you won't see attenuation of the response.

London: It could be or it could be, as Dr Heinemann said, that we are measuring effects on activity in related, non-nicotinic systems that impinge upon systems with nicotinic receptors. The retina contains lots of kainate receptors. These are localized to cell bodies, and we just heard that kainate receptors don't show desensitization.

Collins: Alternatively, it would not be a good idea to have a nicotinic receptor in a visual system that easily desensitized—wouldn't that lead to blindness?

Steinbach: Just because the metabolic effect persists for 120 minutes, it doesn't mean that the receptor didn't desensitize. For example, if there were a giant Ca^{2+} entry, there could be persistent effects on activation of protein kinase C. It might be interesting to try to block the nicotinic response with mecamylamine at 45 minutes and then see if this metabolic enhancement persists or not. This would show whether it is persistent receptor activation or a secondary result of the initial activation. It is not clear that the persistence is directly connected to the receptors.

Clarke: Thinking about the 2-deoxyglucose effects, these are so huge, presumably you could work at the single cell level with [^{3}H]deoxyglucose. That might show exactly which cells are changing their metabolism in response to nicotine.

London: This would be a good idea. However, the single cell approach has some problems in quantitation.

References

Dam M, London ED 1984 Glucose utilization in the Papez circuit: effects of oxotremorine and scopolamine. Brain Res 295:137–144

Freund RK, Jungschaffer DA, Collins AC, Wehner JM 1988 Evidence for modulation of gabaergic neurotransmission by nicotine. Brain Res 453:215–220

London ED, Connolly RJ, Szikszay M, Wamsley JK, Dam M 1988 Effects of nicotine on local cerebral glucose utilization in the rat. J Neurosci 8:3920–3928

London ED, Fanelli RJ, Kimes AS, Moses RL 1990a Effects of chronic nicotine on cerebral glucose utilization in the rat. Brain Res, in press

London ED, Broussolle EPM, Links JM et al 1990b Morphine-induced metabolic changes in human brain. Studies with positron emission tomography and [fluorine 18] fluorodeoxyglucose. Arch Gen Psychiatry 47:73–81

London ED, Cascella NG, Wong DF 1990c Cocaine-induced reduction of glucose utilization in human brain. A study using positron emission tomography and [fluorine 18] fluorodeoxyglucose. Arch Gen Psychiatry, in press

Takayama H, Majewska MD, London ED 1989 Interactions of noncompetitive inhibitors with nicotinic receptors in the rat brain. J Pharmacol Exp Ther 253:1083–1089

General discussion II

Adaptive and cognitive aspects of the response to nicotine

Gray: I would like to present results relating to two effects of nicotine administration: adaptive changes in catecholamine systems, and changes in cognitive performance.

Dr Fuxe's paper addressed adaptation, particularly in dopaminergic and noradrenergic pathways in brain. Stephen Mitchell, Michael Brazell and Michael Joseph in my group have evidence for different patterns of adaptation in noradrenergic and dopaminergic systems.

An injection of 0.8 mg/kg sub-cutaneously of nicotine causes dopamine release in the nucleus accumbens. At this dose there is no dopamine release in the caudate (Brazell et al 1989). The same dose releases noradrenaline in the hippocampus and this is blocked by mecamylamine but not by hexamethonium. These were all measured by *in vivo* intracerebral microdialysis. We also get a response, which we have not measured by dialysis but by other means, in the hypothalamus; this is due to the release of noradrenaline from the ascending dorsal noradrenergic bundle, not from the ventral bundle (Mitchell et al 1990).

We have measured the chronic effects in two ways. The first is by dopa accumulation after inhibition of dopa decarboxylase. We give the animals 28 days of daily injections of saline or 0.8 mg/kg nicotine, followed by an acute challenge with either saline or nicotine. Dopa accumulation after injection of an inhibitor of dopa decarboxylase gives a measure of catecholamine synthesis in the regions concerned. We see no change either acutely or chronically in the caudate; in the nucleus accumbens there is an equivalent increased dopa accumulation after either an acute dose on one day or chronic administration for 28 days. This is also the case in the hypothalamus. In the hippocampus there is sensitization of the dopa accumulation response after chronic injections of nicotine (Mitchell et al 1989).

So there is a regional specificity, such that after 28 days of nicotine the response to an acute nicotine challenge, as measured by dopa accumulation, is increased in the hippocampus only. This specificity applies both to the system concerned (noradrenergic not dopaminergic) and to the terminal region concerned (hippocampus not hypothalamus).

We also looked at the effects of this injection regime on tyrosine hydroxylation. In the caudate, accumbens and hypothalamic regions there were no changes after either the acute or the chronic regimes. In the hippocampus,

147

tyrosine hydroxylase activity does not change after an acute dose of nicotine, but after 28 days of nicotine there is activation whether there is a challenge with saline or nicotine at that time (Joseph et al 1990). So there appears to be a selective adaptation in locus ceruleus terminals, but only in those that go to the hippocampus.

We now believe that the mechanism of these effects may involve enzyme induction, followed by axonal transport from the cell bodies. Katherine Smith (Smith & Joseph 1989) has shown that tyrosine hydroxylase activity after periods of daily nicotine injection initially increases in the locus ceruleus and then disappears. Increases in tyrosine hydroxylase activity follow later in terminal regions, first in the hypothalamus (at about 21 days from the start of the injection regime) and then in the hippocampus (at about 28 days). Thus the difference between the hypothalamus and hippocampus, when either dopa accumulation or tyrosine hydroxylase activity is measured after 28 days of nicotine injections, may reflect the time course of axonal transport to these two regions, rather than absolute differences between them.

These effects closely resemble those observed by Zigmond et al (1974) in response to reserpine and cold stress: adaptation taking the form of increased synthesis of tyrosine hydroxylase in the cell body region of the locus ceruleus, which then travels to the terminals. I believe they will turn out to be very important for our understanding of the chronic effects of nicotine.

I now wish to present a second set of results, concerning the cognitive effects of nicotine. We have been looking at rats that have had damage to the forebrain cholinergic projection system produced in one of two ways (Arendt et al 1989). We inject the excitotoxin, ibotenate, into the medial septal area and into the nucleus basalis, destroying the cholinergic projections to both hippocampus and neocortex, or we give our animals alcohol (20% v/v) to drink for six months. Though neither of these methods is selective for cholinergic neurons, both produce about a 50% fall in choline acetyltransferase levels in the neocortex and the hippocampus. We test these animals in the radial-arm maze, which can test four kinds of memory: reference memory and working memory in both a spatial and a non-spatial task. We get a profound and enduring deficit in the animal's capacity to perform any one of these tasks.

Helen Hodges has found that doses of nicotine that have no effect in control animals on any of the types of memory (0.05 and 1.0 mg/kg s.c.) greatly improve the performance, particularly in working memory in the spatial task, of the ibotenate-lesioned animals (Hodges et al 1990). So there is an enhanced sensitivity to nicotine, which has a beneficial effect. Gemma Jones has shown in a clinical study that you can get similar effects in patients suffering from Alzheimer's disease (Sahakian et al 1989). The enhanced sensitivity to nicotine in the lesioned animals is not just an artifact of poor baseline performance, because there is also increased sensitivity to mecamylamine, which makes performance worse.

Again there is a dose of mecamylamine which makes the lesioned animals worse, while having no effect on controls.

We have exactly the same kind of data for animals that have been rendered memory-impaired with chronic alcohol. One should not forget that nicotine has some very useful properties in affecting cognitive performance, as well as giving rise to the dependence problem that is foremost in our minds.

Iversen: The changes in tyrosine hydroxylase in the adrenergic neurons are particularly fascinating. They might represent the sort of change that you would be looking for in terms of a mechanism of dependence. Dick Zigmond in my lab used different provoking stimuli, a single dose of reserpine caused an adaptive increase in the tyrosine hydroxylase activity in the locus ceruleus; just putting the animals in the cold room for a few hours had the same effect. There is an elevated expression of tyrosine hydroxylase, both the enzyme and the mRNA. The enzyme gradually gets transported from the cell body to the terminal but it can take up to three weeks (Zigmond 1979).

This is a very interesting example of biochemical memory; an event in the animal's life that doesn't have any impact biochemically on the relevant part of the neuron (the part which makes the catecholamine and secretes it in the cortex or the hippocampus) until 2–3 weeks later. Similarly, in chronic drug treatment, after withdrawal of the drug that type of change would take a long time to work itself out of the system. So there are one or two examples in brain where we do understand slow adaptive neurochemical changes.

Gray: We have shown that you don't have to give the nicotine for 28 days, seven days is sufficient (Smith & Joseph 1990); you may have to do it only once.

Rose: Ed Levin in my group has shown that chronic nicotine will improve performance in the radial-arm maze, but the increase in performance develops over two weeks (Levin et al, in press). If you take away the nicotine, the improved performance persists for another two weeks—this is a potential mechanism.

Fuxe: I like these differential effects on the noradrenaline neurons. Within the hypothalamus there are also differential effects on these noradrenaline neuronal systems. After chronic stimulation with nicotine you can maintain enhancement of noradrenaline utilization exclusively in the periventricular hypothalamic and preoptic systems, while the other hypothalamic noradrenaline receptors develop tolerance. So there are discrete differences, even within the hypothalamus and the preoptic area. The periventricular noradrenaline systems are uniquely responsive throughout the chronic nicotine treatment period. This emphasizes that although many of them may originate from the same nor-adrenaline cell groups, they show differences which may be related to differential regulation of the nicotinic receptors belonging to different but adjacent hypothalamic noradrenaline nerve terminals.

Balfour: We have been looking at the release and the extracellular levels of dopamine in the nucleus accumbens. Jeffrey Gray has shown that there is no change in the biosynthesis, but there are increases in the extracellular levels evoked by nicotine. These increases are greater if you pretreat the animals with nicotine.

We showed that chronic nicotine decreases selectively the amount of 5-hydroxytrypatamine (5HT) in the hippocampus. It also decreases the biosynthesis and produces adaptive changes in tryptophan uptake, such that there is reduced tryptophan uptake in the hippocampus. More recently we have shown that that also occurs in human brain. The levels of 5HT and 5-hydroxy-indole-3-acetic acid (5HIAA) are reduced in the hippocampus of humans who smoke cigarettes. This again is a regionally selective effect, suggesting that some of the changes you see in response to nicotine in experimental animals do relate to what happens in the human smoker.

Gray: I am impressed by the report of reduced 5HT and 5HIAA levels in the human smokers. However, for reasons which we don't understand, we never in our experiments have seen any change in measures of serotonergic function. We've looked at extracellular 5HIAA levels by dialysis and by voltammetry (Brazell et al 1987, 1989). We have also looked at 5HTP accumulation in parallel experiments with the dopa accumulation technique (Mitchell et al 1989). So there must be something different between our methods.

Schwartz: I think the pathways may be even more complicated. Ken Kellar and I and other people have found presynaptic sites using lesion studies in many of these areas. If nicotinic receptors are mediating release of neurotransmitters and hormone releasing factors in all of these areas, that increases the complexity of the control of turnover of a particular transmitter in that pathway. It is another area of control that has to be considered. I agree that there is this important possibility of local control over the terminals. However, we were misled when we first saw the difference between the hypothalamic response to 28 days nicotine and the hippocampal response. We had already demonstrated that these were both functions of the ascending noradrenergic projection from the locus ceruleus. It now looks like it is not a difference in local regulation, but the time it takes the enzyme to travel from the cell body to the terminal region. We haven't resolved this issue and local regulation is entirely possible.

Collins: Jeffrey, the increase in tyrosine hydroxylase activity can be accomplished via two mechanisms. The initial, rapidly acting one involves phosphorylation of the enzyme, which is cAMP dependent. This leads to an increase in activity and a decreased K_m for a reduced pteridine co-factor. The second mechanism is an increase in the amount of enzyme owing to an increase in the amount of mRNA. Do you have any idea which of these you are measuring?

Gray: We plan to investigate the possibility of enzyme induction by measuring the mRNA. However, in Katherine Smith's work, we saw quite a different pattern of change in the ventral tegmental area, A10, and substantia nigra, A9 (Smith & Joseph 1990). There is an increase in tyrosine hydroxylase activity at three days after injection which then disappears very rapidly. The increase we saw in the locus ceruleus is there at seven days; that in the other regions occurs much later. We see no increase in the activity of tyrosine hydroxylase in any of the terminal regions served by the dopaminergic projections. So it seems likely at this stage that there is short-term activation of tyrosine hydroxylase in dopaminergic cell bodies, whereas in the locus ceruleus there is enzyme induction.

Collins: Has anyone used a phosphodiesterase inhibitor and looked at the effects of that on tyrosine hydroxylase activity in those brain regions?

Fuxe: We used phosphodiesterase inhibitors such as caffeine (Corrodi et al 1972) and looked at dopamine utilization in the brain but that was in the striatum and forebrain regions. We found a considerable reduction of dopamine utilization with caffeine, which is the opposite effect to that seen with nicotine.

Clarke: It seems that the enzyme takes an awfully long time to reach the axon. Is it going by slow axonal transport or is the synthesis of the mRNA delayed?

Iversen: It's not too surprising. These are very small diameter unmyelinated fibres. The rate of axoplasmic transport in those fibres is slow, and from the locus ceruleus in the hindbrain to the frontal cortex is quite a long way.

Gray: Zigmond's original experiments showed a very good correlation between the time of increased tyrosine hydroxylase activity and the distance from the locus ceruleus to the relevant terminals. In the cerebellum the response appears very shortly after the increase in tyrosine hydroxylase activity in the locus ceruleus, presumably because it has a very short distance to travel.

Fuxe: Tyrosine hydroxylase is not transported via the fast flow, because it is not associated with granules. It probably goes with the bulk flow of cytoplasm, which moves at 1 mm/day.

References

Arendt T, Allen Y, Marchbanks R et al 1990 Cholinergic system and memory in the rat: effects of chronic alcohol, embryonic basal forebrain transplants and excitotoxic lesions of cholinergic projection system. Neuroscience 33:435–462

Brazell MP, Gray JA, Joseph MH, Mitchell SN 1987 In vivo voltammetric detection of increased extracellular ascorbate and DOPAC after acute nicotine. 3rd British Electrochemical Detection Meeting, Cambridge

Brazell MP, Mitchell SN, Gray JA 1989 Nicotine stimulated dopamine synthesis release and metabolism in vivo. Br J Pharmacol 96:339P

Corrodi H, Fuxe K, Jonsson G 1972 Effects of caffeine on central monamine neurons. J Pharm Pharmacol 24:155–158

Hodges H, Allen Y, Sinden J, Lantos PL, Gray JA 1990 Cholinergic-rich transplants alleviate cognitive deficits in lesioned rats, but exacerbate response to cholinergic drugs. Prog Brain Res, 82:347–358

Joseph MH, Peters SL, Prior A, Mitchell SN, Brazell MP, Gray JA 1990 Chronic nicotine administration increases tyrosine hydroxylase selectively in the rat hippocampus. Neurochem Int, in press

Levin E, Lee C, Rose JE, Reyes A, Ellison G, Jarvik M, Gritz E 1990 Chronic nicotine and withdrawal effects on radial-arm maze performance. Behav Neural Biol 53:269–276

Mitchell SN, Brazell MP, Joseph MH, Alavijeh MS, Gray JA 1989 Regionally specific effects of acute and chronic nicotine administration on rates of catecholamine and 5-hydroxytryptamine synthesis in rat brain. Eur J Pharmacol 167:311–322

Mitchell SN, Brazell MP, Schugens MM, Gray JA 1990 Nicotine-induced catecholamine synthesis after lesions to the dorsal or ventral noradrenergic bundle. Eur J Pharmacol, in press

Sahakian BJ, Jones GMM, Levy R, Gray JA, Warburton DM 1989 The effects of nicotine on attention, information processing and short-term memory in patients with dementia of the Alzheimer type. Br J Psychiatry 154:797–800

Smith KM, Joseph MH 1989 Regionally selective effects of chronic nicotine on rat brain tyrosine hydroxylase activity: a time course study. Br J Pharmacol 98:696

Smith KM, Joseph MH 1990 Contrasting effects of chronic nicotine on tyrosine hydroxylase activity in noradrenergic and dopaminergic neurones. Br J Pharmacol, in press

Zigmond RE 1979 Tyrosine hydroxylase activity in noradrenergin neurons of the locus coernleus after reserpine administration: sequential increase in cell bodies and terminals. J Neurochem 32:23–29

Zigmond RE, Schon F, Iversen LL 1974 Increased tyrosine hydroxylase activity in the locus coeruleus of rat brain stem after reserpine treatment and cold stress. Brain Res 70:547–552

Mesolimbic dopamine activation—the key to nicotine reinforcement?

Paul B. S. Clarke

Department of Pharmacology and Therapeutics, McGill University, 3655 Drummond St Room 1325, Montreal, Canada H3G 1Y6

Abstract. The mesolimbic dopaminergic system appears to mediate the rewarding effects of certain stimulant drugs, such as (+)amphetamine. Autoradiographic mapping techniques have revealed that these neurons are potential targets for nicotine, since they possess nicotinic receptors located on their cell bodies and terminals in rat brain. Functional studies are consistent with this proposal: nicotine can increase the firing rate of these neurons, and nicotine-induced dopamine release has been demonstrated *in vitro* and *in vivo*. The locomotor stimulant effect resulting from the acute administration of nicotine is accompanied by, and appears to be dependent upon, activation of mesolimbic neurons. Likewise, destruction of this system appears to attenuate the acute rewarding effects of intravenous nicotine in rats. Thus, when administered intermittently, nicotine, like certain other stimulant drugs, may activate the mesolimbic dopamine system, and this action may contribute to the tobacco habit.

1990 The biology of nicotine dependence. Wiley, Chichester (Ciba Foundation Symposium 152) p 153–168

Scientists and clinicians widely agree that people continue to smoke cigarettes primarily in order to self-administer nicotine for its central actions. Animal studies have shown that nicotine acts at many sites in the central nervous sytem (CNS). One such target is the mesolimbic dopamine system, which appears to mediate the rewarding effects of certain stimulant drugs such as (+)amphetamine and cocaine. This paper highlights evidence from my work and that of others which suggests that activation of mesolimbic dopaminergic neurons may contribute to the reinforcing effects of nicotine.

Evidence that nicotine is reinforcing

Laboratory animals will voluntarily self-administer a number of drugs that humans abuse (e.g. stimulants and opiates), and will not self-administer agents that humans do not usually consume. Nicotine is no exception, and intravenous self-administration of nicotine has been demonstrated in a number of mammalian species, including humans (reviewed by U.S. Surgeon General 1988). For example, in a recent study (Corrigall & Coen 1989), rats readily learned to obtain intravenous infusions of nicotine by pressing a lever during daily one hour sessions, and stable responding was acquired within a few weeks. Very few responses were made on a second, 'non-drug' lever which was not linked to the infusion pump. Rats responded fastest for intermediate doses of nicotine (0.01 and 0.03 mg/kg/infusion), and a substantial amount of drug (up to 0.5 mg/kg) was self-administered within a single session. Responding was greatly reduced by substitution of saline for nicotine. Responding was also reduced by pretreatment with the centrally acting nicotinic antagonist mecamylamine, but not by systemic administration of the quaternary antagonist hexamethonium; this result constitutes weak evidence for a central site of action of nicotine, since the doses of hexamethonium used may not have been sufficient to block the peripheral actions of nicotine. This study highlights an important gap in our knowledge: although the majority of nicotine's behavioural effects in animals appear to be of central origin (Clarke 1987a), there has been no convincing test to determine whether this is true for the reinforcing effects of nicotine in animals.

Certain other drugs produce rewarding effects by enhancing mesolimbic dopamine transmission

The mesolimbic dopamine (DA) system comprises a population of dopamine-secreting neurons which have their cell bodies in the midbrain and which project principally to two forebrain regions—the nucleus accumbens and the olfactory tubercle. Several drugs, of which (+)amphetamine and cocaine are the best studied, can produce reinforcing effects in animals by enhancing the activity of this system (see review by Wise & Rompre 1989). The key evidence for this conclusion is as follows. Intravenous self-administration of (+)amphetamine and cocaine is reduced by prior administration of dopamine receptor antagonists or by destruction of mesolimbic dopaminergic neurons. Both (+)amphetamine and cocaine act at the DA terminal to increase the extracellular concentration of this neurotransmitter within the nucleus accumbens, and microinfusion of these drugs directly into the accumbens can have rewarding consequences that are mediated via DA receptors. In addition, animals will work hard to receive intermittent electrical stimulation of brain sites which results in increased mesolimbic DA activity. Most studies have examined the role of the nucleus accumbens in reward; recent evidence suggests that the other major mesolimbic DA projection, namely that to the olfactory tubercle, probably contributes little to DA-mediated reward (Clarke et al 1989). In summary, it appears that increased DA outflow from terminals in the nucleus accumbens is intrinsically rewarding, and that agents which promote this should be rewarding too.

Nicotine can enhance mesolimbic dopamine transmission

Radioligand binding studies have identified a population of sites which bind nicotinic agonists with high (nanomolar) affinity, and these sites appear to represent the predominant receptor type mediating the effects of smoking nicotine (Clarke 1987b). Lesion experiments combined with autoradiography show that these nicotinic receptors are associated with mesolimbic DA neurons on both cell bodies (within the ventral tegmental area) and terminals (nucleus accumbens, olfactory tubercle) (Fig. 1; Clarke & Perk 1985).

Immunohistochemical studies have identified nicotinic receptor-like immunoreactivity within presumed mesolimbic DA cell bodies and in terminal structures (Swanson et al 1987, Deutch et al 1987). *In situ* hybridization histochemistry has shown that neurons within the ventral tegmental area synthesize significant amounts of the mRNA (and thus presumably of the protein) of the genes which encode the subunits of nicotinic receptors (Wada et al 1989). Although not demonstrated, it seems likely that these neurons are dopaminergic.

The electrophysiological effects of nicotine on individual mesolimbic DA neurons have been investigated. In one study in anaesthetized rats, mesolimbic DA neurons were not excited by systemic administration of nicotine, although the drug did promote a bursting pattern of firing (Grenhoff et al 1986). In another study, nicotine reduced neuronal activity in rats that were under general anaesthesia, but greatly excited these cells in paralysed, locally anaesthetized subjects (Mereu et al 1987).

Nicotine can release DA from isolated nuclear accumbens tissue *in vitro*, and graded responses have been observed at 0.1 μM and above, that is, within the range of nicotine concentrations expected to occur in the brains of cigarette smokers (Rowell et al 1987).

Acute administration of nicotine to rats also increases DA outflow from the nucleus accumbens *in vivo*. This has been most directly demonstrated by the technique of intracranial microdialysis, which permits sampling of extracellular fluid in a brain region of interest. Using this technique, Imperato et al (1986) showed that doses of nicotine relevant to changes in behaviour, administered subcutaneously, increased extracellular DA levels. This was interpreted as an increase in DA release. The effect was blocked by prior administration of the centrally active antagonist mecamylamine, but not by hexamethonium. Once again, this argues only very weakly for a central action of nicotine, since it is not at all certain that the dose of hexamethonium administered was sufficient to block the peripheral actions of nicotine.

Several groups have reported that acute exposure to nicotine also increases other, less direct, *in vivo* indices of DA utilization in rats. For example, Fuxe et al (1986) showed that short-term exposure to cigarette smoke increased the disappearance of DA in rats which had been treated with a DA synthesis inhibitor; this effect was prevented by filtering out the nicotine from the smoke,

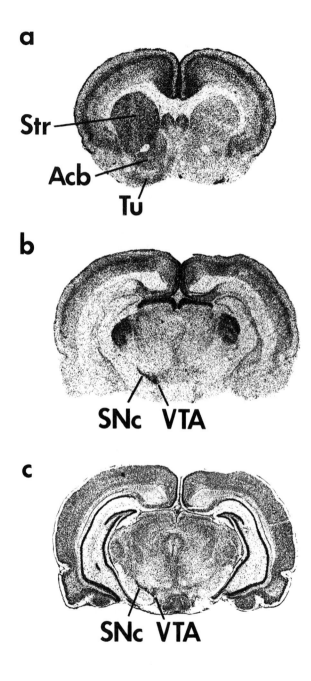

or by pretreating the animals with mecamylamine. The effect of nicotine v
confined to the anterior nucleus accumbens and lateral posterior olfactory

Nicotine-induced activation of mesolimbic DA neurons affects behaviour

Clearly, acute administration of nicotine can result in increased DA outflow
from the mesolimbic system in rats. Activation of this system, for example by
psychomotor stimulant drugs such as (+)amphetamine, tends not only to be
rewarding but also to increase locomotor activity; both phenomena appear to
involve the DA projection to the nucleus accumbens rather than to the olfactory
tubercle (Clarke et al 1988a, 1989), but it is not known whether exactly the same
population of DA neurons subserves both functions.

Acute administration of nicotine exerts a locomotor stimulant effect in rats
through a direct central action (Clarke & Kumar 1983b). This effect is more
pronounced in animals which have received the drug several times previously
(Clarke & Kumar 1983a,b). Therefore, in order to investigate whether
mesolimbic DA activation underlies the locomotor stimulant effect of nicotine,
we first pre-exposed rats to daily nicotine injections (Clarke et al 1988b). Next,
each rat was tested in order to demonstrate an acute locomotor stimulant effect
of nicotine. A few days later, subjects received a single subcutaneous injection
of saline or nicotine and were killed 30 minutes later for biochemical assay of
DA terminal areas (including olfactory tubercle and nucleus accumbens). The
first experiment provided only equivocal evidence for mesolimbic DA activation,
as assessed by metabolite:transmitter ratios—(−)nicotine (0.2–0.8 mg/kg s.c.)
significantly increased homovanillic acid:DA ratios in the olfactory tubercle and
a similar effect was seen in the accumbens, but dihydroxyphenylacetic acid:DA
ratios were not significantly altered. In subsequent experiments, rats were treated
with the (−)aromatic acid decarboxylase inhibitor NSD-1015 in order to inhibit
the conversion of dihydroxyphenylalanine (dopa) to DA, and DA utilization was
measured by dopa:DA ratios. (−)nicotine stimulated locomotor activity, and
increased dopa:DA ratios in the olfactory tubercle and the nucleus accumbens
(Fig. 2). Both the behavioural and neurochemical effects were significantly dose
related (0.1–0.4 mg/kg) and stereoselective (− > + isomer). In a final
experiment, neurochemically selective destruction of mesolimbic DA neurons
abolished the locomotor stimulant effect of (−)nicotine (0.4 mg/kg s.c.) when

---

FIG. 1. Autoradiographs (a,b) of [³H]nicotine binding in frontal sections of rat
brain, following unilateral (right side) destruction of mesolimbic and nigrostriatal
dopaminergic neurons. The lesion reduced [³H]nicotine binding in dopaminergic
terminal areas (including nucleus accumbens, Acb) and in dopaminergic cell body areas
(e.g. ventral tegmental area, VTA). The loss of dopaminergic cell bodies can be seen
in the corresponding Nissl stained section (c). Str, striatum; Tu, olfactory tubercle; SNc,
substantia nigra pars compacta. (From Clarke & Pert 1985.)

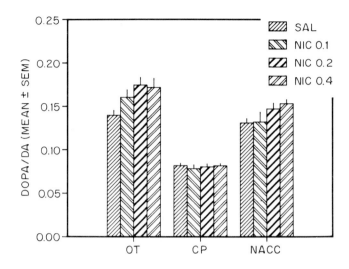

FIG. 2. Effects of (−)nicotine on an indirect index of dopamine utilization (dopa:dopamine ratios) in rats pretreated with NSD-1015. Nicotine (0.1–0.4 mg/kg s.c.) increased this index in mesolimbic terminal regions (nucleus accumbens, olfactory tubercle) but not in the caudate/putamen. $n = 6$–12 (From Clarke et al 1988b.)

tested two weeks after surgery (Fig. 3). The nicotinic response showed some signs of recovery at four weeks after surgery, possibly as a consequence of neuronal regeneration and/or compensatory postsynaptic alterations in sensitivity to dopamine. The lesion resulted in a substantial (89%) depletion of DA in the accumbens and olfactory tubercle. This study suggests that in rats which have been chronically but intermittently pre-exposed to the drug, the acute locomotor stimulant effect of nicotine is not only accompanied by, but *dependent* upon, activation of mesolimbic DA neurons.

Chronic effects of nicotine on mesolimbic DA system activity

Habitual cigarette smoking provides pharmacologically significant levels of nicotine on a 24 hour basis (U.S. Surgeon General 1988). In addition, individual cigarette puffs are hypothesized to deliver intermittent 'boli' of nicotine to the brain, although there is no direct evidence for this (Russell & Feyerabend 1978). Attempts to model the pharmacokinetics of nicotine in animals should probably take into account both of these components. As an added complication, there is evidence both in animals and in humans for the occurrence of acute and chronic tolerance to nicotine (U.S. Surgeon General 1988).

All the studies reviewed above have involved the acute administration of nicotine to animals which were free of drug at the time of testing. The literature on animal studies suggests that chronic continuous administration of nicotine

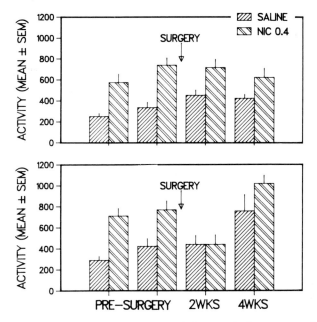

FIG. 3.   Effects of mesolimbic dopamine depletion on the locomotor stimulant effect of ($-$)nicotine (0.4 mg/kg s.c.). Each rat received two pairs of tests with saline and with nicotine before and after surgery. Locomotor activity was measured in photocell cages. Subjects received intra-accumbens infusion of 6-hydroxydopamine (lower panel) or saline (upper panel). $n = 8$–9 (From Clarke et al 1988b.)

can have effects on behaviour and DA function which are different and even opposite from those seen after multiple intermittent exposure. For example, although acute administration of nicotine robustly increases locomotor activity in a dose-related manner in rats pre-exposed to the drug on a daily basis (e.g. Clarke & Kumar 1983a), chronic (two week) infusion of nicotine via osmotic minipumps reduced locomotor activity compared to saline-treated control rats (Grunwald et al 1988). In another study, acute administration of nicotine (0.1 mg/kg s.c.) to drug-naive animals clearly increased *in vitro* tyrosine hydroxylase activity in nucleus accumbens tissue; chronic (two week) nicotine infusion produced appreciable plasma nicotine levels (48 ng/ml) but did not significantly alter the activity of this enzyme (Carr et al 1989). Taken together, these and other studies indicate that chronic continuous infusion of nicotine can result in either tolerance or reverse-tolerance, and that the conditions promoting acute versus chronic forms of tolerance are poorly understood.

The rewarding effects of nicotine may also result from mesolimbic DA activation

As noted above, animals given restricted access to intravenous nicotine will readily self-administer the drug. Moreover, acute subcutaneous administration of nicotine, at doses which would be accumulated intravenously during a self-administration session, activates mesolimbic DA neurons. It seems likely, therefore, that rats which are self-administering nicotine are activating the mesolimbic DA system. To date, this has not been demonstrated directly.

In a recent study (W. A. Corrigall, K. B. J. Franklin and P. B. S. Clarke, in preparation), we investigated whether bilateral destruction of this system would reduce nicotine self-administration in rats. Subjects were trained to work for intravenous infusions of nicotine (0.03 mg/kg), and a stable baseline of responding was established over a number of days. They were then randomly allocated to lesion and sham groups for surgery, and were infused under general anaesthesia with the neurotoxin 6-hydroxydopamine (or vehicle) into the nucleus accumbens. When tested 3–4 days after surgery, the lesioned animals responded at around 25% of their pre-surgery baseline rates, whereas sham-operated animals were little affected. Post mortem tissue analysis revealed a substantial (93%) depletion of DA in the accumbens. Two additional observations suggest that the lesion-induced reduction in response rates was not a result of motor impairment: firstly, lesioned rats were still capable of responding for food at rates comparable to baseline response rates for nicotine infusion; secondly, motor deficits seen after 6-hydroxydopamine lesions are typically associated with substantial ($>50\%$) depletion of the nigrostriatal DA projection to the overlying caudate/putamen, but this structure was depleted by only 25%.

Conclusion

The presence of nicotinic receptors on mesolimbic DA neurons in rat brain makes this neuronal system a natural target for activation by nicotine, and acute administration of nicotine does stimulate DA outflow from this system. This action appears to account for the acute locomotor stimulant and acute rewarding effects of the drug in rats. However, chronic nicotine administration does not always mimic the behavioural and neuropharmacological effects of acute administration. Indeed, because acute and/or chronic tolerance tends to develop with chronic continuous administration of nicotine, it is unclear whether animals would continue to respond for nicotine if it were available on a 24 hour basis. In this context, it is worth recalling that smokers often report a greater impact from the first cigarette of the day than from subsequent ones (Henningfield 1984). Thus, it is conceivable that DA activation is more important in the intermittent smoker than in the heavy smoker. Ultimately, though, whether or not nicotine activates mesolimbic DA neurons in humans, and whether or not such an action underlies the smoking habit, cannot be answered with currently available techniques.

Acknowledgements

The author's work described here has been supported by the Medical Research Councils of the UK and Canada and by NIMH.

References

Carr GD, White NM 1986 Anatomical dissociation of amphetamine's rewarding and aversive effects: an intracranial microinjection study. Psychopharmacology 89:340–346

Carr LA, Rowell PP, Pierce WM 1989 Effects of subchronic nicotine administration on central dopaminergic mechanisms in the rat. Neurochem Res 14:511–515

Clarke PBS 1987a Nicotine and smoking: a perspective from animal studies. Psychopharmacology 92:135–143

Clarke PBS 1987b Recent progress in identifying nicotinic cholinoceptors in mammalian brain. Trends Pharmacol Sci 8:32–35

Clarke PBS, Kumar R 1983a The effects of nicotine on locomotor activity in non-tolerant and tolerant rats. Br J Pharmacol 78:329–337

Clarke PBS, Kumar R 1983b Characterisation of the locomotor stimulant action of nicotine in tolerant rats. Br J Pharmacol 80:587–594

Clarke PBS, Pert A 1985 Autoradiographic evidence for nicotine receptors on nigrostriatal and mesolimbic dopaminergic neurons. Brain Res 348:355–358

Clarke PBS, Jakubovic A, Fibiger HC 1988a Anatomical analysis of the involvement of mesolimbocortical dopamine in the locomotor stimulant actions of d-amphetamine and apomorphine. Psychopharmacology 96:511–520

Clarke PBS, Fu Ds, Jakubovic A, Fibiger HC 1988b Evidence that mesolimbic dopaminergic activation underlies the locomotor stimulant action of nicotine in rats. J Pharmacol Exp Ther 246:701–708

Clarke PBS, White NM, Franklin KBJ 1989 6-Hydroxydopamine lesions of the olfactory tubercle do not alter (+)-amphetamine-conditioned place preference. Behav Brain Res 36:185

Corrigall WA, Coen KM 1989 Nicotine maintains robust self-administration in rats on a limited-access schedule. Psychopharmacology 99:473–478

Deutch AY, Holliday J, Roth RH, Chun LLY, Hawrot E 1987 Immunohistochemical localization of a neuronal nicotinic acetylcholine receptor in mammalian brain. Proc Natl Acad Sci USA 84:8697–8701

Fuxe K, Andersson K, Härfstrand A, Agnati LF 1986 Increases in dopamine utilization in certain limbic dopamine terminal populations after a short period of intermittent exposure of male rats to cigarette smoke. J Neural Transm 67:15–29

Grenhoff J, Aston-Jones G, Svensson TH 1986 Nicotinic effects on the firing pattern of midbrain dopamine neurons. Acta Physiol Scand 128:351–358

Grunwald F, Schrock H, Theilen H, Biber A, Kuschinsky W 1988 Local cerebral glucose utilization of the awake rat during chronic administration of nicotine. Brain Res 456:350–356

Henningfield JE 1984 Behavioral pharmacology of cigarette smoking. In: Thompson E, Dews PB (eds) Advances in behavioral pharmacology. Academic Press, New York vol 4:131–210

Imperato A, Mulas A, Di Chiara G 1986 Nicotine preferentially stimulated dopamine release in the limbic system of freely moving rats. Eur J Pharmacol 132:337–338

Mereu G, Yoon K-WP, Boi V, Gessa GL, Naes L, Westfall TC 1987 Preferential stimulation of ventral tegmental area dopaminergic neurons by nicotine. Eur J Pharmacol 141:395–399

Rowell PP, Carr LA, Garner AC 1987 Stimulation of [^{3}H]dopamine release by nicotine in rat nucleus accumbens. J Neurochem 49:1449–1454

Russell MAH, Feyerabend C 1978 Cigarette smoking: a dependence on high-nicotine boli. Drug Metab Rev 8:29–57

Swanson LW, Simmons DM, Whiting PJ, Lindstrom J 1987 Immunohistochemical
    localization of neuronal nicotinic receptors in the rodent central nervous system. J
    Neurosci 7:3334–3342
U.S. Surgeon General 1988 The health consequences of smoking: nicotine addiction,
    U.S. Department of Health and Human Services
Wada E, Wada K, Boulter J et al 1989 Distribution of alpha2, alpha3, alpha4, and beta2
    neuronal nicotinic receptor subunit mRNAs in the central nervous system: a
    hybridization histochemical study in the rat. J Comp Neurol 284:314–335
Wise RA, Rompre PP 1989 Brain dopamine and reward. Annu Rev Psychol 40:191–225

DISCUSSION

Collins: Twice today we have compared (+) and (−) nicotine, Paul's data and
Eydie London's data, and we didn't see 10-fold differences in dose–response curves.

Clarke: It's true that I didn't have a full dose–response comparison between
the isomers, but as far as we could tell the ratio was more than 10.

Russell: Do you suggest that the initial depressant effect of nicotine on
locomotor activity was due to its action at the Renshaw cell in the spinal cord?

Clarke: Certainly nicotine stimulates Renshaw cells but not motoneurons.
One can show that certain reflexes are greatly depressed by nicotine in the spinally
transected rat.

Russell: Your results show that the rats get tolerant to the initial depressant
effect on locomotor activity. However, smokers do not become tolerant to the
inhibitory effect of nicotine on tendon reflexes, which is attributed to its action
at Renshaw cells.

Clarke: I don't know that human cigarette smokers are not tolerant, they
are obviously not totally tolerant.

Russell: Domino's work on the stretch reflexes shows exquisite responsiveness
of recently deprived human smokers to that effect of nicotine (Domino & von
Baumgarten 1969).

Clarke: Yes, but what would the effect be in a non-smoker?

Gray: Did you show that the projection from the pedunculopontine nucleus
goes both to the substantia nigra and to A10 or just to the substantia nigra?

Clarke: Just to the substantia nigra. I didn't look at the A10 nucleus. It is
hard to study the inputs to A10 with neuroanatomical tracing techniques because
there are many fibres of passage coursing through this general area.

Gray: So that input at present is unknown?

Clarke: Yes, but there is no guarantee that all nicotinic cholinoceptive
receptors in the brain receive a cholinergic input.

Gray: But you did see the receptors?

Clarke: Yes.

Collins: I am perplexed by the self-administration studies that you did. In
the lesion experiments followed by nicotine self-administration, did you train
the animals to press a lever for nicotine before making the lesion and then test
whether there is still self-administration?

Clarke: Yes, I only did the lesions and neurochemistry. Bill Corrigall did the behavioural parts of these experiments. The animals were trained to press for food to get them used to pressing a lever. Then they were fitted with intravenous catheters and they were trained to a stable baseline of responding for nicotine. Then there were three baseline days.

Henningfield: How long was there after the reinforcement?

Clarke: There was a one minute period of time-out after each infusion.

Rose: I am not convinced by your argument that because the rates of food self-administration were higher than those for nicotine in the lesioned animals they would therefore have responded to nicotine, if it was reinforcing. For instance, if you paralysed both my legs, I might crawl out of the room for food but not to get a cup of coffee. The animals could have found nicotine just as rewarding after the lesion, but because of some motor impairment they would not respond for nicotine, whereas they would respond for a more potent reinforcer like food. One could equate the rate of self-administration in advance with rates of responding for negative reinforcement versus positive reinforcement. Then you could see whether the rates of responding for negative reinforcement persisted but the nicotine self-administration was abolished.

Clarke: That's a good test to do.

Stolerman: This approach is extremely valuable, because in contrast to many of the other presentations, including my own, we are seeing a direct measure of a behavioural basis for nicotine intake. Nearly all the other responses have been rather indirectly related to drug-seeking behaviour and craving.

Paul, what do you think about the overall importance of the mesolimbic dopamine in relation to nicotine reward? Do you regard this as the main mechanism or is it the only one we know about?

Clarke: I think it's the only bit we know about. It may contribute to human smoking, but there may be many reasons why people smoke, at both the psychological and neurobiological levels. We don't know whether this dopamine release even occurs in humans. The studies that I described have all been with one single injection or repeated chronic intermittent dosing. The effect with chronic continuous infusion can be totally different. Someone who is dosing themselves on a 24 hour basis with nicotine from cigarette smoking may not experience these effects at all.

Collins: A number of studies with self-administration of other reinforcing agents, for example opiates, indicate that if you give a receptor antagonist to an animal that has been pre-trained to the drug, shortly after administration you see 'bursting', an increase in activity. However, the animal later perceives that this is no longer giving it the boost it is looking for and it quits. You didn't see that in a lesioned animal, which confuses me.

Clarke: I didn't show you the data broken down over time within each test session that would have allowed you to see whether or not there was such an extinction burst. Secondly, I don't believe that occurred. Thirdly, you don't always see an extinction burst, it depends on the drug. For nicotine, Bill Corrigall reported that less than half the animals showed an extinction burst when they were pretreated with mecamylamine (Corrigall & Coen, 1989). If you have a drug that has aversive effects as well as rewarding effects and take away the rewarding effects, you need not see an extinction burst.

Svensson: Pert & Chiueh (1986) reported that microinjections of nicotine into discrete brain regions had different effects on locomotor activity. Injection of nicotine into the ventral tegmental area caused locomotor stimulation, whereas injection into the nucleus accumbens did not. Could you comment on that? What could be the relative importance of nicotine receptors on cell body regions versus terminal regions as regards the behavioural stimulant action of nicotine?

Clarke: It's true what you say. These authors used cytisine rather than nicotine. The problem is that putting cytisine into a structure like the accumbens, which is a little bigger than the ventral tegmental area, may cause desensitization as the drug spreads as well as activation. I believe that the response you see to nicotine is always going to be a balance of activation and desensitization. Maybe smokers are constantly fighting a battle to maximize their activation and minimize their desensitization. Cytisine does not produce locomotor activity readily when injected into the accumbens, but I don't think that necessarily means that systemic nicotine doesn't act that way.

Svensson: The nicotinic receptors on the terminals may represent non-innervated receptors, but those in the ventral tegmental area may well be different, according to your results. Innervated receptors and non-innervated receptors may show differential responses when you treat them chronically with agonists.

Clarke: I make no claims that the ventral tegmental area dopamine neurons have a cholinergic input. I don't think there is any evidence for whether or not the nicotinic receptors in the accumbens are cholinergically innervated.

Gray: All these lovely experiments show that nearly every drug that is self-administered by animals and people causes dopamine release in the nucleus accumbens. The initial reaction is that one has found the final common pathway. But these systems are also part of normal reinforced behaviour.

The mesolimbic dopaminergic pathway is part of an overall behavioural approach system, as we heard from Dr London. She only showed the mesolimbic part, but that is integrated with the nigrostriatal system, and with a variety of other structures in the basal ganglia, thalamus and cortex. These interrelated structures constitute a ramified system whose function, in general terms, is to direct the animal towards the things it needs (food, water, etc) and away from danger (Gray 1990). One of the things that can become a rat's goal is self-administration of a drug. So, it may simply be that when we see dopamine release in the nucleus accumbens, we see exactly what we would see, for example, when the animal negotiates a maze to find a more conventional goal, such as food or water.

Then we get caught up in these political issues about what is an addiction and what is not an addiction. Maybe we should make a distinction between drugs that act directly to cause dopamine release in the accumbens and have very powerful reinforcing effects, such as amphetamines, and a compound like nicotine that acts indirectly.

Iversen: That's a very important point. If you have a rat that is trained to self-administer nicotine, can you switch to any of these other drugs that release dopamine?

Stolerman: It is my understanding that animals trained to self-administer one abused drug often switch to other abused substances when these are offered as alternatives. I would expect this to apply to nicotine as well.

Henningfield: When cocaine and nicotine are directly compared in the same paradigm, nicotine is a somewhat weaker reinforcer, although it is a powerful reinforcer, nonetheless. This is in marked contrast to caffeine, for example, which has not been clearly shown to maintain self-administration behaviour in animals.

Gray: Is there a good correlation between the degree to which a substance is self-administered and the degree to which it causes dopamine release in the nucleus accumbens?

Stolerman: There is evidence that this is not the case. The idea that all abused drugs produce their positive reinforcing effects by releasing dopamine in the mesolimbic system has been popularized by the work of Di Chiara & Imperato (1988). This hypothesis has now been substantially modified (Di Chiara 1989). The difficulties with the original hypothesis included findings that a benzo-diazepine decreased dopamine release instead of enhancing it. However, dopamine is clearly implicated in the reinforcing effects of psychomotor stimulants and probably those of nicotine as well, as we heard from Paul Clarke.

Collins: George Koob has argued that if dopamine was the only story, apomorphine would be the most reinforcing drug known to man. Dopamine receptor agonists might be extremely abusable and yet they appear not to be, so the story is more complicated.

Iversen: If apomorphine was not a powerful emetic, maybe it would be an abused drug!

Clarke: The mesolimbic system probably is involved in goal-directed reward. Nevertheless, if you lesion the system to the extent that I did, the rats still eat. They may lose a little weight but they are not seriously food deprived. They locomote perfectly well, perhaps 20% less than the control animals. Drugs which increase dopamine in the system, such as cocaine, apparently nicotine and possibly alcohol, do seem to be rewarding and there is some evidence that it is this action within the mesolimbic dopaminergic system that is responsible for their rewarding effects.

Henningfield: A drug's ability to produce a 'high' is neither necessary nor sufficient for it to be a reinforcer for people or animals. Chronic drug addicts often say they need their daily dose to feel normal, not to get high. Moreover, highly tolerant individuals may not even be capable of strong euphoric responses, but they still take the drug.

I would like to ask Dr Clarke, was there a shift to the right in the dose–response curve? Was the overall reinforcing effect diminished?

Clarke: We don't know because we only used a single dose of nicotine.

Fuxe: One problem with regard to reward and nicotine and other drugs that produce dependence is that we do not really consider the entire pattern of changes within the nucleus accumbens. Each of those rewarding agents probably produces a unique pattern of changes in the afferents to the accumbens, both dopamine afferents and, for example, glutamate fibres from various cortical areas. Thus, the afferent signal which comes out of this accumbens network must be the integrated response to a number of changes, including those in interneurons in the accumbens. We have to look upon the nucleus accumbens in a more global fashion to get a better understanding of the euphoric response.

Henningfield: But the euphoric response itself is a complex integrated response. It just happens to be a little better assay for abuse potential than is, for example, heart rate elevation.

Rose: What bothers me is that caffeine is probably the most commonly self-administered drug in the world, yet it is not a potent releaser of dopamine in the nucleus accumbens, it is only a mild euphoriant and it is only weakly self-administered by animals. Are there any data on the action of caffeine in the nucleus accumbens? If it does not affect the accumbens, that means there are persuasive reasons for self-administering stimulants that do not produce a local action in the nucleus accumbens. That relates to nicotine, because it is not clear that at any time from the acquisition of the smoking habit onwards, a pronounced euphoria is a major part of the subjective experience. I know you can get euphoria under some conditions, but what is known about the natural history of euphoria maintaining initiation of cigarette smoking?

Iversen: You could constrain caffeine into the dopamine theory if you tried hard, if you believe that it works partly by phosphodiesterase inhibition. One of the dopamine receptors in brain is the adenylate cyclase-linked D1 receptor, so the phosphodiesterase could be making the released dopamine more effective.

Rose: It also should inhibit adenosine receptors and thereby facilitate release.

Russell: Another slight problem for this hypothesis of the mesolimbic release of dopamine as a mechanism for reward and reinforced behaviour is the action of new 5HT3 antagonists which are being studied as potential treatments for schizophrenia. These damp down activity in the mesolimbic dopamine system fairly specifically and cause less disturbance of the nigrostriatal system. Schizophrenia is not necessarily associated with euphoric or good feelings, yet schizophrenics seem to need their mesolimbic dopamine systems damped down a bit. This could mean that neither overactivity nor hypoactivity of that system is reinforcing, and that just the right amount of activity or the right kind of activity is what is wanted.

Iversen: Could you say a little more about the idea that the mesolimbic dopamine system is the reward and pleasure centre of the brain and the final common pathway by which many psychostimulant drugs of abuse mediate their actions.

Clarke: Clearly not all rewarding drugs work through activating the mesolimbic dopamine system, for example, benzodiazepines are self-administered but they decrease dopamine release. I personally think that cocaine, amphetamines, and probably nicotine, do produce rewarding effects by increasing extracellular dopamine when given acutely. Whether this is true when nicotine is given chronically is a different matter entirely. Whether this occurs in humans is again an unsolved question. I wouldn't want to pretend that there aren't other systems, but it does seem that the drugs I mentioned gain access to reward circuitry at the level of the mesolimbic dopaminergic system.

Iversen: I have never had the opportunity of comparing all these drugs myself, but I believe them to be different! How do you explain that? Are you saying that the rewarding properties of each of those drugs are really the same?

Clarke: It seems they may have something in common.

Rose: One analogy is that between different reinforcing aspects of behaviours, which presumably use those endogenous pathways, such as food reward or sexual reward. I don't think you can substitute food for sex or vice versa under most circumstances. The same could be true for different drugs—although they activate pathways in the same region, there may be important distinctions.

Svensson: Many years ago there was a clinical study in Uppsala, Sweden by Professor Gunne. He tried to block the euphoriant action of amphetamines in humans by administrating α-methyltyrosine. This blocks the effect of amphetamines in animals and it certainly blocked the euphoriant and stimulant action of amphetamine in humans as well. That would suggest that this is an effect related to brain catecholamines.

Iversen: But did it stop the smokers smoking?

Svensson: The initial reaction of the smoker would be to use higher doses of nicotine to overcome such treatment. α-methyltyrosine cannot be used at high doses because of renal toxicity.

Secondly, I don't think these drugs are all doing the same thing or are perceived as doing the same thing. People can smoke heavily and they remain essentially normal. Their behaviour doesn't get out of hand in the same way as with cocaine, for example.

There are two possible contributing factors. One is that there is a down-regulation of nicotine intake and you really feel sick if you exceed a certain limit. This doesn't seem to happen with cocaine or amphetamines, despite the fact that you may even have cerebral bleeding. The second is that with nicotine you maintain the normal impulse-generating functioning of the dopamine system; you don't shut off the firing. With cocaine or amphetamine something different happens: you block uptake and with a feedback mechanism you turn off the firing. That is a much more artificial situation; the synapses will be continuously exposed to dopamine. In that sense I think nicotine is a much more deviously designed drug, because it feels normal.

References

Corrigall WA, Coen KM 1989 Nicotine maintains robust self-administration in rats on a limited-access schedule. Psychopharmacology 99:473–478

Di Chiara G 1989 Role of mesolimbic dopamine in drug-induced psychomotor activation and reward: permissive versus active. Behav Pharmacol 1 (suppl 1):25

Di Chiara G, Imperato A 1988 Drugs abused by humans preferentially increase synaptic dopamine concentrations in the mesolimbic system of freely moving rats. Proc Natl Acad Sci USA 85:5274–5278

Domino EF, von Baumgarten AM 1969 Tobacco, cigarette smoking and patella reflex depression. Clin Pharmacol Ther 10:72–79

Gray JA 1990 The neuropsychology of temperament. In: Angleitner A, Strelau J (eds) Exploration in temperament. Plenum Press, in press

Pert A, Chiueh CC 1986 Effects of intracerebral nicotinic agonists on locomotor activity: involvement of mesolimbic dopamine. Soc Neurosci Abstr 12:917

Effect of nicotine on dynamic function of brain catecholamine neurons

Torgny H. Svensson, Johan Grenhoff and *Göran Engberg

Department of Pharmacology, Karolinska Institutet, P.O. Box 60 400, S-104 01 Stockholm, *Department of Pharmacology, University of Göteborg, P.O. Box 33 031, S-400 33 Göteborg, Sweden

Abstract. Burst firing in the mesolimbocortical dopamine (DA) neurons, originating in the ventral tegmental area (VTA), is facilitated by systemic administration of nicotine. Pharmacological results show that bursting in VTA-DA cells is critically dependent on a tonic, excitatory amino acid drive, probably originating from the medial prefrontal cortex. Cold inactivation of the prefrontal cortex caused pacemaker-like firing of VTA-DA cells, an effect partly antagonized by systemic nicotine. Clinically, hypofrontality has been associated with negative symptoms in chronic schizophrenia and with chronic alcoholism. Thus, smoking may provide a means to partially restore the dynamics of the VTA-DA system in such disorders. Intravenous nicotine also induces a selective activation of bursting in noradrenaline neurons of the pontine nucleus locus ceruleus. Pharmacological and physiological experiments clearly suggest that this effect is indirect, e.g. peripherally elicited and relayed to the locus ceruleus through its excitatory amino acid input from the paragigantocellular nucleus. The locus ceruleus activation is rapid in onset, dose dependent, short lasting and can be repeated within minutes. This effect of nicotine, which would imply an instant coping response, may be relevant to nicotine dependence, particularly in depressive states.

1990 The biology of nicotine dependence. Wiley, Chichester (Ciba Foundation Symposium 152) p 169–185

Successive reports of the US Surgeon General over the past 25 years have identified tobacco smoking as the single largest preventable cause of morbidity and mortality in the United States and, probably, in the Western world. Moreover, compelling evidence now exists that regular smoking is a form of drug addiction to nicotine. The power of the nicotine dependence is illustrated by several surveys showing that at least three out of four smokers wish to quit, yet only one in four men and one in three women succeed in stopping permanently before the age of 60. Thus, understanding the brain mechanisms involved in nicotine addiction must be a central task for medical research. The emerging evidence that pharmacological treatment, e.g. nicotine substitution therapy, can significantly improve the outcome in smoking cessation programmes (for a review, see Jarvik & Henningfield 1988) underlines the necessity for further neuropharmacological research in this area. Non-addictive treatment strategies would be especially advantageous. Thus, identification of the physiological mechanisms involved in mediating the desired effects of nicotine in the brain is of particular importance.

This paper focuses on nicotine's stimulatory action on brain catecholamine neurons, i.e. the dopamine (DA)-containing cells of the ventral tegmental area (VTA), which give rise to the so-called mesolimbic DA system, and the noradrenaline (NA)-containing cells of the pontine nucleus locus ceruleus (LC), since the VTA-DA system seems to be critically involved in the reinforcing effect of nicotine (Grenhoff & Svensson 1989, Clarke, this volume). Moreover, the LC activation by nicotine may be highly significant for its vigilance enhancing capacity (see below). Apart from characterizing these effects of nicotine in brain, we attempt to identify putative dysfunctional states of such key neuronal cell populations in brain, which may aggravate the prognosis in smoking cessation programmes. Such results may also shed more light on the neurobiology of nicotine dependence.

Methods

In the present experiments, computer-assisted, conventional single-cell recording methodology was used in the chloral hydrate anaesthetized male rat (Grenhoff et al 1986). This technology allows recording of extracellular action potentials from units in the VTA or the LC with a high time resolution, which detects drug effects on a subsecond time level. Temporal distribution of spikes was analysed by interspike time interval histograms (ISH) of 256 bins with bin widths of 1–8 ms simultaneously executed by an Apple II computer. A burst onset was recognized when an interspike interval shorter than 80 ms occurred, and a burst termination was recognized at the next interval exceeding 160 ms. Firing rate and burst firing were calculated within the program. Burst firing was quantified by the burst percentage, i.e. the ratio between spikes in bursts and the total number of spikes of an ISH. In addition, the variation coefficient of an ISH was employed to study the regularity of cell firing pattern (Werner & Mountcastle 1963). The variation coefficient is the ratio between the standard deviation and the mean interval value of an ISH, expressed as a percentage.

The ventral tegmental area dopamine cells: physiology and clinical aspects

The mesolimbic (mesolimbocortical) DA system is critically involved in drive and normal, reward-motivated behaviour (see Fibiger & Phillips 1986). Generally, two major functional modes of these cells appear: single spike firing and burst firing (see e.g. Grenhoff et al 1986). Studies in awake primates have shown that midbrain DA cells respond to rewarding sensory stimuli by short-lasting burst responses (Schultz 1986, Nishino et al 1987, T. Ljungberg, personal communication 1989). Since impulse-mediated terminal release of DA is exponentially related to the frequency of discharge (Gonon 1988), such bursting responses of the DA cells imply a dramatic increase in DA release, probably acting as a 'Go' signal for behaviour.

Recently, we have shown that administration of kynurenic acid, an antagonist of excitatory amino acids without intrinsic activity, induces profound regularization of firing of the VTA-DA neurons and virtual abolition of burst firing (Grenhoff et al 1988). Moreover, cold inactivation of the medial prefrontal cortex of the rat had the same effect, i.e. the cells fired in a pacemaker-like mode similar to what is seen in a brain slice preparation (Svensson & Tung 1989). Thus, all normal variation and bursting had disappeared, although the average firing rate did not change. Inactivation of the prefrontal cortex had no effect on LC firing (Svensson & Tung 1989). Clearly, VTA-DA cells firing in this fashion would not allow normal behaviour driven by rewarding environmental stimuli. As a consequence, learning should also be impaired in association with such DA dysfunction. The mechanism behind the VTA-DA cell dysfunction caused by experimental inhibition of the prefrontal cortex is likely to involve inhibition of an aspartate-containing pathway to the VTA from the medial prefrontal cortex (Christie et al 1985). Interestingly, functional inactivation of the frontal/prefrontal cortex is seen clinically in a subgroup of schizophrenics and correlates to so-called negative symptoms. This hypofrontality has also been observed in chronic alcoholics (see Ingvar 1987). Such patients or individuals suffer from a clear deficit in self-guided behaviour and severely impaired motivational behaviour.

The ventral tegmental area dopamine cells:
effect of nicotine and some other drugs

Systemic administration of nicotine induces a significant activation of VTA-DA cells, particularly burst activity (Grenhoff et al 1986; Fig. 1). As discussed by Clarke (this volume), this effect of nicotine may represent the critical effect of nicotine in brain as regards its reinforcing action. The stimulation of VTA-DA cells is probably executed at nicotinic receptors on the VTA-DA cells (see Grenhoff & Svensson 1989). Interestingly, only DA cells which showed spontaneous bursting responded with increased bursting to systemic nicotine administration, whereas single spike firing cells only responded with increased rate of single spike firing (Grenhoff et al 1986). Thus, the normal quality of discharge within the DA cell population seemed to be maintained.

In our most recent experiments we have found that systemic administration of nicotine in doses relevant to behaviour (0.17 mg/kg base i.p.) induces a partial, but significant, reversal of the dysfunction of VTA-DA cells caused by

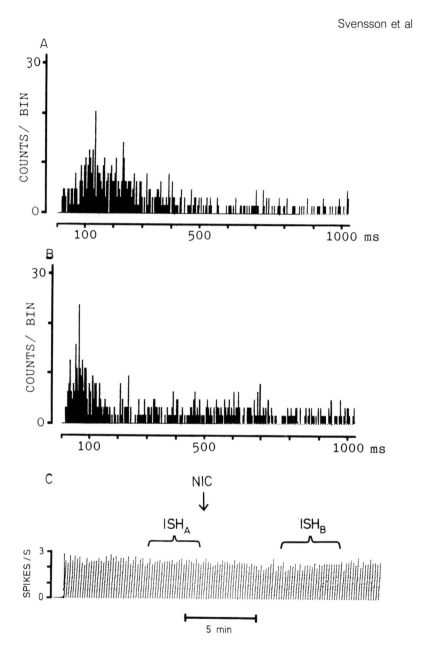

FIG. 1.   Effect of nicotine (0.17 mg/kg base i.p.) on the firing pattern of a VTA-DA cell.
(A) An interspike time interval histogram (ISH) recorded before nicotine. Firing rate
2.37 Hz, burst firing 26%. (B) Recorded 10 minutes after nicotine, this ISH shows an
increased burst firing, reflected as the emergence of a peak to the left in the ISH, representing the short intervals within bursts. Firing rate 2.10 Hz, burst firing 43%. (C) The
specific change in firing pattern is not revealed by the simultaneous pen chart recording
of the firing rate. ISHs in (A) and (B) were recorded in the periods indicated by the brackets.

experimental hypofrontality in rats (Tung et al 1990; Fig. 2). Thus, a significant amount of bursting was maintained by nicotine in spite of the inactivation of the prefrontal cortex. The firing rate of the VTA-DA cells was not altered by either this inactivation or administration of nicotine.

Even more effective in blocking the VTA-DA cell dysfunction caused by experimental hypofrontality was ritanserin, a potent 5-hydroxytryptamine (5-HT$_2$) receptor antagonist (Svensson et al 1989b). No change in either bursting or variation coefficient of the VTA-DA neurons was obtained by inactivation of the prefrontal cortex in rats treated with ritanserin. Similar results were obtained with amperozide, a novel atypical neuroleptic drug (Grenhoff et al 1990), which, like ritanserin (Svensson et al 1989b), in clinical trials has been found to improve motivation and drive, with some effect on negative symptoms in schizophrenia. Amperozide is also a highly potent 5-HT$_2$ antagonist (see Grenhoff et al 1990). Thus, restoration or normalization of VTA-DA cell dysfunction caused by hypofrontality may be related to the clinical improvement of normal motivational behaviour.

Excessive smoking in certain schizophrenics may therefore represent a form of attempted self-medication. The same principle may apply to smoking in chronic alcoholics, in whom a specific and long-lasting reduction in functional activity of the prefrontal cortex has been observed (Ingvar 1987).

It follows that drugs which block 5-HT$_2$, such as ritanserin or amperozide, might have a role in smoking cessation programmes, particularly for psychiatric patients suffering from chronic schizophrenia or advanced alcoholism.

Locus ceruleus noradrenaline cells: physiology

The pontine nucleus LC gives rise to the largest central NA network, amounting to about 70 per cent of all NA in the brain of primates. It ascends, for example, to the cerebral cortex and limbic areas and is generally considered to be directly involved in maintaining vigilance. The LC cells are highly responsive to various sensory stimuli of salient nature, both from the external environment and from the internal environment, the latter being mediated via various peripheral somatosensory, cardiopulmonary and visceral afferents (for reviews see Foote et al 1983, Svensson 1987). Thus, phasic activation of LC neurons associated with novel and challenging environmental stimuli appears to be an alerting response that improves discriminatory functions and the capacity to cope; it could therefore be regarded as a central component of the classical defence reaction (see Bloom 1979, Svensson 1987).

Locus ceruleus noradrenaline cells: effects of nicotine and other drugs

Three decades ago, Burn (1960) proposed that the central stimulation caused by nicotine, which includes enhanced vigilance, is mediated in part by central

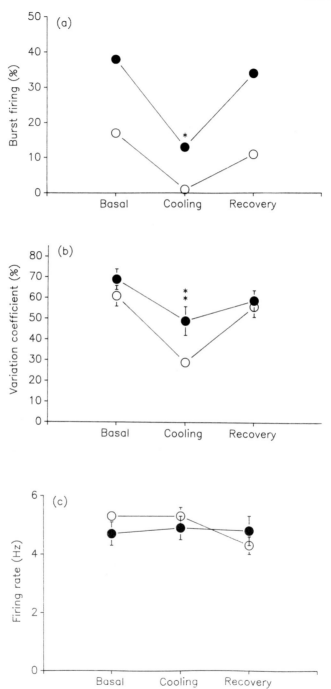

release of NA. The same year Comroe (1960) proposed that most of the actions of nicotine, including central stimulation, might be elicited by stimulation of peripheral afferents.

More recent experiments, employing single cell recording technology, confirm and unite these two hypotheses. Intravenous administration of nicotine in small doses induces a selective activation of burst activity in NA neurons of the LC (Tung et al 1989). LC activation cannot be produced by local micro-iontophoretic application of nicotine onto LC cells, in contrast to the stimulation by microiontophoretically applied acetylcholine. The latter effect is completely blocked by muscarinic antagonists (Svensson & Engberg 1980, Engberg & Svensson 1980). The LC activation by systemic nicotine is extremely rapid in onset, dose dependent, short lasting and can be repeated within minutes (Svensson & Engberg 1980). It is an indirect effect, a notion which is supported by the following findings: the activation is blocked by neonatal capsaicin treatment, which causes a fairly selective degeneration of primary sensory afferents (Hajos & Engberg 1988). It is also blocked by administration of hexamethonium or chlorisondamine, which block peripheral but not central nicotinic receptors (Hajos & Engberg 1988). Pretreatment with kynurenic acid abolishes the effect of nicotine on LC neurons (Engberg 1989, Tung et al 1989; Fig. 3). Thus, a direct effect of systemic nicotine on these cells can be excluded. Interestingly, kynurenic acid also abolished spontaneous burst firing of the LC neurons and induced a pacemaker-like, highly regular activity (Svensson et al 1989a). This effect is probably caused by antagonism of a tonically active excitatory amino acid input from the paragigantocellular nucleus (Ennis & Aston-Jones 1988). Microinjection of a local anaesthetic into this nucleus attenuates the LC activation by systemically administered nicotine (Chen & Engberg 1989). Available evidence thus clearly indicates that the LC stimulation by nicotine is indirect and mediated via release of excitatory amino acids onto the LC cells (Tung et al 1989).

The LC stimulation caused by intravenously injected nicotine showed an average delay of onset of 1.7 seconds and, in some experiments, LC neurons were excited during the injection of nicotine, which lasted for one second (Fig. 4). Given the systemic circulation time in the rat (about 20 seconds), this result provides unequivocal physiological evidence for a peripheral site of action of nicotine for its LC stimulatory action. Consequently, the stimulation of the

---

FIG. 2. Firing pattern of VTA-DA neurons before, during and after prefrontal cortex inactivation by local cooling in saline-treated control ($\bigcirc$, $n = 13$) and nicotine-treated rats (0.17 mg/kg base, i.p.; $\bullet$, $n = 8$). (a) Changes in burst firing. Note absence of burst firing during cooling in control group. (b) Changes in regularity of firing. The decreased variation coefficient in the saline-treated controls represents regularization. (c) Firing rate. No significant differences were observed. $**P < 0.01$, $*P < 0.05$ between control and nicotine-treated group.

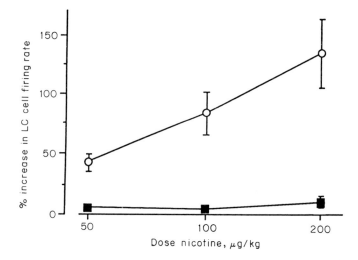

FIG. 3.   Effect of nicotine on the firing rate of noradrenergic locus ceruleus neurons
in untreated controls (○) and animals pretreated with the excitatory amino acid antagonist
kynurenic acid (■) (1 µmol i.c.v., 10–30 minutes). Mean ± SEM, $n = 4$–16.

LC by nicotine may be elicited, for example, via stimulation of peripheral C-
fibre afferents. The marked sensitivity of such afferents, e.g. in the cardiopulmonary region, to nicotine (see Ginzel 1988) agrees with this view. Thus,
the observation of arousal in an electroencephalogram in less than lung-
to-brain circulation time following cigarette smoke inhalation (Murphree et al
1967) may in part be related to peripherally induced LC activation by nicotine.

Locus ceruleus noradrenaline cells: clinical aspects

The activation of the LC by nicotine allows an instant coping response in brain,
with literal finger-tip control executed by the smoker. Since the reinforcing unit
in smoking is the short-lasting puff (Russell 1988), the instant LC response might
be significant for smoking behaviour. Rose et al (1984, 1985) found that local
anaesthesia of the airways caused significant reduction in cigarette-induced
reward. The peripheral origin of the nicotine-induced LC stimulation is clearly
consonant with this contention.

Recent results have shown that priming electrical stimulation of the LC for
short periods, aimed at simulating phasic, vigilance-related LC activation, causes
facilitation of memory retrieval in the rat (Sara & Devauges 1988). Thus, the
phasic activation of the LC by systemic nicotine administration may underlie
reported effects of smoking or nicotine on learning and memory (see Wesnes
& Warburton 1983).

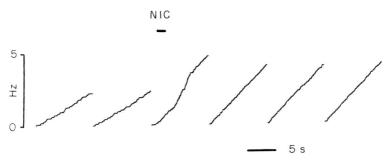

FIG. 4. Cumulative rate record showing the effect of nicotine (50 µg/kg i.v.) on the firing rate of a noradrenergic locus ceruleus cell. Injection period indicated by horizontal bar. The excitatory response can be detected during the intravenous injection.

Generally, the LC activation by nicotine may be highly significant for some of the desirable effects of nicotine, such as enhanced vigilance and discriminatory capacity, ability to cope and reported positive effects on learning and memory.

Recent information indicates that a previous history of depression severely impairs the already normally poor prognosis for cessation of smoking (Glassman et al 1988). The instant coping response provided through the LC activation by nicotine may, clearly, be particularly attractive for depressed or depression-prone individuals. Consequently, treatment with antidepressants, which frequently seem to facilitate central noradrenergic neurotransmission, as evidenced by down-regulation of β-adrenergic receptors in brain (see Svensson 1983), may prove advantageous to counteract nicotine dependence in such individuals. Other drugs, such as α_2-adrenoceptor antagonists, which activate the LC, may also be of interest in this regard.

Conclusions

1. The stimulation of brain catecholamine neurons by systemically administered nicotine is probably critically important for the reinforcing action of nicotine, as well as its central stimulatory action.

2. In both the VTA-DA cells and the LC NA neurons, the nicotine-induced stimulation includes burst activation, i.e. the physiologically most efficient type of neuronal activity as reflected in neurotransmitter release.

3. Whereas the VTA-DA cell stimulation is probably executed directly on nicotine receptors in the VTA, the LC activation is indirect; it is peripherally elicited and relayed onto the LC by release of excitatory amino acids via the input from the paragigantocellular nucleus. Thus, phenomena such as tolerance and dependence may be quite different in these two brain nuclei.

4. In an experimental model of clinical hypofrontality, a condition observed in certain chronic schizophrenics or advanced alcoholics, the VTA-DA cells display a specific dysfunctional state marked by pacemaker-like firing and an absence of burst firing.

5. Nicotine administration can partly but significantly antagonize the VTA-DA cell dysfunction induced by experimental hypofrontality. Thus, excessive smoking in such clinical conditions may represent a form of attempted self-medication.

6. Drugs known to affect positively normal motivational behaviour in individuals with so-called hypofrontality, such as $5HT_2$ receptor antagonists, restore VTA-DA cell dysfunction caused by hypofrontality more effectively than does nicotine. Consequently, such drugs may have clinical potential in the treatment of severe nicotine dependence.

7. The moralistic explanation of excessive smoking, i.e. lack of personal control over motivational behaviour, may have its neurobiological basis in impaired influence from the frontal/prefrontal cortex over the dynamics of the VTA-DA cells.

8. Dysfunctional states of the VTA-DA cells, whether caused by mental disorder or drug abuse, may serve as a biologically based negative reason to continue even excessive smoking, i.e. to sustain strong nicotine dependence, once established.

9. Stimulation of the noradrenergic LC cells by nicotine may, unfortunately, even in normal individuals be a positive reason to smoke because of the enhanced vigilance, intellectual processing, and improved memory retrieval that it produces. These effects may be of particular importance for initiating nicotine dependence.

Acknowledgements

The original work reviewed here was supported by grants from the Council for Tobacco Research-USA, Inc. (grant no. 2192), the Swedish Medical Research Council (project nos. 04747 and 7484), Svenska Tobaks AB, Torsten och Ragnar Söderbergs Stiftelser, and Karolinska Institutet.

References

Bloom FE 1979 Norepinephrine mediated synaptic transmission and hypotheses of psychiatric disorders. In: Meyer E et al (eds) Research in the psychobiology of human behavior. Johns Hopkins University Press, Baltimore, p 1–11
Burn JH 1960 The action of nicotine on the peripheral circulation. Ann NY Acad Sci 90:81–84
Chen Z, Engberg G 1989 The rat nucleus paragigantocellularis as a relay station to mediate peripherally induced central effects of nicotine. Neurosci Lett 101:67–71
Christie MF, Bridge S, James LB, Beart PM 1985 Excitotoxin lesions suggest an aspartatergic projection from rat medial prefrontal cortex to ventral tegmental area. Brain Res 333:169–172
Clarke PBS 1990 Mesolimbic dopamine activation—the key to nicotine reinforcement? In: The biology of nicotine dependence. Wiley, Chichester (Ciba Found Symp 152) p 153–168
Comroe JH 1960 The pharmacological action of nicotine. Ann NY Acad Sci 90:48–51

Engberg G 1989 Nicotine induced excitation of locus coeruleus neurons is mediated via release of excitatory amino acids. Life Sci 44:1535–1540

Engberg G, Svensson TH 1980 Pharmacological analysis of a cholinergic receptor mediated regulation of brain norepinephrine neurons. J Neural Trans 49:137–150

Ennis M, Aston-Jones G 1988 Activation of locus coeruleus from nucleus paragigantocellularis: a new excitatory amino acid pathway in brain. J Neurosci 8: 3644–3657

Fibiger HC, Phillips AG 1986 Reward, motivation, cognition: psychobiology of mesotelencephalic dopamine systems. In: Bloom FE (ed) Handbook of Physiology, Section I: The Central Nervous System, p 647–675

Foote SL, Bloom FE, Aston-Jones G 1983 Nucleus locus coeruleus: new evidence of anatomical and physiological specificity. Physiol Rev 63:844–914

Ginzel KH 1988 The lungs as sites of origin of nicotine-induced skeletomotor relaxation and behavioral and electrocortical arousal in the cat. In: Rand MJ, Thurau K (eds) The pharmacology of nicotine. IRL Press, Oxford, p 269–292

Glassman AH, Stetner F, Walsh BT et al 1988 Heavy smokers, smoking cessation, and clonidine. Results of a double-blind, randomized trial. J Am Med Assoc 259: 2863–2866

Gonon FG 1988 Nonlinear relationship between impulse flow and dopamine released by rat midbrain dopaminergic neurons as studied by in vivo electrochemistry. Neuroscience 24:19–28

Grenhoff J, Svensson TH 1989 Pharmacology of nicotine. Br J Addict 84:477–492

Grenhoff J, Aston-Jones G, Svensson TH 1986 Nicotinic effects on the firing pattern of midbrain dopamine neurons. Acta Physiol Scand 128:351–358

Grenhoff J, Tung C-S, Svensson TH 1988 The excitatory amino acid antagonist kynurenate induces pacemaker-like firing of dopamine neurons in rat ventral tegmental area in vivo. Acta Physiol Scand 134:567–568

Grenhoff J, Tung C-S, Ugedo L, Svensson TH 1990 Effects of amperozide, a putative antipsychotic drug, on rat midbrain dopamine neurons recorded in vivo. Pharmacol Toxicol 66, Suppl 1: 29–33

Hajos M, Engberg G 1988 Role of primary sensory neurons in the central effects of nicotine. Psychopharmacology 94:468–470

Ingvar D 1987 Evidence for frontal/prefrontal cortical dysfunction in chronic schizophrenia: the phenomenon of "hypofrontality" reconsidered. In: Helmchen D, Henn FA (eds) Biological perspectives of schizophrenia. Wiley, Chichester, p 202–211

Jarvik ME, Henningfield JE 1988 Pharmacological treatment of tobacco dependence. Pharmacol Biochem Behav 30:279–294

Murphree HB, Pfeiffer CC, Price LM 1967 Electroencephalographic changes in man following smoking. Ann NY Acad Sci 142:245–260

Nishino H, Ono T, Muramoto K, Fukuda M, Sasaki K 1987 Neuronal activity in the ventral tegmental area (VTA) during motivated bar press feeding in the monkey. Brain Res 413:302–313

Rose JE, Zinser MC, Tashkin DP, Newcomb R, Ertle A 1984 Subjective response to cigarette smoking following airway anesthetization. Addict Behav 9:211–215

Rose JE, Tashkin DP, Ertle A, Zinser MC, Lafer B 1985 Sensory blockade of smoking satisfaction. Pharmacol Biochem Behav 23:289–293

Russell MAH 1988 Nicotine intake by smokers: are rates of absorption or steady-state levels more important? In: Rand MJ, Thurau K (eds) The pharmacology of nicotine. IRL Press, Oxford p 375–403

Sara SJ, Devauges V 1988 Priming stimulation of locus coeruleus facilitates memory retrieval in the rat. Brain Res 438:299–303

Schultz W 1986 Responses of midbrain dopamine neurons to behavioral triggering stimuli in the monkey. J Neurophysiol 56:1439–1461

Svensson TH 1983 Mode of action of antidepressant agents and ECT—adaptive changes after subchronic treatment. In: Angst J (ed) The origins of depression: current concepts and approaches. Dahlem-Konferenzen 1983. Springer, Berlin, p 367–383

Svensson TH 1987 Peripheral, autonomic regulation of locus coeruleus noradrenergic neurons in brain: putative implications for psychiatry and psychopharmacology. Psychopharmacology 92:1–7

Svensson TH, Engberg G 1980 Effect of nicotine on single cell activity in the noradrenergic nucleus locus coeruleus. Acta Physiol Scand Suppl 479:31–34

Svensson TH, Tung C-S 1989 Local cooling of pre-frontal cortex induces pacemaker-like firing of dopamine neurons in rat ventral tegmental area in vivo. Acta Physiol Scand 136:135–136

Svensson TH, Engberg G, Tung C-S, Grenhoff J 1989a Pacemaker-like firing of noradrenergic locus coeruleus neurons in vivo induced by the excitatory amino acid antagonist kynurenate in the rat. Acta Physiol Scand 135:421–422

Svensson TH, Tung C-S, Grenhoff J 1989b The 5-HT$_2$ antagonist ritanserin blocks the effect of pre-frontal cortex inactivation on rat A10 dopamine neurons in vivo. Acta Physiol Scand 136:497–498

Tung C-S, Ugedo L, Grenhoff J, Engberg G, Svensson TH 1989 Peripheral induction of burst firing in locus coeruleus neurons by nicotine mediated via excitatory amino acids. Synapse 4:313–318

Tung C-S, Grenhoff J, Svensson TH 1990 Nicotine counteracts dopamine cell dysfunction induced by pre-frontal cortex inactivation. Acta Physiol Scand, in press

Werner G, Mountcastle VB 1963 The variability of central neural activity in a sensory system, and its implications for the central reflection of sensory events. J Neurophysiol 26:958–977

Wesnes K, Warburton DM 1983 Smoking, nicotine and human performance. Pharmacol Ther 21:189–208

DISCUSSION

Clarke: You ended your talk suggesting that drugs which increase the activity of the locus ceruleus could be used as therapy for people giving up smoking. Clonidine has been used in such therapies, but, if I remember rightly, clonidine decreases the firing rate of those neurons.

Svensson: The efficacy of clonidine in smoking cessation programmes is a relatively recent observation. Clonidine is given when people are still smoking, for perhaps the last week before they stop, and for a few weeks subsequently. This may dampen emotional hyperreactivity and such things. I think that if you give clonidine to smokers for a long time, it might actually promote smoking. It is a very complicated issue; it is even more complicated because clonidine also affects dopaminergic cells (Grenhoff & Svensson 1989).

Rose: The efficacy of clonidine in helping people to abstain from smoking may depend on whether part of the reinforcement derived from nicotine is activation as opposed to suppression of the locus ceruleus.

Henningfield: This discussion presupposes that clonidine is effective in achieving abstinence from smoking: that has yet to be demonstrated in a properly controlled clinical trial.

Iversen: Isn't there a claim that fluoxetine, the 5HT uptake inhibitor, might also have beneficial effects? Would that be hard to reconcile with your argument that 5HT blockers could be useful?

Svensson: No, I don't think so for several reasons. One is the recent observations of Alexander Glassman from Columbia University. He has found that a previous episode of depression seriously impairs the already poor prognosis of smoking cessation programmes. If people have a previous history of depression or affective disorder the prognosis is effectively zero. He also reported that treatment with anti-depressants significantly improves the prognosis under such conditions.

London: Antidepressants, particularly those that block 5HT (serotonin) uptake, may play a more global role than in smoking and depression. They may influence impulse control. A number of studies have suggested that alcoholism is a defect in impulse control (e.g. Edwards & Gross 1976), and the deficit may be ameliorated by promoting serotonergic activity (Lopez-Ibor 1988, Gorelick 1989).

Gray: What do you think is the anatomical basis for the action of a serotonergic agonist on the VTA cells?

Svensson: There are numerous possibilities. Interestingly, the effect of serotonin on a given cell may differ, and be either excitatory or inhibitory, depending on the pre-existing condition of the membrane. So it's very hard to predict the mechanism of action of an agonist at present.

Gray: So your argument was based on the fact that ritanserin has been reported to be an anti-psychotic, rather than on an anatomical hypothesis?

Svensson: The logic here is very simple. In spite of 25 years of research, there is no unequivocal evidence for a disturbance of DA function in schizophrenia. At the same time, 25 years of experience suggest that the only thing anti-psychotic drugs have in common is blocking D2 receptors. That has led many people to speculate what could be the fundamental problem. People have said there might be other systems in brain, which is a possibility. Nevertheless, DA appears interesting.

It has been suggested that there might be some sort of dysfunction of the system. Our idea was to analyse the function and the dynamics of the system and see what is the consequence of experimental hypofrontality on the DA cells. We see there is a dysfunction. Logically, this might help to explain some of these negative symptoms, such as lack of drive, lack of interest, lack of sensory reward, etc.

5HT blockers also do something clinically and there is mounting evidence for a real effect on negative symptoms. In parallel, there is a reversal of the DA cell dysfunction. We tried nicotine in our model, because of the excessive smoking habits of schizophrenics. It seems to have a partial ritanserin-like effect on the DA cells. Thus, if you replace nicotine in those patients with ritanserin or risperidone or amperozide, they may do even better and smoke less.

Gray: In the observation that schizophrenics smoke a lot more than other people, there is one possible artifact. Most schizophrenics now would be on DA receptor blockers. Therefore, could the higher rate of smoking be an attempt, not to self-medicate for the schizophrenia, but to overcome the effects of the prescribed DA receptor blockers?

Svensson: When these patients are admitted to hospital they are not taking medication. I think that almost all psychotics smoke heavily. There might be some point to your suggestion, though. For example, we have looked at the ability of haloperidol to reduce the functional deficit of the DA cells caused by hypofrontality. Haloperidol doesn't work well; you have to block serotonin 2 receptors and not DA receptors. That's why drugs such as risperidone or amperozide, which block both types of receptor, might be more useful in this case than the ordinary neuroleptics which block D2 receptors.

Colquhoun: I know nothing of psychiatry but it seems odd to discuss complicated reasons why schizophrenics might smoke more than other people when there are plenty of simple reasons, for example, they have more time!

Svensson: I don't think it is as simple as that. This is the same as when people used to say smoking is just a psychological habit.

Rose: Schizophrenics have been compared with patients suffering from other psychiatric disorders, in conditions where factors such as institutionalization were controlled for (Hughes et al 1986). The schizophrenic patients smoke much more than patients with anxiety or major depressive disorders.

London: I wonder if the increased smoking behaviour is not just a non-specific increase in substance abuse or a response to sensation seeking in schizophrenics.

Svensson: This is a known phenomenon; there is an increased substance abuse in schizophrenics as regards central stimulants, including amphetamines. There is a report from van Kammen & Boronow (1988) that chronic schizophrenics with an abundance of negative symptoms actually benefit from amphetamines.

Collins: Tom Crowley at the University of Colorado has been investigating the association between cocaine use and smoking. The results show that cocaine users are very heavy users of tobacco; they report two people who smoke only when they are on cocaine. The suggestion that DA receptor blockers are going to facilitate smoking is not entirely consistent with cocaine also facilitating smoking. Clearly, it's a very complicated issue.

London: I don't know that cocaine facilitates smoking. Perhaps it's just that substance abusers are heavy smokers.

Russell: There is a strong correlation between smoking and drug and alcohol abuse, and between smoking and psychiatric disorders generally. The rates of smoking are higher in all these conditions. Early smoking is a common precursor of subsequent drug use, but I don't think these relationships are necessarily due to pharmacological factors.

Svensson: We have heard from Dr Gray that nicotine will increase release of noradrenaline from nerve terminals and that is a different action from the one at cell bodies. The latter effect, which has a rapid onset, is similar to that of a noxious stimulus. Given that stimulation of the locus ceruleus causes induction of tyrosine hydroxylase, this rapid activation might be important for such a long-term effect on a system. Release of noradrenaline from nerve terminals may not necessarily influence tyrosine hydroxylase, but increased neuronal activity may do so. For that reason this effect might be interesting with respect to long-term effects on the noradrenergic system. It does not mean that you are blocking all the effects of nicotine on the noradrenergic system. You could test such an hypothesis by giving chlorisondamine to patients for one month to see if that affects the outcome in smoking cessation.

Russell: I would like to shift to your ideas that the effect of nicotine on the locus ceruleus might be mediated by peripheral receptors. They agree with Ginzel's work on the EEG effects of nicotine occurring before nicotine has time to reach the brain. He postulated the presence of receptors in the lung. Your work shows that if you destroy sensory receptors with capsaicin, you don't get the rapid nicotine effect on the locus ceruleus. Some of the sensory receptors that nicotine could get at rapidly are those in the aortic and carotid bodies, and others in and around the heart. These seem to contain specific nicotinic cholinergic receptors. Are there other sensory receptors in the skin and other places that may be stimulated in a direct nicotine-specific way?

Many of the behavioural effects of nicotine are blocked by mecamylamine but not by nicotinic blockers that act only peripherally. How does that observation fit the theory that peripheral nicotine stimulation is important?

Svensson: This rapid effect of nicotine may be important for long-term changes, for example, enzyme induction, as already mentioned. It may also be that some people would smoke in spite of mecamylamine treatment.

Rose: To answer the first of Dr Russell's questions: we have put (+) and (−) stereoisomers of nicotine on the tongue. The naturally occurring (−)nicotine is much more potent and irritating to tongue, so these receptors may be present in many areas.

Russell: What happens if you give a blocker mouthwash?

Rose: Rinsing the tongue with mecamylamine blocks this effect (Jarvik & Assil 1988). I would like to argue that the lungs are probably the most important locus for those peripheral actions of nicotine. We have shown that anaesthetizing airways locally blocks a great deal of the satisfaction of smoking a cigarette, even when the smoker gets the same amount of nicotine as they would otherwise (Rose et al 1985). Conversely, stimulating those regions with citric acid or with nicotine-containing aerosols, which focus the stimulation on the airways while delivering insignificant systemic levels of nicotine, also satisfies the craving for a cigarette to a much greater extent than do larger systemic nicotine levels which do not stimulate the pulmonary regions (Rose 1988, Rose & Behm 1987, Rose & Hickman 1988, Behm et al 1990, Rose et al 1990).

I don't know whether you do get repeated locus ceruleus activation by repeated nicotine administration, but in the human smoker is it possible that eventually you would get desensitization and that might translate into some sort of tranquilizing effect? Alternatively, the effect could be one of increased vigilance, as you suggested. Clearly those peripheral receptors are important in the human smoker. Clinically, it implies that perhaps the reason that, for instance, nicotine chewing gum produces only modest success rates in smoking cessation isn't necessarily that the rate of nicotine administration is not as fast as from inhaled cigarette smoke but rather that this important stimulation of the respiratory tract receptors does not occur.

Russell: Is it more than just a conditioned reflex?

Rose: It may be an unconditioned effect of nicotine on peripheral receptors, as suggested by Dr Svensson and by Ginzel & Eldred (1977), who showed that nicotinic agents can induce somatic muscle relaxation in the lung. In addition, the sensory cues in smoke may become conditioned reinforcers, particularly the peripheral irritation caused by nicotine in the lung, because it is such a strong signal for the CNS effects that follow nicotine inhalation.

References

Behm F, Levin ED, Lee YK, Rose JE 1990 Low-nicotine smoke aerosol reduces desire for cigarettes. J Subst Abuse, in press

Edwards G, Gross MM 1976 Alcohol dependence: provisional description of a clinical syndrome. Br Med J 1:1058–1061

Ginzel KH, Eldred E 1977 Reflex depression of somatic motor activity from heart, lungs and carotid sinus. In: Paintal AS, Gill-Kumar P (eds) Krogh centenary symposium on respiratory adaptations, capillary exchange and reflex mechanisms. University of Delhi, p 359–395

Gorelick DA 1989 Serotonin uptake blockers and the treatment of alcoholism. In: Galanter M (ed) Recent developments in alcoholism. Plenum Publishing Corporation, New York, vol 7:267–281

Grenhoff J, Svensson TH 1989 Clonidine modulates dopamine cell firing in rat ventral tegmental area. Eur J Pharmacol 165:11–18

Hughes JR, Hatsukami DK, Mitchell JE, Dahlgren LA 1986 Prevalence of smoking among psychiatric outpatients. Am J Psychiatry 143:993–997

Jarvik ME, Assil K 1988 Mecamylamine blocks the burning sensation of nicotine on the tongue. Chemical Senses 13:213–217

Lopez-Ibor JJ Jr 1988 The involvement of serotonin in psychiatric disorders and behaviour. Br J Psychiatry 153 (suppl 3):26–39

Rose JE 1988 The role of upper airway stimulation in smoking. In: Pomerleau OF, Pomerleau CS (eds) Nicotine replacement: a critical evaluation. Alan R Liss, New York, p 95–106

Rose JE, Behm FM 1987 Refined cigarette smoke as a means to reduce nicotine intake. Pharmacol Biochem Behav 28:305–310

Rose JE, Hickman C 1988 Citric acid aerosol as a potential smoking cessation aid. Chest 92:1005–1008

Rose JE, Tashkin DP, Ertle A, Zinser MC, Lafer RL 1985 Sensory blockade of smoking satisfaction. Pharmacol Biochem Behav 23:289–293

Rose JE, Levin ED, Behm F, Adivi C, Schur C 1990 Transdermal nicotine facilitates smoking cessation. Clin Pharmacol Ther 47:323–330

van Kammen DP, Boronow JJ 1988 Dextro-amphetamine diminishes negative symptoms in schizophrenia. Int Clin Psychopharmacol 3:111–121

Pharmacokinetic considerations in understanding nicotine dependence

Neal L. Benowitz

Clinical Pharmacology Unit of the Medical Service, San Francisco General Hospital Medical Center, and the Department of Medicine and Langley Porter Psychiatric Institute, University of California at San Francisco, California 94143, USA

Abstract. The pharmacokinetic and pharmacodynamic characteristics of a drug are important determinants of whether users become dependent on it and of the temporal patterns of drug use. Characteristics of cigarette smoking, which produces a high degree of dependence, and the use of nicotine gum, which has a relatively low risk of dependence, are compared. Nicotine from tobacco smoke is rapidly absorbed and transferred into the brain. This results in high brain concentrations and intensive psychological effects, with relatively little development of tolerance. The smoker may titrate the level of drug and associated psychological effects of nicotine. Thus, smoking provides a nearly optimal situation for behavioural reinforcement. Chewing nicotine gum results in slow absorption of nicotine, leading to lower levels of nicotine in the brain and substantial time for development of tolerance. Thus, the intensity of effect is less and the onset of effect is delayed from the onset of dosing, providing less opportunity for behavioural reinforcement. Pharmacokinetic and pharmacodynamic modelling techniques have been applied to these processes and used to assess the implications for understanding the daily smoking cycle.

1990 The biology of nicotine dependence. Wiley, Chichester (Ciba Foundation Symposium 152) p 186–209

Pharmacokinetic and pharmacodynamic characteristics of a drug are important determinants of whether its use generates dependence, the temporal patterns of drug use, and the level of drug use. To understand better the pharmacokinetic factors that promote drug dependence, I would like to compare cigarette smoking, which produces a high degree of dependence, and the use of nicotine gum, which has a relatively low risk of nicotine dependence (Hughes 1988).

The pharmacology of nicotine dependence will be discussed in relation to four processes: (1) absorption of nicotine into the body, (2) distribution of nicotine within the body, (3) pharmacological effect of nicotine on target organs, and (4) translation of pharmacological effect into behaviour.

Absorption of nicotine

Nicotine is a tertiary amine composed of a pyridine and a pyrrolidine ring. It is a weak base with a pKa of 8.0, soluble both in water and in lipids. At physiological pH, about 31% of nicotine is not ionized and readily crosses cell membranes. The pH of tobacco smoke is important in determining the absorption of nicotine from different sites within the body. The pH of smoke from flue-cured tobaccos found in most cigarettes is acidic. At this pH, most of the nicotine is ionized and does not rapidly cross membranes. As a consequence, there is little buccal absorption of nicotine from cigarette smoke, even when it is held in the mouth. In contrast, nicotine gum is buffered to an alkaline pH to facilitate absorption of nicotine through the mucous membranes of the mouth.

Tobacco smoke is inhaled into the lungs, from which it is absorbed into the systemic circulation. Absorption of nicotine is facilitated by a huge alveolar surface area, thin alveolar epithelial and endothelial layers, and an extensive capillary bed. As a result of these anatomical factors, nicotine moves rapidly from the alveolar spaces into the systemic circulation. Also of importance is that pulmonary capillary blood flow is high, representing passage of the entire blood volume through the lung every minute. Thus, drugs that are absorbed are carried quickly to various parts of the body and to target organs. After absorption through the lungs, blood concentrations of nicotine rise quickly and peak at the completion of cigarette smoking (Fig. 1).

The absorption of nicotine from nicotine polacrilex gum or smokeless tobacco is gradual, with blood levels peaking at the end of the chewing or snuff-taking period. In addition to absorption through the buccal mucosa, a considerable amount of nicotine is swallowed while chewing nicotine gum (Benowitz et al 1987). Nicotine that is swallowed is also absorbed but undergoes presystemic metabolism by the liver so that its bioavailability is relatively low (about 30%).

The kinetics of absorption of nicotine can be examined in detail using the technique of deconvolution (Benowitz et al 1988). The procedure involves administration of nicotine intravenously to determine its disposition kinetics and then measurement of blood levels of nicotine after absorption from cigarette smoke or nicotine gum (Fig. 1). The deconvolution technique estimates the input rate of nicotine at various times using observed concentrations of nicotine after any route of administration and the disposition function resulting from a particular intravenous dose. The results, shown in Fig. 1B, indicate that nicotine is absorbed very rapidly from cigarette smoke, and that absorption is complete when the person stops smoking. In contrast, input from the nicotine gum or smokeless tobacco has a small time lag, peaks and declines during the 30 minute period of chewing or snuff taking, then continues for more than 30 minutes after oral nicotine use has stopped. The prolonged absorption is probably related to absorption of swallowed nicotine.

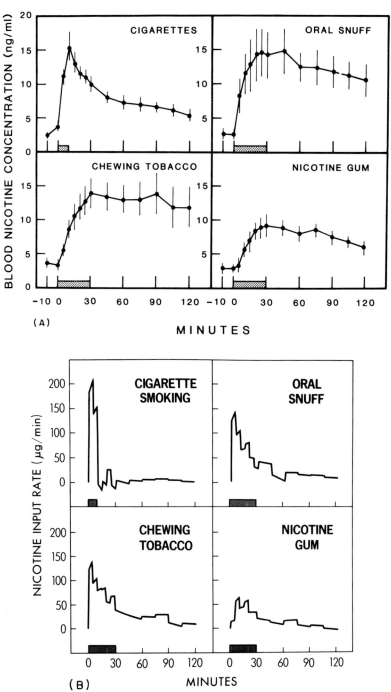

The analysis described above is based on data from 10 research subjects (Benowitz et al 1988). However, absorption of nicotine varies considerably, both in extent and rate, among people. Smoking behaviour is complex and the dose of a drug delivered to the circulation is influenced by how the individual smokes. The intensity, duration and number of puffs, depth of inhalation, degree of mixing of smoke with air, and other factors influence the dose. In one study, the range of intake of nicotine was 10–80 mg/day or 0.4–1.6 mg per cigarette (Benowitz & Jacob 1984). Thus, the smoker has considerable latitude in adjusting the dose to desired levels.

Similarly, absorption of nicotine from gum depends on how the gum is chewed, how much nicotine is swallowed and the local environment in the mouth. Absorption of nicotine varied threefold in one study of gum chewers, all of whom chewed 10 pieces of gum, each for 30 minutes, daily (Benowitz et al 1987). Gum chewers may be able to adjust the dose of nicotine obtained from the gum by altering how they chew or how much nicotine they swallow, but since absorption is slow and persists even after the chewing stops, adjustments of the dose cannot be as precise as when smoking cigarettes.

Distribution of nicotine

Smoking is a unique form of systemic drug administration in that entry into the circulation is through the pulmonary rather than the portal or systemic venous circulations. Entry via the lung influences the rate and pattern of delivery of drugs to body organs. For example, nicotine can be expected to move quickly from inhaled cigarette smoke to the brain. It is estimated that it takes 19 seconds or less from the start of a puff to the delivery of nicotine to the brain (Table 1). This estimation assumes a two second puff, negligible time for diffusion of nicotine across alveolar membranes, and negligible time for movement from the arterial blood into the brain.

Brain concentrations decline quickly as nicotine is distributed to other body tissues. Using partition coefficients (the ratio of drug concentration in tissue to that in blood at steady state) derived from experiments in rabbits, with organ weights and rates of blood flow taken from people, one can devise perfusion models to simulate the concentrations of nicotine in various organs after smoking a cigarette (Fig. 2).

Concentrations of nicotine in arterial blood and the brain increase sharply following exposure, then decline over 20 to 30 minutes as nicotine is redistributed

---

FIG. 1.(A)   Blood concentrations during and after cigarette smoking for nine minutes (1–1⅓ cigarettes), oral snuff (2.5 g), chewing tobacco (average 7.9 g), and nicotine gum (two 2 mg pieces). Average values for 10 subjects ($\pm$ SEM). (B) Nicotine absorption rate profiles, estimated by the point-area deconvolution method, during and after cigarette smoking, oral snuff, chewing tobacco, and nicotine gum. Shaded bars above time axis indicate period of tobacco or nicotine gum exposure. (From Benowitz et al 1988.)

TABLE 1 Estimates of the timing of the effects of nicotine after inhalation

Parameter	Time in seconds
Puff time	2.0
Pulmonary circulation time	7.5
Left ventricle to cerebral circulation	~ 1.0
Brain transit time	8.5
Total circulation time	19.0

Estimates derived from Mapleson (1973).

to other body tissues, particularly skeletal muscle. Venous blood concentrations, reflecting outflow of nicotine from body tissues, are predicted to be considerably lower than arterial concentrations for the duration of the infusion and for several minutes afterwards. This discrepancy has been observed in rabbits after rapid intravenous injection of nicotine (Porchet et al 1987) and in people after cigarette smoking (Henningfield et al 1989). It is seen from Fig. 2 that the ratio of nicotine in the brain to that in venous blood is highest during and at the end of the exposure period, and gradually decreases as the elimination phase is entered. The importance of this disequilibrium between venous and arterial concentrations with respect to pharmacodynamic studies is discussed in a later section.

In contrast to inhalation, the oral route of absorption is expected to result in a gradual increase in concentrations of nicotine in the brain, with relatively little arterial–venous disequilibrium.

In summary, inhalation of drugs allows for rapid transfer into the arterial circulation and into the brain. This provides for the possibility of rapid behavioural reinforcement from smoking and enables the smoker to control precisely the concentrations of nicotine in the brain, and hence to modulate pharmacological effects. Oral absorption results in gradual passage into the brain and provides less opportunity for behavioural reinforcement.

To understand better the reinforcement process, one must examine the relationship between levels of nicotine in the body and effects on the brain.

Pharmacodynamics of nicotine

Nicotine binds to specific receptors in the brain and affects cerebral metabolism in the areas of specific binding (London et al 1985). Nicotine is known to have a complex dose–response relationship. In experimental preparations low doses of nicotine cause ganglionic stimulation and high doses cause brief stimulation followed by ganglionic blockade. This biphasic response is observed in the intact organism as well, although the mechanisms are far more complex. With regard to central nervous system effects, Ashton has provided evidence that nicotine exerts biphasic actions in humans (Ashton et al 1980). Examination of the

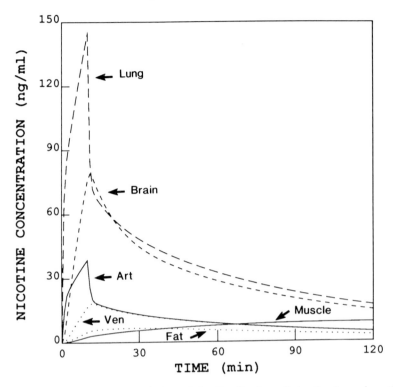

FIG. 2. Perfusion model simulation of the distribution of nicotine in various tissues after infusion of 1.5 mg of nicotine into the lung compartment over 10 minutes. The dose, route and dosing regimen were intended to mimic smoking a cigarette. Typical human organ weights and blood flows, and partition coefficients from rabbits were used for the simulation.

contingent negative variation (CNV, a component of the evoked electro-encephalogram potential) showed that low doses of nicotine increased the amplitude of the CNV, whereas high doses decreased it. It was proposed that low doses produced arousal or increased attention and vigilance, while higher doses produced relaxation and reduced stress. Presumably, the smoker, by titrating the level of nicotine in the brain, can achieve the desired mental state.

The time course of nicotine absorption strongly influences its actions, although it is not clear whether this is a result of a more rapid rate of rise or higher absolute levels of nicotine in the brain. We and others have found that heart rate acceleration, which reflects the level of sympathetic neural discharge and is a sensitive physiological response, correlates with the magnitude of subjective effect (Rosenberg et al 1980, West & Russell 1987). Heart rate acceleration appears to be mediated by the central nervous system either through actions on chemoreceptor afferent pathways or via direct effects on the brainstem.

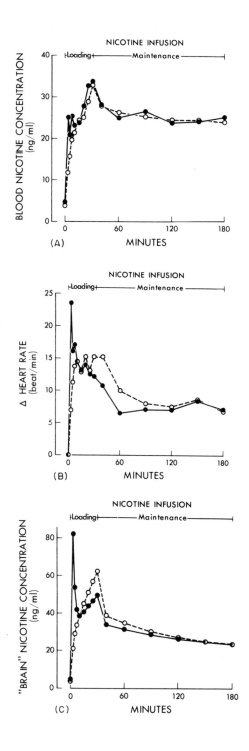

With repeated intravenous injections of nicotine, using doses calculated to simulate cigarette smoking, heart rate acceleration and subjective effects were greatest with the first series of injections and then declined with successive injections (Rosenberg et al 1980).

To examine the importance of rate of dosing in determining the effects of nicotine, and the relationship between effects and brain levels of nicotine, we compared the consequences of rapid and slow infusions of nicotine, followed by a maintenance infusion for 150 minutes (Porchet et al 1987). The study was performed in seven volunteer smokers who had abstained from smoking overnight. Forearm venous blood concentrations of nicotine were not markedly different with the two infusion rates except for the first five minutes, when the increase in blood concentration was greater with rapid infusion (Fig. 3). Peak concentrations were seen at 30 minutes, falling to a steady-state value during the maintenance infusion, and were similar for both infusions. During the slower infusion, heart rate increased slowly, peaking at 30 minutes, and subjective effects were minimal. After rapid infusion heart rate increased much more quickly and to a greater level, and was associated with transient dizziness and euphoria. Subsequent to both types of infusion heart rate declined toward the baseline value and plateaued over the last 120 minutes.

Of particular note are the early peak in heart rate without a corresponding peak in venous nicotine concentration, and a late peak (30 minutes) in venous nicotine concentration without a late peak in heart rate. Possible explanations for the former are the rapid development of tolerance and that the concentration of nicotine in the target site, i.e. the brain, equilibrates with arterial blood faster than with the concentration at the sampling site, i.e. venous blood. If the latter explanation is correct, concentrations of nicotine in the brain during the rapid infusion should be much greater than those measured in the venous blood.

Using pharmacokinetic data derived from this study and studies in rabbits, and using a physiological model, concentrations of nicotine in the human brain during rapid and slow infusions can be predicted (Fig. 3). The predicted brain concentrations follow a time course, at least initially, similar to that observed for the heart rate response. Brain concentrations and heart rate acceleration tended to change in parallel. These observations are consistent with the explanation that, after rapid dosing, venous blood levels underestimate arterial and brain levels, resulting in apparent or 'distributional' tolerance.

FIG. 3.   Pharmacodynamics of nicotine. (A) Average blood nicotine concentration. (B) Increase in heart rate. (C) Predicted mean 'brain' concentrations of nicotine. On the rapid loading day (●), each of the seven subjects received 17.5 µg/kg/min nicotine for 1.5 minutes, then 1.75 µg/kg/min for 30 minutes; on the slow loading day (○), 2.5 µg/kg/min for 30 minutes. Maintenance infusion on both days was 0.35 µg/kg/min from 30–180 minutes (Porchet et al 1987).

In summary, for drugs that rapidly enter and act upon the brain, drug dosing by inhalation results in higher brain concentrations and greater psychological effects than when the same dose is given by routes with slower absorption. The possibility of titrating the level of a drug in the brain to achieve a desired mental state is therefore facilitated by inhalation compared with oral dosing. This may explain why inhaling nicotine is preferred over the oral route of administration.

Tolerance to nicotine

In the rapid intravenous nicotine study described above, it was observed that there was a late (30 minute) peak in venous nicotine concentrations, but no late peak in heart rate (Fig. 3). This observation cannot be explained by distributional tolerance, but rather suggests the development of true tolerance. Tolerance is defined as when, after repeated doses, a given dose of a drug produces less effect. Pharmacodynamic tolerance can be further defined as when a particular concentration of a drug at a receptor site (in the intact organism approximated by the concentration in the blood) produces less of an effect after exposure to the drug than it did before.

Studies in animals demonstrate rapid development of tolerance to many effects of nicotine, although tolerance may not be complete (Marks et al 1985). Smokers know that tolerance develops to some effects of smoking. Smoking one's first ever cigarette is commonly associated with dizziness, nausea and/or vomiting, effects to which the smoker rapidly becomes tolerant. Smoking a cigarette after 24 hours of abstinence increases heart rate, whereas smoking an identical cigarette during a day's smoking fails to increase heart rate (West & Russell 1987).

These and other findings indicate that tolerance is gained rapidly, possibly within minutes (tachyphylaxis). Tolerance is lost, at least to some degree, after overnight abstinence. To characterize the time course of tolerance development and regression, we conducted a study in which subjects received paired intravenous infusions of nicotine, separated by different time intervals (Porchet et al 1988) (Fig. 4). Despite higher blood concentrations, heart rate acceleration and subjective effects were much less when a second infusion was given at 60 or 120 minutes after the first infusion. At 210 minutes, the response was fully restored.

The pharmacodynamics was modelled using a pharmacokinetic–pharmacodynamic model (Porchet et al 1988) (Fig. 5). This incorporates the features that the degree of tolerance increases as the concentration of drug in the effector organ (C_e) increases and tolerance decreases as the time between exposures decreases. Thus, the greater the exposure to a drug, the greater the tolerance, but tolerance is less if the exposure was longer ago. The model incorporates a mathematical construct such that a theoretical metabolite which is a competitive inhibitor of the action of nicotine is formed from nicotine, and that metabolite is eliminated at a rate K_{ant0}. Such modelling indicates a half-life

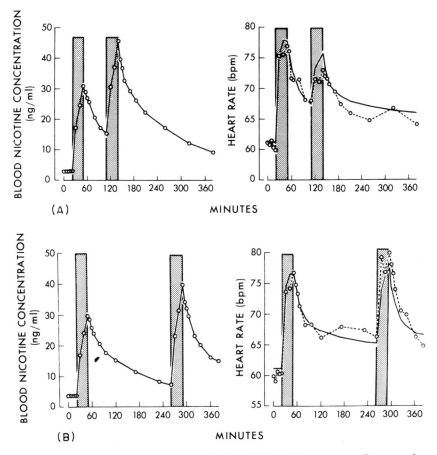

FIG. 4. Mean blood concentrations of nicotine (left) and the corresponding mean heart rate (right) in eight subjects after two 30 minute intravenous infusions of 2.5 µg/kg/min of nicotine separated by 60 minutes (A) or 210 minutes (B). The shadowed area indicates the periods during which nicotine was infused. The solid line shows the fit of the model to the heart rate data (Porchet et al 1988).

of development and regression of tolerance of 35 minutes. Thus, after three half-lives (one and one-half to two hours) of steady-state exposure, nearly all the tolerance that will ultimately develop will have developed and, conversely, one and one-half to two hours after the last cigarette nearly full sensitivity to nicotine will be regained. The estimate of S, the slope of the linear relationship between the effect on heart rate and the concentration, was 1.31 beats/min/ng/ml. C_{ant50}, the concentration of the hypothetical antagonist that results in loss of 50% of the maximal effect due to tolerance, was 7.7 ng/ml. E_0, the value of the baseline effect, was 61.2 beats/min. The implications of a C_{ant50} value of

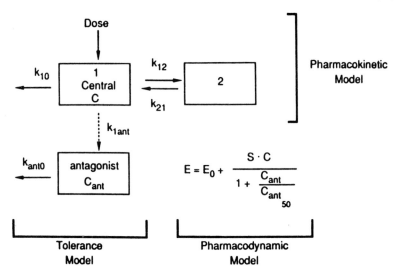

FIG. 5. Diagram of the pharmacokinetic and pharmacodynamic model for nicotine tolerance. k_x represents the intercompartmental and elimination rate constants; C, concentration of the agonist; C_{ant50}, concentration of this antagonist that results in loss of 50% of the maximal effect due to tolerance. E, effect; E_0, baseline effect; S, slope of linear relationship between effect and concentration (Porchet et al 1988).

7.7 ng/ml is that at a typical steady-state blood nicotine level of 30 ng/ml, tolerance will have reduced the effect to about 20% of the value that would have been achieved without the development of tolerance. Because tolerance develops so quickly, the rate of drug dosing influences the magnitude of effect. That is, the faster the administration, the less time there is to develop tolerance and the greater the effect for any given dose or maximal level.

A full model of the pharmacokinetics and pharmacodynamics of nicotine, incorporating both the distributional and the tolerance levels, has been presented by Sheiner (1989) (Fig. 6). The model was used to compare the effects of cigarette smoking and nicotine gum used throughout the day. Pharmacokinetic data from intravenous infusions, cigarette smoking and chewing nicotine gum, as presented previously, were used in the model. A simulation was performed for smoking one cigarette per half hour for 16 hours (30 cigarettes) and chewing one 2 mg piece of gum per hour for 16 hours (16 pieces). The dose of nicotine systemically absorbed from each cigarette and from each piece of gum was set at 1 mg.

As seen from Fig. 6, heart rate is predicted to accelerate more slowly and with lesser increments when chewing nicotine gum than when smoking a cigarette. This is a consequence of the slower input of nicotine from chewing, such that levels of nicotine in the brain are lower and tolerance develops during the input process, thereby decreasing the maximal response. At the end of the day, the response to each cigarette or piece of gum is blunted owing to

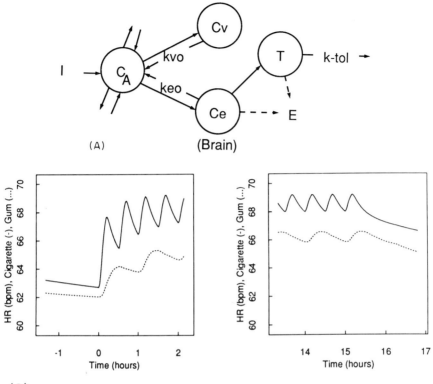

FIG. 6. (A) Pharmacokinetic–pharmacodynamic model incorporating distributional and tolerance features. Drug input (I) into arterial blood (drug concentration $= C_A$) and subsequent distribution to venous blood (C_V) and the effect site (C_e), the brain. The drug effect (E) is determined by C_e and T, the latter a hypothetical entity ('metabolite') to which tolerance is proportional (the same as C_{ant} in Fig. 5) The venous blood and effect sites are modelled as homogeneous compartments with first order transfer (rate constants $= k_{vo}$ and k_{eo}, respectively) to the arterial compartment. The 'inhibitory metabolite' acts on the effect site and is lost by a first order process (rate constant $= k_{tol}$). (From Sheiner 1989.) (B) Simulation of heart rate response to daily intake of cigarettes (—) or nicotine gum (----) versus time of day made with the model shown in (A). Parameters given in the text. The intake begins after overnight abstinence (left) and ceases with sleep (right). (From Sheiner 1989.)

development of tolerance. Assuming that psychoactive effects of nicotine parallel heart rate acceleration, one may see that the first cigarette of the day will provide the most intense stimulation, while later in the day stimulation will be minimal, and smoking may become motivated primarily by avoidance of abstinence symptoms. Nicotine gum chewing never achieves the impact of cigarette smoking, but, particularly later on in the day, may provide a cushion against abstinence symptoms.

In summary, tolerance develops rapidly to the effects of nicotine. The kinetics of tolerance are such that tolerance may develop and regress in cycles throughout the day. The interval at which users smoke cigarettes may be influenced by two factors: the rate of distribution of nicotine out of the brain after a particular dose of the drug and the kinetics of regression of tolerance to effects of nicotine. Rapid rate of dosing, as by inhalation, produces high levels of nicotine in the brain, resulting in the maximal drug effect with the least extent of development of tolerance. A slow rate of dosing, as obtained by chewing nicotine gum, produces lower levels of nicotine in the brain and allows for substantial development of tolerance, with a lesser intensity of drug effect with each dose.

Pharmacokinetics and pharmacodynamics of drug dependence

The reinforcing properties of a drug are strongest when a psychoactive effect, usually a pleasant one, follows in close temporal proximity the self-administration of a drug. Considering pharmacokinetic and pharmacodynamic factors, the drug should enter the bloodstream rapidly and move rapidly from the bloodstream into the brain. The appearance of the drug in the brain should be temporally associated with the desired psychological effects. If the effect of a drug is delayed after appearance of the drug in the brain or if tolerance to the drug effect has developed, the drug is less likely to be reinforcing.

That the user can easily control the dose of the drug and modulate the resultant psychoactivity would be expected to strengthen the reinforcing nature of the drug. As discussed previously, nicotine obtained by cigarette smoking demonstrates these characteristics, as do other drugs of abuse which are inhaled, such as crack cocaine or marijuana, and drugs which are intravenously injected, such as heroin and cocaine. Nicotine derived from nicotine gum is slowly absorbed and is not expected to be as reinforcing.

Tolerance is most likely to develop to the effects of a drug when its receptors are continuously exposed to the drug. Frequent and sustained dosing and/or a long half-life of a drug would favour development of tolerance. The half-life of nicotine in the brain following a single dose exposure is short, probably about 10 minutes in humans, owing to redistribution out of the brain to other body tissues. Some degree of tolerance does develop rapidly (tachyphylaxis), even after brief exposures. Such tolerance also regresses relatively quickly (half-life of 35 minutes), and a smoker may learn that smoking a cigarette at particular intervals is more reinforcing than smoking more frequently.

With repetitive dosing, levels of nicotine build up in the body (and in the brain) in accordance with the elimination half-life of two hours. Thus, there is substantial accumulation of nicotine in the brain and an increasing general level of tolerance throughout the day. Presumably, however, smoking individual cigarettes still results in peaks of nicotine in the brain, which overcomes the underlying level of tolerance and produces some of the desired effects. Chewing nicotine gum is less likely to overcome tolerance and produce any degree of stimulation.

Withdrawal symptoms are most likely to occur when there has been a sustained effect of a drug on the brain and then the drug quickly disappears. Thus, rapid exit from specific brain regions would favour more severe withdrawal symptoms. Nicotine, as it is taken by cigarette smokers, exhibits both of these characteristics. Owing to repetitive dosing, the brain is exposed to nicotine for prolonged periods of time such that neuroadaptation occurs during the smoking day. When exposure is terminated, nicotine rapidly exits the brain and withdrawal symptoms are experienced. It is likely, therefore, that relief of withdrawal symptoms plays an increasingly important role in determining smoking behaviour as the day progresses. Nicotine gum, by generating relatively constant levels of nicotine in the brain, would be expected to reduce the severity of nicotine withdrawal symptoms, which is consistent with clinical observations.

Nicotine and the daily smoking cycle

The pharmacokinetic and pharmacodynamic considerations discussed thus far help us to understand the development of nicotine dependence, human cigarette smoking behaviour and the adverse effects of cigarette smoking. The daily smoking cycle can be conceived as follows. The first cigarette of the day produces substantial pharmacological effects, primarily arousal, but at the same time tolerance begins to develop. A second cigarette may be smoked later, at a time when the smoker has learned there is some regression of tolerance. With subsequent cigarettes, there is accumulation of nicotine in the body, resulting in a greater level of tolerance and withdrawal symptoms become more pronounced between successive cigarettes. Transiently high brain levels of nicotine after smoking individual cigarettes may partially overcome tolerance. But the primary (euphoric) effects of individual cigarettes tend to lessen throughout the day. Overnight abstinence allows considerable resensitization to actions of nicotine. Because of the dose-response and tolerance characteristics, habitual smokers need to smoke at least 15 cigarettes and consume 20 to 40 mg nicotine per day to achieve the desired effects of cigarette smoking and minimize withdrawal discomfort throughout the day.

Acknowledgements

Supported in part by US Public Health Service grants DA02277, CA32389, and DA01696. These studies were carried out in part in the General Clinical Research Center (RR-00083) with support of the Division of Research Resources, National Institutes of Health.

References

Ashton H, Marsh VR, Millman JE, Rawlins MD, Telford R, Thompson JW 1980 Biphasic dose-related responses of the CNV (contingent negative variation) to i.v. nicotine in man. Br J Clin Pharmacol 10:579–589

Benowitz NL, Jacob P III 1984 Daily intake of nicotine during cigarette smoking. Clin Pharmacol Ther 35:499–504

Benowitz NL, Jacob P III, Savanapridi C 1987 Determinants of nicotine intake while chewing nicotine polacrilex gum. Clin Pharmacol Ther 41:467–473

Benowitz NL, Porchet H, Scheiner L, Jacob P III 1988 Nicotine absorption and cardiovascular effects with smokeless tobacco use: comparison with cigarettes and nicotine gum. Clin Pharmacol Ther 44:23–28

Henningfield JH, London E, Benowitz NL 1989 Arterio-venous differences in plasma concentrations of nicotine after cigarette smoking. J Am Med Assoc, in press

Hughes JR 1988 Dependence potential and abuse liability of nicotine replacement therapies. In: Pomerleau OF, Pomerleau CF (eds) Progress in clinical and biological research. Alan R. Liss, New York, p 261–277

London ED, Connolly RJ, Szikszay M, Wamsley JK 1985 Distribution of cerebral metabolic effects of nicotine in the rat. Eur J Pharmacol 110:391–392

Mapleson WW 1973 Circulation-time models of the uptake of inhaled anesthetics and data for quantifying them. Br J Anaesth 45:319–334

Marks MJ, Stitzel JA, Collins AC 1985 Time course study of the effects of chronic nicotine infusion on drug response and brain receptors. J Pharmacol Exp Ther 235:619–628

Porchet HC, Benowitz NL, Scheiner LB, Copeland JR 1987 Apparent tolerance to the acute effect of nicotine results in part from distribution kinetics. J Clin Invest 80:1466–1471

Porchet HC, Benowitz NL, Scheiner LB 1988 Pharmacodynamic model of tolerance: application to nicotine. J Pharmacol Exp Ther 244:231–236

Rosenberg J, Benowitz NL, Jacob P III, Wilson KM 1980 Disposition kinetics and effects of intravenous nicotine. Clin Pharmacol Ther 28:516–522

Sheiner LB 1989 Clinical pharmacology and the choice between theory and empiricism. Clin Pharmacol Ther 46:605

West RJ, Russell MAH 1987 Cardiovascular and subjective effects of smoking before and after 24 h of abstinence from cigarettes. Psychopharmacology 92:118–121

DISCUSSION

Iversen: So the reason humans set light to tobacco, as opposed to chewing it, is that to get the maximum beneficial effect one needs this sudden transient increase of nicotine in the brain?

Benowitz: For a psychoactive drug that has to get into the brain quickly for maximum pharmacological effect, smoking is the most efficient way to use it. This is why the smoking of crack and cocaine has become so popular.

West: The main issue with respect to dependence is the extent to which heart rate is a model for other effects of smoking that might be motivational or dependence inducing. It is interesting that you cite in support of this assumption the link observed between the subjective effects of smoking a cigarette after a certain period of abstinence and a heart rate effect. But the subjective effects we observed, that we associated with a heart rate rise, were aversive effects—primarily dizziness and nausea. That doesn't necessarily mean those aversive effects are not also linked with potentially rewarding effects. We have to accept that different physiological systems, as well as behavioural systems, are subject to tolerance in different ways. The question might be, why not use, for example, peripheral vasoconstriction, which doesn't appear to be subject to acute tolerance.

Benowitz: You are right that the biggest challenge in this sort of research is to identify responses that relate to the reinforcing effects of nicotine. To my knowledge there are no studies that measure continuous variable responses to nicotine in the same way as we have measured heart rate. If we can find such responses, we will be in a much better position to clarify the differences in the extent and rate of development of tolerance in different organ systems.

Gray: Could diurnal rhythm be a confounding factor? The baseline on the heart rate graph was going down towards the end of the day in the people who didn't receive nicotine. There was a slightly smaller effect of nicotine towards the end of the day, so there could be an artifact due to a shift of the baseline from which you start or to the way the system responds later in the day rather than earlier. Could you exclude that as an alternative account?

Benowitz: There is circadian pattern in heart rate whether people are smoking or not. But the first cigarettes of the day, when the blood levels of nicotine are rising most sharply, produce a big shift in heart rate. Thereafter heart rate follows the same circadian pattern, whether a person smokes or not. If the heart rate increased in proportion to the blood nicotine concentration, one would expect the heart rate in people smoking to diverge progressively from the circadian pattern, at least for the first 6–8 hours, until plateau concentrations of nicotine in the blood are achieved. That was not the case.

Gray: I accept the point about the beginning of the day, but if tolerance were developing, I would expect to see the two curves come closer steadily over the day. What actually occurs is that the curves approach each other only as the control curve starts going down towards the end of the day, as though the system changes its reactivity at that time.

Benowitz: The explanation according to our pharmacodynamic model is that complete tolerance never develops. The response becomes attenuated to about 20% of the maximum response, then that level of response persists as steady-state blood concentrations of nicotine are maintained. Our data are consistent with the prediction that only partial tolerance to nicotine is developed.

Colquhoun: You mentioned the 1957 Katz & Thesleff desensitization scheme, but I wasn't clear how you incorporated that into your model. Where did you get the numbers for that scheme to put into your calculations? And were you using the scheme in the way in which it was originally proposed, to describe receptor desensitization, or as an empirical description of any unspecified type of tolerance?

Benowitz: No, we developed the pharmacokinetic–pharmacodynamic model first. However, mathematically our model simplifies to the same 1957 desensitization model. The data that we used to generate the parameters of our model were blood concentration of nicotine and heart rate responses over time.

Colquhoun: How are these estimated?

Benowitz: We didn't fit the receptor model, we fitted a mathematical model based on the pharmacokinetics and pharmacodynamics. We used blood levels of nicotine and heart rate values that we measured in our patients. Those data were used to generate the parameters for our model. My reference to the receptor desensitization model was just to make the point that mathematically both models reflect the same sort of process. I did not suggest that there is an actual metabolite acting as a receptor antagonist.

Colquhoun: So you took data where the blood concentration of nicotine was more or less constant and looked at the heart rate response and that essentially gave the parameters for this model? What aspect of the data would give you information on that tolerance parameter?

Benowitz: We modelled three sets of paired infusions. Information about tolerance is obtained by examining the extent of recovery of response to nicotine with different intervals separating paired infusions of the drug.

Russell: Are you concerned by the fact that your half-life for tolerance is 1/4 of the elimination half-life of nicotine in plasma? You have developed your model on the basis of the rates of regression of tolerance with three isolated injections separated by longer than smokers would normally separate their cigarettes: a 60 minute interval before the second dose, then 110 minutes before the third for maximal response. Accumulation doesn't really come into the picture in your model, whereas we know that smokers smoke more frequently and show considerable accumulation of nicotine due to the elimination half-life of two hours. I am a bit worried about your modelling from that point of view, because you are implying that tolerance is regressing while sufficient nicotine is still there to occupy the receptors.

The second aspect is that your portrayal of nicotine as a single dose from a cigarette is wrong. People take about 10 puffs from a cigarette, which are sufficiently widely spaced in time for the nicotine to have got to the brain between puffs. Rand (1989) has measured arterial levels between puffs. He shows that just after the very first puff, the arterial concentration of nicotine exceeds 100 ng/ml. Then it will go right down again until the next puff. So your model does not represent what's happening. I think it's probable that the brain equilibrates rapidly with these boli. That is why Stalhandske (1970) showed that after rapid intravenous injection the brain:blood ratio of nicotine was 5.6:1, whereas after intraperitoneal injection it was 3:1. In your model it was about 3:1.

Benowitz: I agree with your comments. I think you misunderstood the model that was used to develop tolerance. On three different days there were paired infusions at different intervals. The half-life of 35 minutes is the half-life of the tolerance effect, assuming that there is no more nicotine in the system. The tolerance half-life is a parameter that is part of the model. It implies that if there is an effect of nicotine in the brain, and there is a sudden marked drop in the concentration of nicotine, the extent of tolerance (that would occur if more nicotine were added to the system) would regress with a half-life of 35 minutes. What we believe occurs in smokers is that initially, while smoking, there are very high levels of nicotine in the brain, but consistent with the distribution half-life of 5–10 minutes, nicotine levels in the brain fall quickly after cessation of smoking.

The 35 minute half-life of tolerance regression is a measure of how long it takes for resensitization of the response system. I agree it's hard to extrapolate directly from this 35 minute estimate to the interval before a person chooses to smoke his or her next cigarette.

In answer to the question about arterial and brain concentration ratios of nicotine: the value of three for the partition coefficient that I presented represents a steady-state value. When you give a rapid injection of nicotine, as Stalhandske did, there is rapid uptake of nicotine into the brain, so in the first minutes after injection there will be a very high brain:blood ratio. That ratio declines quickly as the nicotine comes out of the brain into the blood and other body tissues.

Russell: It didn't fall off quickly, it came down at a proportionate rate; the high ratio was maintained for a full hour.

Benowitz: If that's true, it means there is some kind of avid binding of nicotine in the brain, such that nicotine is not easily released into the blood. Assuming that nicotine distribution into the brain occurs according to the law of mass action, the concentration of nicotine in the brain will be proportional to the partition coefficient and the concentration gradient of nicotine between the blood and the brain. As soon as the brain concentration exceeds that of the blood, nicotine should start coming out of the brain. If nicotine does persist at high levels in the brain, it suggests that there is very tight binding.

Rose: Your conclusion would be that in the morning hours the smokers are smoking predominantly for the positive reinforcing stimulant effects; later in the day they smoke to alleviate withdrawal. But if that's true, then a continuous all day infusion should lead to a dramatic reduction in smoking. Tolerance would develop from the infusion in the morning, which should dampen the positively reinforcing effects of smoking cigarettes. In the afternoon, the high levels would alleviate withdrawal, so why are they still smoking at 75% of their baseline levels?

Benowitz: That's an interesting question. It is constructive to compare our data on intravenous nicotine administration and cigarette smoking to those of Mike Russell. He has given subjects short-term infusions of nicotine and looked at the rise in plasma levels of nicotine after smoking a cigarette. The smokers titrated the amount of nicotine in the body very well, and did not overshoot this level of nicotine when smoking. However, with a long infusion, such as was administered to our subjects, people become totally tolerant to the effects of the infused nicotine, including the toxic effects. At this time, when tolerance is fully developed, it is not clear what motivates them to smoke.

Rose: The reinforcement derived from the local perception of nicotine or smoke in the respiratory tract, including the taste, aroma and tracheobronchial sensations, may contribute to maintenance of smoking behaviour.

Henningfield: Similar observations have been made with opioids. A study by the Addiction Research Center in the US showed that volunteers given access to hydromorphine continued to take it at high levels, even when given 100 mg methadone per day. We have also observed that people given the opportunity to take intravenous nicotine often report that during a three hour session the effects of nicotine diminished to negligible levels—yet they continued to take the injections.

Grunberg: In considering a therapeutic strategy, it seems to me that we should encourage people to smoke one cigarette first thing in the morning and then put on a nicotine patch or chew nicotine gum. To take it a step further, one could use something like the nicotine nasal spray first thing in the morning or only for the first hour, and then go to the steady-state approach.

Benowitz: Yes, that approach is logical. The concept of combining an aerosol with a transdermal nicotine preparation is being evaluated. It will be a challenge to work out the optimal dosing regimen for smoking cessation therapy.

Iversen: Do you want to replace nicotine too satisfactorily? Won't people then be dependent on the aerosol?

Rose: Wouldn't people be likely to keep using the nasal aerosol throughout the day?

Benowitz: The use of nicotine aerosols would be expected to have the same dependence liability as cigarette smoking. People might well use the aerosols throughout the day.

Schwartz: Could you devise a model for the changes in smoking habits during the day imposed by environmental restrictions? At Duke Medical Center, smoking is banned inside all of the medical school buildings and there are a large number of people who smoke only before they come to work, at lunch and when they leave. How might this change the reinforcement property and motivation over a long-term period?

Benowitz: I have no data on such changes. Dr Shiffman has been studying the 'chipper' population—people who smoke only five or less cigarettes per day (Shiffman et al 1989). Working with him we found that the levels of nicotine in the blood, after allowing for the number of cigarettes they smoke, are the same in people who smoke five a day as in those who smoke 30 a day. 'Chippers' seem to get a greater effect from each cigarette than do regular smokers, which you would expect because their cigarettes are smoked at longer intervals.

Russell: In teenagers who are just learning to smoke, and smoking 3–4 cigarettes a week, the saliva concentrations indicate that the amount of nicotine taken in per cigarette is similar to that taken in by regular smokers. So although they are smoking very infrequently, the actual kick they get from an individual cigarette is probably greater, since there is less short-term tolerance.

Collins: Neal, your results are reminiscent of some studies Ian Stolerman did 10–14 years ago where he showed that pretreatment with a low dose of nicotine caused an acute reduction in the sensitivity to a subsequent nicotine challenge. Ian was measuring a locomotor response.

We have looked at this acute desensitization phenomenon (Miner & Collins 1988, deFiebre & Collins 1988, 1989). We examined desensitization to nicotine-induced seizures. The experimental protocol was to pretreat an animal with a low dose of nicotine, then construct dose–response curves for nicotine-induced seizures. Pretreatment shifts the dose–response curve to the right. The dynamics of that process are very similar to what you have just reported; the half-life is approximately the same.

We have recently found, however, that removal of the animals adrenal gland prevents this acute behavioural desensitization. Have you looked at steroids in your subjects? Because steroids may be responsible for the desensitization that you observe.

Benowitz: We haven't looked at steroids. We plan to look at factors that influence the kinetics of tolerance, including steroid treatment.

Stolerman: I would be interested in your views on chronic tolerance to nicotine, the continuous level of tolerance that may be present in cigarette smokers. It seems to me that you are studying the superimposition (perhaps every day) of relatively short-lasting increases in tolerance of a more acute nature on this chronic tolerance. How long does this chronic tolerance last in people? In animal studies (Stolerman, this volume), we found that it could be very long lasting.

Benowitz: We've looked at what I would call intermediate tolerance. If a smoker abstains overnight or for a week, then is given an infusion of nicotine, the effects after a week of abstinence are greater than those observed after overnight abstinence (Lee et al 1987). That's not surprising because blood levels of nicotine are still 3–4 ng/ml after overnight abstinence. A regular daily smoker is never completely nicotine free, so there is always some degree of tolerance.

But the longer term tolerance, especially to some of the toxic effects like nausea, may persist for years. Many people who have given up smoking for years, then start again do not experience the same nausea that they did with their first cigarette.

Stolerman: Are those people tolerant or do they simply remember how to regulate their dose of nicotine?

Clarke: From your model could you predict, in the presence of a steady-state concentration of nicotine in the body, the relationship between the effect of nicotine and the steady-state concentration of the nicotine?

Benowitz: You could calculate it. The problem in humans is that there is a very narrow tolerable dose range for nicotine, at least in acute studies. With prolonged infusions, it may be possible to study a wider range of concentrations. For example, in our 14 hour infusion studies, the level of nicotine in the blood of our subjects could reach 30 ng/ml or more, but the subject was not able to tell whether they were receiving nicotine or saline.

Clarke: Is it possible that someone smoking, say 70 cigarettes a day, and inhaling could in fact be desensitizing 99% of their receptors, and therefore experiencing very little effect of nicotine?

Benowitz: I have wondered about that. There is a precedent with high dose methadone treatment, where you can block the euphoric effects of intravenous heroin. It is theoretically possible to get blood levels of 100 ng/ml of nicotine chronically, for example using transdermal applications.

Colquhoun: Obviously, to determine this relationship experimentally would be preferable, but surely the parameters that you have fitted to the model must imply the position of such a curve?

Benowitz: That's true. I haven't done that.

West: When smokers are trying to give up cigarettes, even those using nicotine chewing gum at quite high doses still experience withdrawal symptoms over the first week or so of abstinence. There is a clear, positive relationship between the amount of gum they use and the severity of their withdrawal symptoms (West et al 1989). The obvious explanation is that they are in some sense more dependent and therefore need more gum. But it is also clear that pretty high, relatively continuous systemic levels of nicotine do not abolish their withdrawal symptoms, and still less their craving. So we should view with caution the idea that a continuous infusion of nicotine or a continuous patch can abolish this cigarette withdrawal syndrome.

London: Would you define the withdrawal syndrome?

West: The classic features are irritability, hunger, restlessness, difficulty concentrating and mood swings.

London: Have true performance decrements been measured?

Gray: There's a large literature on the psychology of dependence which shows you can't trust reported withdrawal symptoms unless there has been a placebo control. We are doing an experiment in which we shift benzodiazepine users onto either further benzodiazepine or a placebo in a double-blind manner. So far neither we nor the patients are able to tell the difference (A. Higgett, P. Hayward, J. Wardle, personal communication). A cigarette smoker who is not smoking but is chewing gum is very sure he is not smoking cigarettes.

West: That's true, but we and others have shown relationships between plasma nicotine concentrations before giving up smoking and severity of withdrawal symptoms, taking account of things like the number of cigarettes they smoke (West & Russell 1985). These are values that the subjects wouldn't be conscious of, so I have reasonable confidence that these measures are not simply expectation effects.

Russell: It is also well established that if you randomly assign people to a placebo or a nicotine-containing gum, those who are getting the active gum experience less severe withdrawal symptoms (West 1984).

Gray: I wasn't questioning the role of the nicotine in the gum. But, when a smoker who doesn't have a cigarette in his hands claims that he has withdrawal symptoms, should that be attributed to the lack of the cigarette or to knowledge of the lack of the cigarette?

Pomerleau: I would like to address a slightly more complicated situation. Imagine two dosing methods, one producing a steady intake of nicotine and another that mimics the sharp rise of plasma nicotine concentration that occurs during cigarette smoking.

Dr Benowitz's model is really one of tolerance to the relief of withdrawal by nicotine, and it doesn't take into account the fact that smokers don't live in an environmental vacuum. If anxiety reduction is a reinforcing event, for example, then situations that enhance anxiety will make smoking under those conditions more reinforcing (see Pomerleau & Pomerleau 1984).

I think some interesting things could be tested in the Benowitz kinetic model. For example, imagine a psychologically sterile environment, in which steady-state plasma nicotine levels are sufficient to relieve withdrawal completely. If you introduced a psychological stressor, I would predict that there would be enhanced self-administration of nicotine, particularly by rapid intake methods, e.g. inhalation.

There are many complications. As Dr Rose mentioned, independently of whatever nicotine provides as a primary reinforcer, events such as upper airway irritation may act as a conditioned stimulus and/or a secondary reinforcer for smoking. This is consistent with the observation that stimulation of upper airways by smoke in the absence of nicotine reduces the desire to smoke nicotine-containing cigarettes (Rose 1988).

Grunberg: Several comments have reminded us that there are interactions between the psychological and biological cues, and others you can elicit through psychosomatic responses. However, although we have concentrated on the biology of nicotine dependence, we have mostly focused on the neurobiology of the positive reinforcing effects of nicotine. Although many of us here work exclusively at the cellular and molecular biology level, it is important that we recognize the number of levels of reinforcement for which we know there probably are no clear data on biological mechanisms.

There has been a certain assumption here that has bothered me. When, for example, Dr Clarke presents some evidence for the importance of the mesolimbic dopaminergic system, if someone in the room can cite that an antagonist for that system doesn't block the entire reinforcing effects of the drug, everybody says that cannot be the mechanism. There is no single mechanism. We know that self-administration is based on some kind of rewarding system: euphoriant effects, changes in performance, behavioural, cognitive, learning and memory. We also know that there are other effects, such as the effect of nicotine on weight control or perceived stress reduction, which contribute to the use of this drug. For each of these phenomena, some aspects may be explained partially by the mesolimbic system, or the locus ceruleus, or general sympathetic nervous system arousal. I am surprised no one has brought up the work of Hans Eysenck, which is clearly relevant here.

We also know that there are other effects: catecholaminergic, serotonergic and cortical steroids (see Collins, Pomerleau & Pomerleau, this volume). In my lab we found changes in the effect of nicotine on circulating insulin concentration (Grunberg et al 1988). We think this is very important in various reinforcing effects, both directly in the brain and indirectly through its effects on body weight regulation.

There is another side to reinforcement that only Dr Benowitz and Dr Rose have mentioned: the biology of negative reinforcement. We need to determine the mechanisms underlying this phenomenon.

We have heard about some interesting studies that suggest a biological basis for nicotine dependence. However, it is critical that we remember that a pharmacological or surgical antagonism which does not significantly alter the behaviour of dependence probably reflects the existence of multiple pathways. We should therefore be careful when proposing mechanisms for dependence and not miss the forest for the trees.

References

Collins AC, Bhat RV, Pauly JR, Marks MJ 1990 Modulation of nicotine receptors by chronic exposure to nicotinic agonists and antagonists. In: The biology of nicotine dependence. Wiley, Chichester (Ciba Found Symp 152) p 68–86

de Fiebre CM, Collins AC 1988 Decreased sensitivity to nicotine induced seizures as a consequence of nicotine pretreatment in long sleep and short sleep mice. Alcohol 5:55–61

de Fiebre CM, Collins AC 1989 Behavioral desensitization to nicotine is enhanced differentially by ethanol in long sleep and short sleep mice. Alcohol 6:45–51

Grunberg NE, Popp KA, Bowen DJ, Nespor SM, Winders SE, Eury SE 1988 Effects of chronic nicotine administration on insulin, glucose, epinephrine, and norepinephrine. Life Sci 42:161–170

Katz B, Thesleff S 1957 A study of the 'desensitization' produced by acetylcholine at the motor end-plate. J Physiol (Lond) 138:63–80

Lee BL, Benowitz NL, Jacob P III 1987 Influence of tobacco abstinence on the disposition kinetics and effects of nicotine. Clin Pharmacol Ther 41:474–479

Miner LL, Collins AC 1988 Effect of nicotine pretreatment on nicotine-induced seizures. Pharmacol Biochem Behav 29:375–380

Pomerleau OF, Pomerleau CS 1984 Neuroregulators and the reinforcement of smoking: towards a biobehavioral explanation. Neurosci Behav Rev 8:503–513

Pomerleau OF, Pomerleau CS 1990 Behavioural studies in humans: anxiety, stress and smoking. In: The biology of nicotine dependence. Wiley, Chichester (Ciba Found Symp 152) p 225–239

Rand MJ 1989 Neuropharmacological effects of nicotine in relation to cholinergic mechanisms. In: Nordberg A et al (eds) Nicotinic receptors in the CNS: their role in synaptic transmission. Progress in Brain Research, Elsevier Science Publishers, Amsterdam, vol 79:3–11

Rose JE 1988 The role of upper airway stimulation in smoking. In: Pomerleau OF, Pomerleau CS (eds) Nicotine replacement: a critical evaluation. Prog Clin Biol Res 261:95-106

Shiffman S, Fischer LB, Zettler-Segal M, Benowitz NL 1989 Nicotine exposure among non-dependent smokers. Arch Gen Psychiatry, in press? details

Stolerman IP 1990 Behavioural pharmacology of nicotine: implications for multiple brain nicotinic receptors. In: The biology of nicotine dependence. Wiley, Chichester (Ciba Found Symp 152) p 3-22

Stalhandske T 1970 Effects of increased liver metabolism of nicotine on its uptake, elimination and toxicity in mice. Acta Physiol Scand 80:222-234

West RJ 1984 Psychology and pharmacology of cigarette withdrawal. J Psychosom Res 28:379-386

West R, Russell MAH 1985 Pre-abstinence smoke intake and smoking motivation as predictors of severity of cigarette withdrawal symptoms. Psychopharmacology 87:334-336

West R, Hayek P, Belcher M 1989 Time course of cigarette withdrawal symptoms while using nicotine gum. Psychopharmacology 99:143-145

Nicotine pharmacodynamics: some unresolved issues

Robert J. West

Psychology Department, Royal Holloway and Bedford New College, London University, Egham, Surrey TW20 0EX, UK

Abstract. This paper focuses on some issues in the field of nicotine pharmaco-dynamics in which widely held suppositions have outstripped the supporting evidence. It considers how far the view that nicotine acts as a stimulant in low doses and as a sedative in higher doses is supported by the data and concludes that within the range of doses ingested by cigarette smokers, only stimulant actions have been reliably observed. It examines evidence for the view that nicotine improves ability to sustain attention and concludes that a positive effect of nicotine not attributable to relief of a withdrawal deficit has yet to be demonstrated. Finally, it considers the issue of physiological tolerance and argues that ideas concerning a role for chronic tolerance in nicotine dependence have yet to be supported empirically. Despite advances in our understanding of nicotine's effects in recent years there is still much work to be carried out before fundamental issues underlying its addictive potential can be resolved.

1990 The biology of nicotine dependence. Wiley, Chichester (Ciba Foundation Symposium 152) p 210–224

Now that there is a consensus that nicotine is addictive (US Department of Health and Human Services 1988), it is increasingly important to examine what it is about the actions of nicotine that underlies this propensity. This involves examining dose–response relationships and issues of tolerance—in other words, the pharmacodynamics of nicotine. Rather than attempt a comprehensive review of nicotine pharmacodynamics, this paper will focus on issues about which assertions and beliefs have tended to outstrip the supporting evidence. In some instances, individual studies will be selected for critical examination. The purpose is not to make light of these studies, rather to recommend caution in interpreting results which we have been too ready to accept and use as a basis for generalizations.

This paper will consider three major areas where more or less widely held beliefs about the effects of nicotine do not as yet have sound empirical backing. In all three, there are potentially important implications for the understanding of cigarette dependence. These areas are: biphasic actions of nicotine on arousal depending on dose and/or concurrent stressors; effects of nicotine on cognitive performance, and the role of chronic tolerance to nicotine in cigarette dependence.

Biphasic effects of nicotine on arousal

The simple form of the hypothesis is that low doses of nicotine stimulate and high doses sedate. This biphasic action is proposed as an explanation for smokers' reports that cigarettes can both pep them up and calm them down (Ikard & Tomkins 1973, Ashton & Golding 1989, US Department of Health and Human Services 1988). This view has followed from a range of studies in animal and human subjects examining the effects of nicotine on physiological measures of arousal. The neurochemical basis often proposed to underlie this biphasic action is the action of nicotine at neuromuscular junctions; when the nicotine molecule first hits the receptor it helps initiate muscular contraction but this is followed by prolonged paralysis possibly due to blocking of subsequent depolarization (Paton & Savini 1968). With high doses one may obtain a net effect of prolonged receptor blockade.

It has not been difficult to show effects of nicotine which may be interpreted as increased activation of the autonomic and central nervous systems or arousal. These include increases in the hormones adrenaline and cortisol as well as desynchronization of the resting electroencephalogram (EEG), increased heart rate, and decreased skin temperature resulting from peripheral vasoconstriction (e.g. Cam & Bassett 1983, Frankenhaeuser et al 1968, Golding 1988, Pickworth et al 1988). Although there has been widespread acceptance of the view that larger nicotine doses have an opposite effect, including statements to this effect in the recent US Surgeon General's report on nicotine addiction (US Department of Health and Human Services 1988), the evidence is far less convincing.

One of the studies most often cited is that of Armitage et al (1969). Second-hand reports of this study variously interpret the findings as showing that low doses of nicotine cause desynchronization of the resting EEG whereas larger doses cause increased synchronization, or alternatively that low doses desynchronize and high doses cause mixed synchronization and desynchronization effects. However, in the study concerned, the dose was not varied. In one experiment the cats were given 2 µg/kg every 30 seconds, whereas in the other they were given 4 µg/kg every minute. In neither experiment were the results subjected to statistical analysis, but the 'mixed stimulant–depressant effect' of the 4 µg/kg dosing schedule could more parsimoniously be considered 'no reliable effect'.

Recent findings have in any case thrown doubt upon the interpretation of all EEG data from smoking studies. Knott (1989) has noted that increased wakeful alertness is often associated with an increase in alpha power rather than a decrease and that when smokers are allowed to smoke their own cigarettes in a manner of their choosing, one observes increased alpha power and decreased theta and delta power. The classic desynchronization of the EEG found in earlier studies, which involved decreased alpha and increased beta, may well have been due to the use of unfamiliar cigarettes or unduly high nicotine ingestion.

Another series of studies cited as showing stimulant effects of nicotine at low doses and sedative effects at high doses is that by Ashton et al (1974, 1980). In one of these studies (Ashton et al 1974), smoking a cigarette was reportedly associated with a change in Contingent Negative Variation (CNV), a build up in electrical potential in anticipation of a stimulus to which a response is required. There was an increase in magnitude in four smokers, a decrease in seven and a 'biphasic' action in four. Although statistical analyses were reported to support the view that these effects were genuine, these involved *post hoc* examination of individual results after removal of the 'sign'. This, together with lack of adequate controls for temporal order effects, means that the findings must be treated with extreme caution. It was briefly reported that similar results were obtained on 11 of the same subjects in a second experiment but details were not given and reference was made to biphasic results within individual subjects, which may equally well be interpreted as lack of reliable results.

The doses of nicotine obtained by subjects from their cigarettes were not measured but it was argued that one possible reason for the results was a biphasic dose–response effect of nicotine. This was based on a negative correlation between extraversion and butt nicotine content and a positive correlation between the magnitude of change in CNV and extraversion.

The effect was examined more systematically in a later intravenous nicotine study (Ashton et al 1980) in which eight subjects were given a range of doses of nicotine intravenously and dose–response curves were plotted. These were interpreted as showing a biphasic relationship, but they could equally well have been interpreted as showing no relationship. A biphasic relationship would involve intermediate points on the curve being, on average, higher than the end points; this was the case in only three or possibly four of the eight subjects. Averaged data were also presented, adjusted to maximize the size of any dose–response relationship by choosing the maxima and minima for each subject. These appeared to show a biphasic effect but the *post hoc* selection of data points throws doubt on the statistical validity of the exercise. It is important to note when evaluating these findings that the dose at which the maximum stimulant effect was apparently observed was around 0.05 mg and the dose at which the greatest sedative effect was observed was 0.4 mg. Given that the average intake from a cigarette is around 1 mg, all of the doses used in the CNV studies were on the low side. It is not reported whether any or all of the subjects in the experiment were smokers and if so whether they had abstained prior to the tests. However, even if they were non-smokers, the dose creating the apparent stimulant effect would be little more than a placebo.

More recently, another theory relating to possible biphasic actions of nicotine has been proposed and gained acceptance. This is that a given dose of nicotine will stimulate in certain conditions and sedate in others. In particular, de-arousing effects of nicotine will be found when subjects are stressed. The most commonly cited study supporting this view is that by Golding & Mangan (1982). In that study smokers (degree of prior abstinence not reported) smoked a cigarette either while being subjected to loud bursts of white noise or while relaxing on a bed. It was reported that skin conductance level and skin conductance response showed stimulant effects (increased conductance) of smoking in the 'sensory isolation' condition but sedative effects (decreased conductance) in the stress condition. In fact, real and sham smoking responses did not differ significantly in the stress condition. Alpha power in the EEG was reported as being significantly decreased by real smoking compared with sham smoking under conditions of sensory isolation, reflecting greater arousal, but increased under conditions of stress. However, the difference between the alpha power during real smoking and sham smoking was not significant in the stress condition. Thus the critical test for a sedative effect did not receive statistical support. The Golding & Mangan data, while suggestive of an effect, could be interpreted in terms of a general increase in arousal caused by smoking which becomes obscured when subjects are already aroused. The difficulty in replicating effects in this area is illustrated by a recent study testing a more elaborate theory, namely that the subjective de-arousing effects of smoking are associated with a relative reduction in activation of the right hemisphere compared with the left hemisphere (Gilbert et al 1989). In that study reduction in alpha power was apparently found only in the right hemisphere during stressful episodes in a film. No effect was found on the left hemisphere, which is where Golding & Mangan (1982) had placed their electrodes.

It appears that the results of the studies most often cited in support of the biphasic action of nicotine on arousal are at best suggestive. Church (1989) in a comprehensive review of the EEG literature has also cast doubt upon the validity of claims that nicotine can have de-arousing effects on the EEG. If a dose–response relationship is to be postulated as a possible factor underlying smoking motivation and smoking dependence, large-scale, carefully controlled studies must be performed in double-blind trials with multiple doses using both smokers and non-smokers. The analysis of the data should be undertaken using predetermined routines, preferably by computer to avoid bias in interpretation, or if they are examined by eye, this should be done 'blind'. All bands within the EEG spectrum should be analysed and a more sophisticated view of arousal adopted, which would include the possibility of both arousal associated with aversive or novel stimuli, and relaxed concentration.

Before leaving the issue of sedative smoking effects, it is worth noting that reference is often made in reviews to animal studies which appear to show that high doses of nicotine have depressant effects. For example, Clarke & Kumar

(1983) showed a dose-dependent reduction in locomotor activity followed by increased activity later in the testing session. Unfortunately, whereas the original authors of these studies are careful to use terms such as 'depressant' to refer to locomotor activity, without implying anything about levels of sympathetic or cortical arousal or psychological sedation, reviews have sometimes taken the word 'depressant' out of context and taken the evidence as support for general sedative effects of nicotine. Yet clearly, locomotor activity can change for any number of reasons, for example it can decrease because of induction of nausea, fright or paralysis. In the case of high nicotine doses, it appears that the effect is characterized by a large and generalized loss of muscle tone. This contrasts with the immobility and rigidity caused by high doses of morphine.

Effect of nicotine on cognitive performance

The second issue to be addressed in this paper is that of the nature and extent of improvements in cognitive performance attributable to nicotine. It has been argued that such effects could be a major factor in why people smoke and could explain why they find it difficult to give up. Foremost among these effects is an enhanced ability to maintain attention over time. This has apparently received support from a wide range of studies in which smokers and non-smokers have variously been asked to smoke cigarettes or use nicotine tablets. The general finding appears to be that under control conditions there is a decrement over time in performance on tasks requiring continuous sustained attention, and nicotine prevents or reduces this decrement (e.g. Tong et al 1977, Wesnes & Warburton 1978).

However, a close examination of the evidence calls into question the conclusions which many now take for granted. There is little doubt that when smokers smoke cigarettes, their ability to sustain attention is better than when they abstain. There is greater doubt about to what extent this is a positive effect rather than alleviation of a withdrawal effect, and also to what extent nicotine is involved. One source often cited is that of Wesnes & Warburton (1978). In their study, subjects had to detect changes in regular movement of a hand around a kind of clock face. Unfortunately, a crucial experiment in which non-smokers were given nicotine tablets failed to show any effect. A subsequent experiment in which nicotine tablets were given to light and heavy smokers revealed a marginally significant effect of the tablets only when one subject had been eliminated on the grounds that he or she was an outlier, i.e. his/her results were different from those of other subjects. This effect of the tablets was for the combined group of heavy and light smokers, but conclusions were drawn as though the result had been observed separately for the light smokers.

Wesnes et al (1983) also reported an effect of nicotine tablets on sustained attention in the clock task described above—this effect being the same in heavy smokers, light smokers and non-smokers. Some important features of this report make it difficult to evaluate the conclusions drawn. The first is that all scores were expressed as decrements from the scores obtained during the first 20 minutes. This leaves open the possibility that baseline scores for the subjects given nicotine were worse than those for the control subjects, so that improvements over time were due to habituation to a stimulus that adversely affected performance. Secondly, if one is to claim specifically that nicotine improves performance in non-smokers, it is necessary to test positively for an effect in this group, not to rely on the absence of a significant difference between effects in groups of heavy smokers, light smokers and non-smokers. Finally, examination of the data indicates that the pattern of the dose–response relationship is irregular. For example, the expected dose-dependent effect is found only in the second of three time periods. In the first there was no difference between responses in the presence or absence of nicotine; in the third results with the 1 mg dose differed from those with the 2 mg and the placebo, which were similar.

A potentially important study following from that just discussed was carried out by Wesnes & Warburton (1984). In that study nicotine tablets of varying doses were given to non-smokers. These subjects then had to detect repetitions of digits presented one at a time over a period of 30 minutes. It was reported that there was a dose-dependent alleviation of a reduction in performance over time. Thus there was no decrement in performance when subjects were given 1.5 mg nicotine tablets, but a substantial reduction when subjects were given a placebo. As with the previous study, the fact that the results were expressed as a difference from baseline (the first 10 minutes on task) makes it impossible to know whether the result was due to a nicotine-induced temporary decrement in performance in the early part of the session. Secondly, the authors used 'hit probability' rather than stimulus sensitivity as a measure of accuracy. It is not clear whether this was attributable to a change in response bias rather than a genuine improvement in performance. Even so, the only significant difference was between subjects given 1.5 mg nicotine and the combined results from those given tablets containing 1 mg, 0.5 mg or no nicotine in the 10 minutes following the baseline period. No significant effects were observed on response times.

Despite the extremely weak nature of the findings, the above studies are frequently cited as evidence for the view that nicotine has a positive enhancing effect on sustained attention. It may turn out that such claims are accurate, but at present they go beyond the data reported in the literature. It is worth noting in relation to this that Snyder et al (1989) have reported reliable decrements in performance on a range of information processing tasks during cigarette abstinence, and that at least some of these show a return to pre-abstinence values within 10 days. This suggests that certain performance enhancements of cigarettes may turn out to be alleviation of a withdrawal effect. On the other hand, West & Hack (in preparation) have found a significant improvement in performance on the Sternberg Memory Search task in smokers who smoked a cigarette without prior abstinence. This would suggest an effect which is not subject to acute or chronic tolerance and from which one would expect no withdrawal rebound. West & Jarvis (1986) have also shown that a 2 mg nasal nicotine solution continued to improve the maximal rate of finger tapping in non-smokers with repeated doses over the course of a day, suggesting little acute tolerance to this effect. This demonstrates performance-enhancing effects of nicotine without prior deprivation and therefore can be postulated as a positive effect rather than merely relief of withdrawal.

Tolerance and nicotine dependence

Tolerance is believed to play a role in drug dependence. One view is that tolerance results in physiological changes so that the drug concerned is eventually taken primarily to stave off a highly dysphoric withdrawal syndrome. A variant on this idea is that there is neuroadaptation leading to disturbance of one or more motivation systems, so that chronic ingestion of the drug accentuates drug seeking and/or desire to use the drug, this effect being independent of other aspects of the withdrawal syndrome. Another possibility is that tolerance acts in a facilitatory manner. Thus it may selectively decrease aversive reactions to moderate or high doses of the drug, leaving users free to enjoy positive effects on which they then come to depend. In addition to the notion of acquired tolerance, there is the concept of constitutional tolerance (or its obverse, sensitivity) to one or more drug effects as a predisposing factor to the development of dependence. This has been proposed with respect to alcohol dependence and might apply to nicotine.

Tolerance to certain effects of nicotine has been carefully studied and much is known about it, most notably the influence of nicotine on heart rate. It is now well established that the increase in heart rate caused by nicotine is subject to acute tolerance, and that this does not simply reflect a ceiling effect. If one plots the hysteresis loop of the rise in heart rate during nicotine infusion and the subsequent fall in heart rate post infusion against plasma nicotine concentrations, one finds that heart rate at a particular plasma nicotine concentration on the downward part of the curve is less than on the upward part (Benowitz et al 1983). Moreover, a subsequent nicotine dose will have reduced efficacy (Porchet et al 1988). Studies have also shown that tolerance to nicotine's effect on heart rate disappears very rapidly during the first 24 hours of abstinence (e.g. West & Russell 1987), indicating that there is little residual chronic tolerance. Further to this, a recent study by West & Hack (in preparation) showed that occasional smokers showed the same profile of heart rate boost when smoking a cigarette on a normal smoking day and after 24 hours abstinence as regular daily smokers. Thus we found evidence of minimal chronic tolerance associated with regular as opposed to occasional nicotine ingestion.

Unfortunately, claims that have been made for a relationship between heart rate tolerance and psychological dependence (Hughes & Hatsukami 1986) are based on a different picture of tolerance. Hughes & Hatsukami found a negative correlation between the heart rate boost per estimated unit of nicotine intake from a cigarette smoked prior to a period of abstinence and the severity of withdrawal discomfort during that period of abstinence. Their interpretation was that withdrawal severity is associated with chronic tolerance developed over a period of months or years of use. However, as just mentioned, tolerance to the heart rate effects of nicotine are primarily acute. In a study by West & Russell (1988), the relationship between heart rate boost from a cigarette smoked after 24 hours abstinence when most or all acute tolerance would have vanished, was *positively* correlated with craving. This was contrary to what one would expect from a chronic tolerance model, but was consistent with the idea of a relationship between constitutional sensitivity to nicotine predisposing to physical dependence. These correlational data suffer from limitations in assessment of nicotine doses obtained from the cigarettes and would need to be replicated using known doses of intravenous nicotine before firmer conclusions could be drawn. In addition, it would be necessary to take into account the fact that different nicotine effects are differentially subject to tolerance. The peripheral vasoconstriction effect does not appear to be subject to tolerance at all (e.g. Benowitz et al 1983). Possibly more important from the point of view of understanding psychological dependence is tolerance to the subjective effects of nicotine. Very little systematic data have been collected to address the issue of acute and chronic tolerance to nicotine's subjective effects. A study by Jones et al (1978) is widely cited but it was not controlled. West & Russell (1988) showed that a considerable amount of tolerance to the dizziness and nausea induced by nicotine disappears after 24 hours' abstinence, suggesting that it is largely of the acute kind. What is required is a series of studies similar in design to those carried out by Benowitz and his colleagues (1983) on heart rate, but using a battery of subjective and performance measures. From the very patchy data so far obtained, it seems unlikely that a simple chronic tolerance model for causation of withdrawal symptoms such as craving will suffice. Examination of individual differences in development of pharmacokinetic tolerance and pharmacodynamic tolerance to nicotine may provide an understanding of why different smokers seek different levels of nicotine from cigarettes and why, even allowing for this, they are differentially dependent on their cigarettes.

Conclusion

It is important to reiterate a point made at the beginning of the paper, that in cases where studies have been picked out for critical examination, the purpose has not been to belittle these. Indeed, it is because they have dealt with important issues imaginatively that they have been widely cited and influential. The point of this paper has been to suggest a more conservative approach to adopting findings in reviews, even though they may appear to confirm existing beliefs.

The studies described provide an excellent beginning for more detailed examination of the issues, which will no doubt help our eventual understanding of cigarette dependence.

References

Armitage AK, Hall GH, Sellers CM 1969 Effects of nicotine on electrocortical activity and acetylcholine release from the cat cerebral cortex. Br J Pharmacol 35:152–160

Ashton H, Golding JF 1989 Smoking: motivation and models. In: Ney T, Gale A (eds) Smoking and human behaviour. Wiley, Chichester p 21–57

Ashton H, Millman JE, Telford R, Thompson JW 1974 The effects of caffeine, nitrazepam, and cigarette smoking on the contingent negative variation in man. Electroencephalogr Clin Neurophysiol 37:59–71

Ashton H, Marsh VR, Millman JE, Rawlins MD, Telford R, Thompson JW 1980 Biphasic dose-related responses of the CNV (contingent negative variation) to IV nicotine in man. Br J Clin Pharmacol 10:579–589

Benowitz NL, Peyton J, Jones R, Rosenberg J 1983 Interindividual variability in the metabolism and cardiovascular effects of nicotine in man. J Pharmacol Exp Ther 221:368–372

Cam GR, Bassett JR 1983 The effect of acute nicotine administration on plasma levels of thyroid hormones and corticosterone in the rat. Pharmacol Biochem Behav 19:559–561

Church RE 1989 Smoking and the human EEG. In: Ney T, Gale A (eds) Smoking and human behaviour. Wiley, Chichester p 115–140

Clarke PBS, Kumar R 1983 The effects of nicotine on locomotor activity in non-tolerant and tolerant rats. Br J Pharmacol 78:329–337

Frankenhaeuser M, Myrsten Waszak M, Neri A, Post B 1968 Dosage and time effects of cigarette smoking. Psychopharmacologia 13:311–319

Gilbert DG, Robinson JH, Chamberlin CL, Spielberger CD 1989 Effects of smoking/nicotine on anxiety, heart rate and lateralization of EEG during a stressful movie. Psychophysiology 26:311–320

Golding J, Mangan GL 1982 Arousing and de-arousing effects of cigarette smoking under conditions of stress and mild sensory isolation. Psychophysiology 19:449–456

Golding JF 1988 Effects of cigarette smoking on resting EEG, visual evoked potentials and photic driving. Pharmacol Biochem Behav 29:23–32

Hughes JR, Hatsukami D 1986 Signs and symptoms of tobacco withdrawal. Arch Gen Psychiatry 43:289–294

Ikard FF, Tomkins S 1973 The experience of affect as a determinant of smoking: a series of validity studies. J Abnorm Psychol 81:172–181

Jones TR, Farrell TR, Herning RI 1978 Tobacco smoking and nicotine tolerance. In: Krasnegor N (ed) Self administration of abused substances: methods for study. NIDA Monograph 20. US Department of Health and Human Services, p 202–208

Knott V 1989 A neuroelectric approach to the assessment of psychoactivity in comparative substance abuse. Paper presented to international workshop on Comparative Substance Abuse, Florence

Paton WDM, Savini EC 1968 The action of nicotine on the motor endplate in the cat. Br J Pharmacol 32:360–380

Pickworth WB, Herning RI, Henningfield JE 1988 Mecamylamine reduces some EEG effects of nicotine chewing gum in humans. Pharmacol Biochem Behav 30:149–153

Porchet HC, Benowitz NL, Sheiner LB 1988 Pharmacodynamic model of tolerance: application to nicotine. J Pharmacol Exp Ther 244:231–236

Snyder FR, Davis FC, Henningfield JE 1989 The tobacco withdrawal syndrome: performance decrements assessed on a computerised test battery. Drug Alcohol Depend 23:259-266

Tong JE, Leigh G, Campbell J, Smith D 1977 Tobacco smoking, personality and sex factors in auditory vigilance performance. Br J Psychol 68:365-370

US Department of Health and Human Services 1988 The health consequences of smoking: nicotine addiction. Report of the Surgeon General

Wesnes K, Warburton DM 1978 The effects of cigarette smoking and nicotine tablets upon human attention. In: Thornton RE (ed) Smoking behaviour: physiological and psychological influences. Churchill Livingstone, Edinburgh, p 131-147

Wesnes K, Warburton DM 1984 Effect of scopolamine and nicotine on human rapid information processing performance. Psychopharmacology 82:147-150

Wesnes K, Warburton DM, Matz B 1983 Effects of nicotine on stimulus sensitivity and response bias in a visual vigilance task. Neuropsychobiology 9:41-44

West R, Jarvis M 1986 Effects of nicotine on finger tapping rate in non-smokers. Pharmacol Biochem Behav 25:727-731

West R, Russell MAH 1987 Cardiovascular and subjective effects of smoking before and after 24 h abstinence from cigarettes. Psychopharmacology 92:118-121

West R, Russell MAH 1988 Loss of acute nicotine tolerance and severity of cigarette withdrawal. Psychopharmacology 94:563-565

West R, Hack S. Subjective and heart rate effects of cigarettes in occasional and regular smokers, in preparation

DISCUSSION

Pomerleau: You have criticized these studies on methodological grounds. Do you think there is no evidence for a biphasic effect of nicotine on behaviour or are you simply saying that the methodological basis for the studies conducted so far is inadequate and therefore it is still an open issue?

West: I think it's an open issue. It is very clear that smokers report that smoking peps them up and calms them down. It is quite possible though that the calming effects represent a relief from withdrawal. A study on school children found an interesting positive correlation between the reported calming effects of their cigarettes and the reported severity of their withdrawal symptoms when they abstained (McNeill et al 1986).

Pomerleau: I tend to be sceptical about that as the sole explanation. We observed subjective changes (reduction in anxiety and pain) after administration of nicotine under conditions in which there was no change in nicotine withdrawal symptoms (Pomerleau 1986). The problem may come from the lack of precision in measurement of subjective states.

Gray: We need to distinguish between two possibilities: 1) that nicotine improves performance because it alleviates withdrawal symptoms, and 2) that nicotine improves performance when performance is bad, and one reason the performance is bad may be that there are withdrawal symptoms getting in the way. There are two examples from our group where there cannot be withdrawal symptoms, but there are clear beneficial effects of nicotine.

One is the example where nicotine had no effect in control animals, but dramatically improved the performance of rats previously impaired by either chronic alcohol or lesions to the forebrain cholinergic projections (Hodges et al 1990). Those animals were not suffering from withdrawal from nicotine.

The second example is the work of Gemma Jones and Barbara Sahakian (Sahakian et al 1989). Using the rapid visual information processing task developed by Wesnes & Warburton (1984), we showed that doses of nicotine (0.4, 0.6 and 0.8 mg subcutaneously) that had no effect in normal elderly or young people improved performance in patients with Alzheimer's disease, particularly signal detection rather than response bias. Like our rats with lesions, these patients have a damaged cholinergic system in the brain, but they are certainly not suffering from nicotine withdrawal.

West: That's a very good point. Again, I don't want to deny the possibility that nicotine has positive enhancing effects, I think we need to make sure that the evidence is on a sound footing. It is a very important issue, that nicotine might be particularly effective in situations where for some reason there is some decrement in performance.

Henningfield: Let me take your critical evaluation of the theory that nicotine enhances cognitive function one step further. There are few data indicating that nicotine is a cognitive enhancer. We do know that performance may suffer in dependent individuals when they are deprived of tobacco, and that these defects can be reversed by administration of nicotine. I am not aware of any drugs that robustly enhance cognitive performance in healthy motivated humans.

Stolerman: There are a small number of studies in animals never previously exposed to nicotine where there is an improvement in performance that looks like enhancement of cognition. These observations cannot be explained as a reversal of an effect due to deprivation of nicotine. They are not due to the animals running around faster; there is clearly something else involved. These effects need to be analysed in more detail.

Dr Svensson showed that an arousal response related to activation of the locus ceruleus noradrenergic system came from a peripheral site of action of nicotine on a sensory receptor. As far as I am aware, the cognitive enhancement effect of nicotine has not been conclusively shown to be of central origin. There is evidence for that view but more work needs to be done.

Russell: Another problem is that most of the human studies of nicotine's effects on cognitive performance have been done in smokers after varying periods of nicotine deprivation. It is therefore not clear how much of the improvement is a primary effect of nicotine, as opposed to reversal of impairment due to nicotine withdrawal.

The number of studies that have also looked at the performance of non-smokers is relatively small. We need more studies looking at performance in non-smokers and comparing them with deprived smokers and non-deprived smokers. The few studies that have done this seem to show the smokers are similar to non-smokers when they are not deprived, and when they are deprived they are worse. There is no evidence that smokers when smoking out-perform non-smokers. This suggests that either smokers are suffering withdrawal when they are deprived or, if it is not a withdrawal effect, they are inherently poor performers and perhaps smoke to overcome this defect.

One can understand how looking for the effects of nicotine in non-smokers is a fairly rare kind of study; people are reluctant to give nicotine to non-smokers. You can't give them cigarettes to smoke, because they wouldn't get the same kind of dosage. But it would be easy to do more tests comparing deprived and non-deprived smokers with non-smokers, which would answer at least part of the question.

Gray: If you use vigilance tasks, such as the rapid visual information processing task of Wesnes & Warburton, you might find that non-smokers and smokers start out differently, even if these are potential smokers who have never smoked. Hans Eysenck (1965, 1981) established both that smokers tend to be more extrovert than non-smokers and that extroverts perform poorly relative to introverts on that kind of task. So the hypothesis that the smoker starts out with a poorer performance in certain kinds of information processing task is probably correct.

Russell: The difference in extroversion scores of smokers and non-smokers is really very small. Hans Eysenck needed huge populations to make it statistically significant. There is enormous overlap of two distribution curves along a scale of extroversion.

Rose: Presumably most of those studies look at people after they have taken up smoking. In one of the few longitudinal studies, Cherry & Kiernan (1978) looked at adolescents before they took up smoking. There were differences in both extroversion and neuroticism between those going on to be smokers and those remaining non-smokers. So it could be that smokers are self-medicating or somehow normalizing the differences due to some original impairment.

Russell: Robert West has done a study which suggests that nicotine may enhance performance of some tasks by non-smokers. He gave a nasal nicotine spray to non-smokers or very long-term ex-smokers and found a clear increase in finger-tapping performance. This effect was blocked by mecamylamine. The other interesting thing about this effect was that it didn't appear to be subject to acute desensitization.

West: We repeated doses over a day and got the same effect time and time again. I would argue that it may be the same with the Sternberg serial memory task. But it has to be remembered that the subjects of the tapping experiment were people who do occasionally take nicotine, they are not completely naive users. I think there may be some difference between totally naive users, in terms of the aversive effects of nicotine, and people who have had experience of nicotine.

Grunberg: Clark Hull (1924) published a finger-tapping study using nicotine and found exactly the same thing. However, we must dismiss that study in the present context, largely because nicotine affects motor activity. Your finger-tapping test may have been better devised than Hull's to separate the effects on motor activity and learning.

George Spilich (1987) tried to replicate David Warburton's work on human cognitive performance in smokers and non-smokers, giving nicotine or a placebo. He included simple learning and complex learning tests. This is critically important from the cognitive psychologist's point of view; we are making too much of one type of test. Spilich's data are very interesting. When he uses a simple cognitive test, similar to that used by Warburton, he observed improved performance in smokers smoking or smokers given nicotine compared to when they were not smoking, which can be interpreted either as enhancement or as alleviation of withdrawal symptoms. He also gets improved performance in the simple test in a non-smoker given nicotine. So from these tests it looks like Warburton is right.

However, when Spilich does the complex cognitive test, he gets completely the opposite. There is decreased performance with nicotine in a non-smoker, and, as Michael Russell suggests, offsetting of some of the tolerance in the smoker. So when we get into performance we have to be careful with extrapolation from animal models to humans, and we have to be careful with the type of tests used.

West: I agree; a major problem with extrapolation from animals to humans is finding comparable tasks and dose levels.

Grunberg: The animal models that are most appropriate for understanding biphasis responses may have little relevance to the range of doses of nicotine experienced by the human smoker.

West: The choice of tasks is critical. I was very impressed by a paper recently from Jack Henningfield's lab (Snyder et al 1989), in which they looked at the performance decrements during abstinence from smoking and the extent to which those could be relieved by nicotine. I think the choice of tasks there was pretty well spot on.

Gray: The correct task is not necessarily just a question of complexity. In our experiments on memory-impaired rats (Hodges et al 1990), the effect of nicotine was very clear in spatial working memory, it was moderate in non-spatial working memory, and it was not present in reference memory. Those tasks didn't differ in difficulty of original learning in that order. So it is the nature of the task that is important. Similarly, in the work Gemma Jones did on patients with Alzheimer's disease (Sahakian et al 1989), the effects found in the same patients at the same time on the rapid visual information processing were significant, but in a task of delayed matching to sample, a visual memory task, she saw no effects at all. Again, the former task was not obviously more complex than the latter. We have to do a lot of dissection of the processes at work.

Grunberg: Spilich first interpreted his results in terms of the complexity of the task. However, one could also interpret these results in terms of Hull's notion of dominant versus subordinate responses, namely that dominant responses are enhanced in particular situations. I believe that studies of nicotine and performance could profit from inclusion of paradigms that examine effects on dominant and subordinate responses, as well as complex versus simple tasks. Animal models could be used to test the effect of particular pharmacological agonists at particular regions of the brain, such as various hippocampal regions, on the performance of these tasks.

Gray: Every other cholinergic manipulation we have carried out in the animal studies in the radial-arm maze has been non-specific with respect to the type of memory affected; only nicotine had a task-specific effect.

Collins: I would like to comment on the difficulties inherent in determining biphasic drug response in heterogenous populations. Your computer-generated dose–response curves reminded me of something that was presented about 20 years ago by Jerry McClearn. Jerry is one of the pioneers in the pharmaco-genetics of alcohol. Jerry looked at different people, usually identical twins, as well as at inbred strains of mice. He found that some twins or some strains of mice show only a depressant response to alcohol over a given dose range. Some strains would show only a stimulatory response over that dose range, and other strains would show a biphasic dose–response curve. In our recent analysis of nicotine response in 19 inbred strains of mice we see the same thing for a number of responses to nicotine: some strains show only a decrease, some strains show only an increase and other strains show the biphasic response. When you average it, there is no overall effect, so we should be cautious about results from population studies.

West: But there's only one way to check that, which is to do it either in groups or in the same individual many times, and that needs to be done.

References

Cherry N, Kiernan KE 1978 A longitudinal study of smoking and personality. In: Thornton RE (ed) Smoking behaviour: physiological and psychological influences. Churchill Livingstone, Edinburgh, p 12–18

Eysenck HJ 1965 Smoking, health and personality. Weidenfeld & Nicholson, London

Eysenck HJ 1981 A model for personality. Springer-Verlag, New York

Hodges H, Allen Y, Sinden J, Lantos PL, Gray JA 1990 Cholinergic-rich transplants alleviate cognitive deficits in lesioned rats, but exacerbate response to cholinergic drugs. Prog Brain Res 82:347–358

Hull CL 1924 The influence of tobacco smoking on mental and motor efficiency. Psychological Monograph 33

McNeill A, West R, Jarvis M, Jackson P, Bryant A 1986 Cigarette withdrawal symptoms in adolescent smokers. Psychopharmacology 90:533–536

Pomerleau OF 1986 Nicotine as a psychoactive drug: anxiety and pain reduction. Psychopharmacol Bull 22:865–869

Sahakian BJ, Jones GMM, Levy R, Gray JA, Warburton DM 1989 The effects of nicotine on attention, information processing and short-term memory in patients with dementia of the Alzheimer type. Br J Psychiatry 154:797–800

Snyder FR, Davis FC, Henningfield JE 1989 The tobacco withdrawal syndrome: performance decrements assessed on a computerized test battery. Drug Alcohol Depend 23:259–266

Spilich GJ 1987 Cigarette smoking and memory: good news and bad news. Presented at the annual convention of the American Psychological Association, New York, August 29

Wesnes K, Warburton DM 1984 Effects of scopolamine and nicotine on human rapid information processing and performance. Psychopharmacology 82:147–150

Behavioural studies in humans: anxiety, stress and smoking

Ovide F. Pomerleau and Cynthia S. Pomerleau

Behavioral Medicine Program, University of Michigan Department of Psychiatry, Riverview Building, 900 Wall Street, Ann Arbor, Michigan 48105, USA

Abstract. Numerous observers have reported that smokers smoke more under stressful conditions. The most frequent explanation is that nicotine reduces anxiety, an intervening variable identified as a negative reinforcer for smoking behaviour. The conditions under which anxiety reduction occurs in response to smoking, however, have not been well defined, nor are underlying mechanisms well understood. There are several possible explanations, including Schachter's theory based on stress-induced changes in urinary pH and the hypothesis of endogenous opioid involvement. The work of Collins and his associates in animals has shown that genetic variations in corticosteroid responsiveness to nicotine are associated with differences in sensitivity to nicotine. Research in our laboratory has extended to humans Collins' findings that sensitivity to nicotine is inversely related to corticosteroid activity. We also found that the combination of a psychological stressor and smoking produced additive effects on cortisol release in humans. These findings suggest a novel way of explaining the interaction between smoking and stress, in that increased nicotine intake in the context of stress may in part reflect behavioural compensation for diminished sensitivity to nicotine when corticosteroid activity is enhanced by the stressor.

1990 The biology of nicotine dependence. Wiley, Chichester (Ciba Foundation Symposium 152) p 225–239

We have been asked to discuss behavioural studies in humans. After considering various ways in which we might narrow this broad area into a manageable topic, we have chosen to focus our attention on the problem of the modulation of anxiety by nicotine—in part because anxiety reduction is held to be a key motive for smoking and nicotine dependence, and in part because recent research in this area shows potential for extending our understanding of reinforcement mechanisms in smoking. The topic seems particularly well suited to a conference on the biology of nicotine dependence, incorporating as it does both biological and behavioural perspectives.

Anxiety reduction and stress-induced smoking

Numerous studies involving surveys and informal monitoring have indicated that smokers smoke more under stressful conditions. These retrospective and impressionistic observations have been confirmed by controlled studies (e.g. Pomerleau & Pomerleau 1987), although the phenomenon seems to depend at least in part on the nature of the stressor and on the topographic measure used as an index of smoking behaviour (see Jarvik et al 1989).

Reduction of anxiety via nicotine self-administration is the principal hypothesis offered to explain reinforcement for smoking in the context of stress. A review of studies in non-human animals using open field tests, the conditioned emotional response, shock avoidance behaviour, *etcetera*, affirms that nicotine can attenuate inferred emotional distress; however, various methodological considerations, such as differences in dosing, rate and mode of nicotine administration, schedule/paradigm used, and species, have made these results difficult to interpret or extrapolate to people (Gilbert 1979). In humans, Schachter et al (1977) reported that aversive shock thresholds increased in proportion to the nicotine content of cigarettes smoked. They speculated that this phenomenon was a manifestation of anxiety reduction caused by nicotine, but no measurements of plasma nicotine or direct assessments of change in subjective state were made. Subsequent studies have demonstrated both antinociceptive and anxiolytic effects for nicotine under controlled conditions, but difficulties in reproducing some of the effects have also been reported (see Jarvik et al 1989).

An unusual approach to the question of nicotine's anxiolytic effects in humans was recently taken by Bennett & Cherek (unpublished paper, annual meeting of the American Psychological Association, August 14, 1989). Reasoning that known anxiolytic compounds generally cause a loss of the characteristic suppression of operant responding in non-human animals when the behaviour is punished, they investigated in human subjects the effects of nicotine administration via tobacco smoke upon behaviour (bar-pressing for monetary reward) suppressed by punishment (contingent monetary loss). They found no evidence of an anti-punishment effect, but rather a nicotine dose-related decrease in punished responding that is consistent with the effects of central nervous system (CNS) stimulants.

An alternative to the anxiety-reduction hypothesis was offered by Schachter (1978), who noted that acidification of urine by a stressor increases the excretion of nicotine; the resulting nicotine withdrawal, he speculated, might be perceived as anxiety and compel replacement of nicotine by increased smoking. This explanation had a certain appeal, since it obviated the necessity of relying exclusively on an intervening variable, anxiety, that was hard to define and harder to measure. Subsequent parametric exploration involving extremes of urinary pH by Rosenberg et al (1980), however, failed to support the hypothesis.

The task of characterizing the relationship between anxiety and smoking is complicated by the possibility of individual differences in susceptibility to anxiety, which can include high trait anxiety and/or frequent exposure to anxiety-provoking situations. The strongest support for the relevance of individual differences comes from a study by Myrsten et al (1975), who selected, from a population of 90 smokers, eight smokers who indicated most unequivocally that they smoked to relieve tension and eight who indicated that they smoked to alleviate boredom or increase arousal. On a monotonous, low-arousal task, the latter group performed better and obtained more gratification from smoking, whereas on a high-arousal task, those who smoked to relieve tension performed better and obtained more gratification.

The ability of nicotine to produce both arousal and sedation poses a special challenge to research on this problem. Nicotine is generally classified pharmacologically as a CNS stimulant. As indicated by Bennett & Cherek's study, as well as the many studies showing its ability to improve various types of motor performance, nicotine's effects often resemble those of a stimulant. Its concomitant ability to produce relaxation has been sufficiently puzzling to become enshrined as 'Nesbitt's paradox' (Schachter et al 1977). The phenomenon was observed in non-human animals some time ago; for example, Silvette et al (1962) noted that lower doses of nicotine stimulated spontaneous activity in rats, whereas higher doses depressed this behaviour. Similarly, Rosecrans (1971) demonstrated that a moderate dose of nicotine produced maximal modulation, with acute administration stimulating a greater amount of spontaneous activity in low-activity rats than in high-activity rats. In humans, the biphasic response—typically involving arousal followed by sedation/calming— has been noted by numerous researchers using both objective and subjective indicators and has been shown to depend on the initial state of arousal, on dose, and, less obviously, on other factors such as degree of dependence (see Pomerleau & Pomerleau 1984).

Possible underlying biological mechanisms

In our attempt to identify underlying mechanisms in the reinforcement of smoking (Pomerleau & Pomerleau 1984), we advanced two possible explanations for nicotine's biphasic effects: (1) in low doses, nicotine from smoking may enhance arousal by stimulating cholinergic and catecholaminergic activity, whereas at higher doses the initial phase of cholinergic activation is followed by sedation or relaxation brought about by cholinergic blockade; (2) at lower doses, the cholinergic catecholaminergic response may predominate, producing arousal, but at higher doses the initial response may be superseded or swamped by a slower and longer-lasting endorphinergic response with calming, opioid-like effects. This second interpretation was suggested by the demonstration of a significant dose–response relationship between nicotine from smoking and β-endorphin in plasma (Pomerleau et al 1983). Further support was derived from a study of the effects of smoking on respiratory drive (mean inspiratory flow rate) in cigarette smokers (Tobin et al 1982); during smoking, respiratory drive was significantly higher than during the pre-smoking period but after smoking it was significantly depressed. Administration of the opioid-blocker naloxone before smoking (at a dose that did not significantly change respiratory drive) had no effect on respiratory stimulation during smoking, but blunted the depression of respiratory drive after smoking.

Attempts to define the role of nicotine-stimulated endogenous opioid activity in the reinforcement of smoking under ordinary circumstances have produced mixed results. Karras & Kane (1980) reported that administration of naloxone resulted in a significant reduction in smoking behaviour in a work setting; these findings were reproduced in the laboratory by Gorelick et al (1989). Similarly, in a preliminary study, Palmer & Berens (1983) reported that naloxone blocked subjective pleasure from smoking. On the other hand, in a parametric study in which naloxone dosage was varied systematically, Nemeth-Coslett & Griffiths (1986) were unable to demonstrate any consistent effect of naloxone on subsequent smoking behaviour or on subjective effects. None of these studies determined plasma nicotine levels, and the exact contribution of nicotine's endogenous opioid response to the reinforcement of smoking is still not known.

We have recently become interested in the possibility that corticosteroid activity may be involved in the phenomenon of increased nicotine intake in stressful situations. Adrenocorticotropic hormone (ACTH), like β-endorphin, is a hypophyseal peptide under the control of corticotropin releasing factor in the hypothalamus and is co-released with β-endorphin in response to either nicotine or stress (see Pomerleau & Pomerleau 1984). Nicotine, in a dose-related manner, has been shown to stimulate release of ACTH in an isolated perfused mouse brain preparation (Marty et al 1985) and to increase the levels of plasma ACTH and corticosterone (a mineralocorticoid with some glucocorticoid activity) *in vivo* in rats (Conte-Devolx et al 1981). In a series of studies on human cigarette smokers, we demonstrated significant, dose-related increases in circulating ACTH and cortisol following the smoking of high-nicotine cigarettes after overnight deprivation (Pomerleau et al 1983, Seyler et al 1984).

More than fifteen years ago, Hall & Morrison (1973) proposed that corticosteroid activity might be involved in mediating interactions between nicotine and anxiety, especially in the context of stress, but the mechanisms by which this might occur were unclear. A series of studies recently conducted by Collins and his colleagues has begun to characterize the nature of that relationship. Using inbred mice, a consistent strain difference in corticosterone stimulation by nicotine was demonstrated (Freund et al 1988); the effect was completely inhibited by mecamylamine, substantiating the involvement of a nicotinic cholinergic receptor. Moreover, strain-specific differences in the endogenous corticosterone response paralleled behavioural and physiological differences in sensitivity to nicotine. Thus, individual differences in responsiveness to nicotine in mice were found to be stable and genetically based.

Pauly et al (1988) conducted a series of related studies on corticosteroid modulation of physiological and behavioural sensitivity to nicotine. After adrenalectomy, though nicotinic cholinergic receptor number was unaffected and nicotine metabolism was unchanged, mice exhibited greatly enhanced sensitivity to the effects of nicotine, with significant dose-related increases in acoustic startle response and decreases in Y-maze activity, heart rate and core temperature. Administration of exogenous corticosterone restored protection from the effects of nicotine in the adrenalectomized animals; the synthetic glucocorticoid, dexamethasone, significantly reduced sensitivity only for core temperature. Administration of corticosterone to non-adrenalectomized animals decreased sensitivity to nicotine still further, strengthening the hypothesis that nicotine's own corticosteroid response (rather than ACTH changes, etc.) reduced the sensitivity of nicotine receptors. Collins and his associates (personal communication) have subsequently found that extended exposure to nicotine produces dose-related decreases in nicotine stimulation of corticosterone, indicating that the nicotinic receptor involved in corticosteroid regulation is also subject to diminution of sensitivity as a result of chronic dosing.

Effect of corticosteroids on nicotine sensitivity in humans

The findings reported by Collins and his colleagues of reduced sensitivity to nicotine under conditions of enhanced corticosteroid activity led us to wonder whether similar effects might occur in humans. De Kloet et al (1987) have observed that in primates, cortisol, an endogenous glucocorticoid, performs most of the functions that corticosterone does in rodents. We manipulated corticosteroid levels by administering dexamethasone and used magnitude of cortisol stimulation by nicotine as a marker of sensitivity to nicotine (Pomerleau & Pomerleau 1990b). We hypothesized that dexamethasone administration, by increasing overall corticosteroid activity, would dampen the cortisol response to nicotine.

In a double-blind, placebo-controlled procedure, five non-depressed (as indicated by scores of less than 19 on the Beck Depression Inventory), male, heavy smokers participated in sessions in which dexamethasone (1 mg) or placebo was administered orally at 23.00 hours the night before a session (order of conditions counterbalanced across subjects). Sessions were in the early afternoon, with *ad libitum* smoking terminated an hour before, and involved the smoking of two high (2.87 mg) nicotine research cigarettes five minutes apart followed by quiet rest. As can be seen in Fig. 1 and Table 1, there was a significant dampening of the cortisol response to nicotine following administration of dexamethasone (despite somewhat higher nicotine intake in that session), indicating diminished sensitivity to nicotine as a result of administration

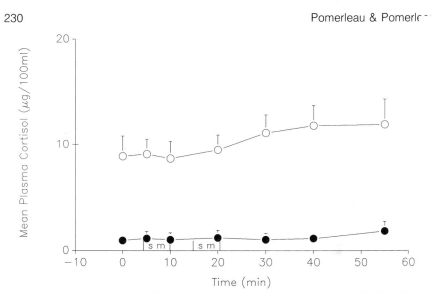

FIG. 1.   Mean plasma cortisol levels before and after smoking two high nicotine (2.9 mg) cigarettes, approximately fourteen hours after administration of placebo (○) or dexamethasone (●) (1 mg); mean ± SEM; $n = 5$. (1 µg/100 ml cortisol equals 27.59 nM.) Cigarettes were smoked in the intervals marked *sm*, i.e. 5–10 minutes and 15–20 minutes after the first measurement.

TABLE 1   Cortisol concentrations in plasma on the day following administration of placebo or dexamethasone[a]

Subject	Placebo Baseline	Placebo Peak	Change	Dexamethasone Baseline	Dexamethasone Peak	Change
1	6.5	9.7	3.2	0.0	0.0	0.0
2	16.2	19.9	3.7	2.0	4.0	2.0
3	7.3	7.4	0.1	0.6	0.7	0.1
4	7.9	14.7	6.8	0.9	4.9	4.0
5	6.5	9.9	3.4	1.3	1.1	−0.2
x̄	8.9	12.3	3.4	1.0	2.1	1.2
SEM	± 1.8	± 2.2	±1.1	±0.3	±1.0	±0.8

[a]Baseline represents plasma concentration of cortisol at the beginning of the experimental session; peak represents the maximal value attained during the session. Cortisol concentrations are given in µg/100 ml; 1 µg/100 ml equals 27.59 nM.

of a synthetic corticosteroid. There was also a trend towards a correlation ($r = 0.796$; $P = 0.053$) between cortisol increases for the dexamethasone and placebo conditions, suggesting characteristic individual differences in response to nicotine. These observations, while consistent with those of corticosteroid modulation of sensitivity to nicotine in animals by Collins and his associates, will need to be repeated in a larger sample of smokers (and non-smokers), using a variety of synthetic corticosteroids and additional physiological and behavioural measures of sensitivity.

Effects of stress and smoking on corticosteroid release

Another recent study in our laboratory (Pomerleau & Pomerleau 1990a) examined the combined effects of stress and smoking upon corticosteroid release. Morse (1989) reported that restraint (a stressor) and repeated acute nicotine dosing produce additive effects on circulating corticosterone in rabbits. We therefore hypothesized that psychological stress and nicotine administration via smoking would produce additive effects.

In a 2×2 factorial, repeated measures design, eight moderate smokers were exposed to stress and/or nicotine in four successive sessions (Latin square order). The stressor was competitive mental arithmetic (serial subtraction of 13 from a four digit starting number, performed aloud for ten minutes for a monetary bonus); the control condition consisted of reading a magazine aloud. Subjects were deprived of cigarettes for half an hour prior to the session. The nicotine condition consisted of the subject's smoking one cigarette of his usual brand (mean 1.04 ± 0.07 mg nicotine); the control condition was sham smoking ('smoking' an unlit cigarette).

There were no significant differences in plasma nicotine increase between the two nicotine conditions (i.e. smoking following mental arithmetic versus smoking following reading aloud). Subjective anxiety was significantly increased in the competitive mental arithmetic condition, confirming that the procedure was psychologically stressful. As can be seen in Fig. 2a, cortisol levels exhibited a secular downward trend during the session, which is normal for late-morning cortisol. To illustrate more clearly the effects of the experimental manipulations, the cortisol levels at each time point in the control condition (reading aloud followed by sham smoking) were subtracted from the comparable time point in each experimental condition, as shown in Fig. 2b. A statistically significant stress effect and a strong trend $(0.10 > P > 0.05)$ towards a nicotine effect on plasma concentrations of cortisol were observed; the two in combination were additive (i.e. there were no significant stress $\times$ nicotine $\times$ time interactions).

These findings suggest that the demonstration of corticosteroid modulation of sensitivity to nicotine in animals is applicable to human self-administration of nicotine via cigarette smoking and that psychological stressors exacerbate the corticosteroid response to nicotine, potentially reducing sensitivity to nicotine still further. Research that systematically examines the order and timing of nicotine administration and of various stressors, monitoring behavioural and physiological sensitivity to nicotine in response to corticosteroid activity in non-humans and humans, should make possible a more complete elucidation of these mechanisms.

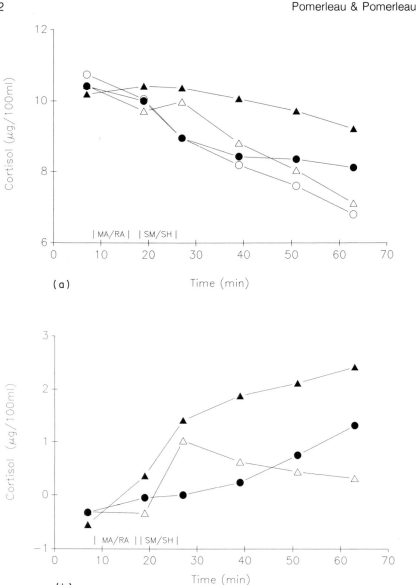

FIG. 2. (a) Plasma cortisol concentrations as a function of time for experimental conditions—mental arithmetic and smoking usual cigarette (MA/SM, ▲), reading aloud and smoking usual cigarette (RA/SM, ●), mental arithmetic and sham smoking (MA/SH, △)—and control condition—reading aloud and sham smoking (RA/SH, ○). (b) Plasma cortisol levels for each time point in the control condition (RA/SH) in (a) were subtracted from the comparable timepoint in each experimental condition to give values for the changes due to nicotine and/or stress. (1 μg/100 ml cortisol equals 27.59 nM.)

Discussion

The observation of increased smoking in the context of stress posed a difficult problem for researchers in the 1970s, because the mechanisms by which stressors could influence smoking were not obvious. Among the solutions offered was the idea that stress induced anxiety, which in turn was relieved by nicotine self-administration. But, as has been mentioned above, the conditions under which anxiety reduction from nicotine administration/smoking does or does not occur are still not well understood (see Jarvik et al 1989). On the one hand, the idea that nicotine-stimulated corticosteroid mechanisms might play a role in the reduction of anxiety is supported by demonstrations that corticosteroids decrease central nervous system excitability by modulating the activity of the γ-aminobutyric acid/benzodiazepine receptor complex (Majewska et al 1986). On the other hand, as a reinforcer for smoking, anxiety reduction following nicotine self-administration in the context of stress may simply be an epiphenomenon, an effect that is frequently associated with but not critical for the maintenance of the behaviour.

The question of endogenous opioid involvement in the reinforcement of smoking behaviour remains open. Research on nicotinic cholinergic modulation of endogenous opioid release has yet to produce findings of sufficient magnitude or consistency to explain stress-induced smoking or anxiety reduction following ordinary smoking. However, the demonstration by Badawy et al (1981) that naloxone restores the corticosteroid response to nicotine after complete adaptation to chronic nicotine administration does indicate that nicotine-stimulated opioid activity may modulate the corticosteroid response to nicotine.

Although the research on corticosteroids described above is still preliminary, we believe that it shows potential for increasing our understanding of various smoking-related phenomena. For example, Collins and his associates have demonstrated that variations in corticosteroid responsiveness are associated with differential nicotine sensitivity, possibly accounting for individual differences that could contribute to susceptibility to reinforcement by nicotine. Finally, the demonstration that nicotine and/or stress cause corticosteroid release provides a novel way of explaining interactions between smoking and stress, for it suggests that increased nicotine intake during exposure to a stressor may represent, at least in part, behavioural compensation for diminished sensitivity to nicotine.

Acknowledgements

Preparation of this chapter was facilitated by a grant from the United States National Cancer Institute (CA 42730). We thank Allan Collins and his co-workers for sharing unpublished findings with us.

References

Badawy AAB, Evans M, Punjani NF 1981 Reversal by naloxone of the effects of chronic administration of drugs of dependence on rat liver and brain tryptophan metabolism. Br J Pharmacol 74:489–494

Conte-Devolx B, Oliver C, Giraud P et al 1981 Effect of nicotine on *in vivo* secretion of melanocorticotropic hormones in the rat. Life Sci 28:1067–1073

De Kloet ER, Ratka A, Reul JM, Sutanto W, Van Eekelen JAM 1987 Corticosteroid receptor types in brain: regulation and putative function. In: Ganong WF et al (eds) The hypothalamic-pituitary-adrenal axis revisted. New York Academy of Sciences, New York, p 351–361

Freund RK, Martin BJ, Jungschaffer DA, Ullman EA, Collins AC 1988 Genetic differences in plasma corticosterone levels in response to nicotine injection. Pharmacol Biochem Behav 30:1059–1064

Gilbert DG 1979 Paradoxical tranquilizing and emotion-reducing effects of nicotine. Psychol Bull 86:643–661

Gorelick DA, Rose JE, Jarvik ME 1989 Effect of naloxone on cigarette smoking. J Subst Abuse 1:153–159

Hall GH, Morrison CF 1973 New evidence for a relationship between tobacco smoking, nicotine dependence and stress. Nature (Lond) 243:199–201

Jarvik ME, Caskey NH, Rose JE, Herskovic JE, Sadeghpour M 1989 Anxiolytic effects of smoking associated with four stressors. Addict Behav 14:379–386

Karras A, Kane JM 1980 Naloxone reduces cigarette smoking. Life Sci 27:1441–1445

Majewska MD, Harrison NL, Schwartz RD, Barker JL, Paul SM 1986 Steroid hormone metabolites are barbiturate-like modulators of the GABA receptor. Science (Wash DC) 32:1004–1007

Marty MY, Erwin VG, Cornell K, Zgombick JM 1985 Effects of nicotine on beta-endorphin, alpha-MSH, and ACTH secretion by isolated perfused mouse brains and pituitary glands, *in vitro*. Pharmacol Biochem Behav 22:317–325

Morse DE 1989 Neuroendocrine response to nicotine and stress: enhancement of peripheral stress responses by the administration of nicotine. Psychopharmacology 98:539–543

Myrsten AL, Andersson K, Frankenhauser M, Elgerot A 1975 Immediate effects of cigarette smoking as related to different smoking habits. Percept Mot Skills 40:515–523

Nemeth-Coslett R, Griffiths RR 1986 Naloxone does not affect cigarette smoking. Psychopharmacology 89:261–264

Palmer RF, Berens A 1983 Double blind study of the effects of naloxone on the pleasure of cigarette smoking (abstract). Fed Proc 42:654

Pauly JR, Ullman EA, Collins AC 1988 Adrenocortical hormone regulation of nicotine sensitivity in mice. Physiol Behavior 44:109–116

Pomerleau CS, Pomerleau OF 1987 The effects of a psychological stressor on cigarette smoking and subsequent behavioral and physiological responses. Psychophysiology 24:278–285

Pomerleau OF, Pomerleau CS 1984 Neuroregulators and the reinforcement of smoking: towards a biobehavioral explanation. Neurosci Biobehav Rev 8:503–513

Pomerleau OF, Pomerleau CS 1990a Cortisol response to a psychological stressor and/or nicotine. Pharmacol Biochem Behav, in press

Pomerleau OF, Pomerleau CS 1990b Dexamethasone attenuation of the cortisol response to nicotine in smokers. Psychopharmacology, in press

Pomerleau OF, Fertig JB, Seyler LE, Jaffe J 1983 Neuroendocrine reactivity to nicotine in smokers. Psychopharmacology 81:61–67

Rosecrans JA 1971 Effects of nicotine on behavioral arousal and brain 5-hydroxy-tryptamine function in female rats selected for differences in activity. Eur J Pharmacol 14:29–37

Rosenberg J, Benowitz NL, Jacob D, Wilson KM 1980 Disposition kinetics and effects of intravenous nicotine. Clin Pharmacol Ther 28:517–522

Russell MAH 1988 Nicotine replacement: the role of blood nicotine levels, their rate of change, and nicotine tolerance. In: Pomerleau OF, Pomerleau CS (eds) Nicotine replacement: a critical evaluation. Alan R Liss, New York, p 63–94

Schachter S 1978 Pharmacological and psychological determinants of smoking. Ann Intern Med 88:104–114

Schachter S, Silverstein B, Kozlowski LT, Perlick D, Herman CP, Liebling B 1977 Studies of the interaction of psychological and pharmacological determinants of smoking. J Exp Psychol 106:3–40

Seyler LE, Fertig JB, Pomerleau OF, Hunt D, Parker K 1984 The effects of smoking on ACTH and cortisol secretion. Life Sci 34:57–65

Silvette H, Hoff EC, Larson PS, Haag HB 1962 The actions of nicotine on central nervous system functions. Pharmacol Rev 14:137–143

Tobin MJ, Jenouri G, Sackner MA 1982 Effects of naloxone on change in breathing pattern with smoking. Chest 82:530–537

DISCUSSION

Henningfield: Has nicotine been compared directly against benzodiazepines in animal models that are standard for evaluating anxiety-avoiding paradigms?

Stolerman: In the classical animal models for anxiety that are very selective for benzodiazepine-like effects, such as punished behaviour in rats, nicotine is inactive. These models are also insensitive to the newer non-benzodiazepine anxiolytic drugs. In some animal models that are sensitive to benzodiazepines but in addition show sensitivity to drugs such as buspirone and ondansetron, nicotine seems to have some efficacy (e.g. Costall et al 1989). However, these models are not so well established and some of them are rather less specific. One exception may be punished behaviour in pigeons (Barrett et al 1986). In this model, nicotine can increase rates of punished responding to 1.5–2.0 times control rates at doses (0.01–0.1 mg/kg) that slightly reduce rates of unpunished responding (J. E. Barrett, personal communication). This effect is qualitatively similar to the effects of many anxiolytic drugs, but considerably smaller in magnitude. However, none of the animal results of which I am aware support the view that nicotine has sedative effects.

Gray: I agree, I know of no reliable evidence from the animal behavioural literature that nicotine could be regarded as an anxiolytic. It may have certain effects in certain tests which look like that, but that would probably be true for any compound. From the overall pattern of effects, I would regard the case for nicotine being an anxiolytic as almost zero. Similarly, I don't think it is an anxiogenic. There was a report by Haroutunian et al (1985), which we replicated, that if you give nicotine after the shock in an avoidance task, you increase the consolidation of the memory of the shock (S. Smith, J. Sinden, personal communication). But one would need a whole pattern of such findings before concluding that nicotine increases anxiety.

Steinbach: We tested the effects of several days exposure to dexamethasone on nicotinic sensitivity of PC12 cells (Ifune & Steinbach 1989). Culturing cells in the presence of 1 μM dexamethasone alone does not enhance or diminish nicotinic responses. However, nicotine blocks the ability of nerve growth factor (NGF) to enhance nicotinic sensitivity. The sensitivity to ACh was assayed after dexamethasone had been washed from the medium; the cells had been exposed to dexamethasone or dexamethasone plus NGF for approximately one week. So it appears that dexamethasone at a micromolar concentration has some effect on expression of functional neuronal nicotinic receptors. We don't know whether receptor number is reduced but there is much less response.

Kellar: Is this due to decreased protein synthesis?

Steinbach: Our control was to look for an increase in Na^+ current density. Dexamethasone had no effect on the ability of NGF to increase Na^+ currents but it completely occluded the ability of NGF to increase nicotinic responsiveness. The cells grew the stubby processes that they grow in the presence of dexamethasone and at least one physiological response was completely normal.

Benowitz: Dr Pomerleau, concerning the cortisol response that you see, an increase of 2 μg/100 ml is very small, smaller than the decrement due to the circadian rhythm.

Pomerleau: We are using a rather crude measure. We are looking at hormones in circulation, which presumably are reaching target receptors, but we don't really know the effect on the target receptor in the context of stress. The response was consistent, but we simply can't say what is a large and what is a small effect at this time.

Benowitz: I am bothered by the dexamethasone paradigm when you are looking at cortisol responses. Dexamethasone will suppress ACTH-mediated cortisol responses in general. Cortisol is not the best measure of response because there is a competition between the suppressing effects of dexamethasone and the stimulating effect of nicotine. Would you expect stimulation of cortisol release by any stimulus in the presence of dexamethasone?

Pomerleau: Stimulation by nicotine might occur through steroidogenesis (Rubin & Warner 1975), independently of suppression of ACTH/cortisol by dexamethasone. I would not have presented these data had not Dr Collins' group developed an animal model that explained these effects more systematically. Dr Collins used adrenalectomized mice and, despite the fact that ACTH levels are sharply increased in these animals, the sensitivity to nicotine in several response systems was inversely related to corticosteroid activity.

Collins: Our results were both very reliable and genotype dependent. Some mouse strains show a profound effect, other mouse strains show effects on some responses and other mouse strains will show no effect. That might explain why $P = 0.053$ in a sample of only five subjects. There is probably variability in terms of responders and non-responders within the human population.

Balfour: I am a little concerned about using corticosterone as a measure of stress. There is no doubt that plasma concentrations of corticosterone go up when animals or humans are stressed. They are also increased in response to many other stimuli. We find that in rats trained to run through mazes, the corticosterone levels can remain relatively high, even when the test is repeated for 25 days (Copland & Balfour 1987). We regard plasma corticosterone more as a measure of arousal than as a measure of stress *per se*. Stress is an arousing stimulus and an increased arousal is one of the ways in which animals or people cope with stressful stimuli.

As far as I know, there is only one fairly weak piece of evidence that corticosterone or cortisol given systemically to animals is anxiolytic (File et al 1979). If it has been converted to something which stimulates GABA transmission, one would expect it to mimic the actions of the benzodiazepines and it doesn't do this.

Pomerleau: I am aware of that. I cited the study by Majewska et al (1986) because I thought it was suggestive and might be worth pursuing. It is possible that as a reinforcer for smoking, anxiety reduction may simply be an epiphenomenon, a non-essential correlate of a more fundamental process.

Schwartz: In collaboration with Dr Maria Majewska, we showed that some of the metabolites of other steroids, dihydroprogesterone and deoxycorticosterone, which are present in brain, have profound effects on GABAergic transmission, both to increase and to decrease. They act more like endogenous barbiturates—anxiolytics or convulsants. That may be independent from what's happening in the periphery.

Grunberg: In my laboratory David Morse (1989) used a rabbit infusion nicotine model similar to Dr Collins' mouse model. He examined similar questions regarding potential biochemical mediators of stress responses. Morse found that a stress stimulus plus nicotine caused greater catecholaminergic and cholinergic effects than did each stimulus alone. This finding is relevant to the anxiolytic effect of nicotine being postulated as a modulation of the relationship between stress and smoking.

Susan Winders in collaboration with Neal Benowitz's lab has used a rat model with chronic infusion of nicotine at various dosages followed by applied stressors. She found that the presentation of the stressor, a rubber band on the leg, in animals exposed for two weeks to continuous nicotine administration resulted in a significant decrease in blood levels of nicotine and a significant decrease in brain levels of nicotine. In the interaction between stress and nicotine, there appear to be multiple mechanisms. The work of Dr Collins and Dr Pomerleau on modification of the nicotinic response by corticosteroids is very interesting, but we are also finding that under stress there is a decrease in the availability of the drug.

Gray: Whatever happened to Stanley Schacter's lovely experiments showing that the increased rate of smoking reported by people when they are anxious can be eliminated if you load them with alkali, affecting the excretion of the nicotine (Schachter et al 1977)?

Grunberg: Latiff et al (1980) tried to develop an animal model based on Schachter's findings. They used a rat self-administration model; there was self-administration of nicotine under different urinary pH conditions, which they then manipulated. When they acidified the urine, there was greater self-administration than under alkaline pH. However, when they did the cross-over design, changing the order of the manipulations, they got a partial replication of Schachter's results, but mostly they showed that behaviour, once established, is not easily changed in a self-administration paradigm. So it ended up being completely controversial.

We used a paradigm from Ian Stolerman's work, in squirrel monkeys (Grunberg et al 1983). We looked at intramuscular injections of nicotine under conditions in which we manipulated the pH of body fluids by intragastric administration of alkali. We found that if we acidified the body fluids then looked at the effect of nicotine on the animal's behaviour in a stimulus shock termination paradigm, we got changes consistent with those seen by Schachter. From that we speculated that what we were getting was not increased urinary excretion of nicotine, but changed transport from blood to brain and changed binding affinity (Grunberg et al 1983, Grunberg & Kozlowski 1986). In the light of recent results, that becomes a testable hypothesis.

Gray: But in humans, does Schachter's finding that the increased smoking seen under stress can be blocked just by changing urinary pH still hold?

Benowitz: Urinary pH is not the right link. Only a very small amount of nicotine is renally excreted. With extreme acidification of urinary pH you can increase excretion to as much as 30% of the total intake of nicotine (Benowitz & Jacob 1985). The stress-induced changes that Schacter described would be expected to change the renal excretion by only a few per cent of the total dose. As Neil Grunberg said, if you systemically acidify or alkalinize the blood, you can change the distribution of nicotine in the body, and that is likely to be the pharmacological link between pH and behaviour.

Gray: Either way, it remains the case that one of the planks for the story that nicotine is an anxiolytic, namely that people smoke more when they are subject to stress, is a weak plank.

Collins: I would argue that the reason people smoke more when they are under stress is because the steroid is blocking the receptor.

Gray: But as far as the story that nicotine is an anxiolytic is concerned, there is still no evidence that people smoke more when they are anxious.

References

Barrett JE, Witkin JM, Mansbach RS, Skolnick P, Weissman BA 1986 Behavioral studies with anxiolytic drugs. III. Antipunishment actions of buspirone in the pigeon do not involve benzodiazepine receptor mechanisms. J Pharmacol Exp Ther 238:1009–1013

Benowitz NL, Jacob PJ 1985 Nicotine renal excretion rate influences nicotine intake during cigarette smoking. J Pharmacol Exp Ther 234:153–155

Copland AM, Balfour DJK 1987 Spontaneous activity and brain 5-hydroxyindole levels measured in rats tested in two designs of elevated X-maze. Life Sci 41:57–64

Costall B, Kelly E, Naylor RJ, Onaivi ES 1989 The actions of nicotine and cocaine in a mouse model of anxiety. Pharmacol Biochem Behav 33:197–203

File SE, Vellucci SV, Wendlandt S 1979 Corticosterone—an anxiogenic or anxiolytic agent. J Pharm Pharmacol 31:300–305

Grunberg NE, Kozlowski LT 1986 Alkaline therapy as an adjunct to smoking cessation programs. Int J Biosocial Res 8:43–52

Grunberg NE, Morse DE, Barrett JE 1983 Effects of urinary pH on the behavioral responses of squirrel monkeys to nicotine. Pharmacol Biochem Behav 19:553–557

Haroutunian V, Barnes E, Davis KL 1985 Cholinergic modulation of memory in rats. Psychopharmacology 87:266–271

Ifune CK, Steinbach JH 1989 Regulation of sodium currents and acetylcholine responses in PC12 cells. Brain Res 506:243–248

Latiff AA, Smith LA, Lang WJ 1980 Effects of changing dosage and urinary pH in rats self-administering nicotine on a food delivery schedule. Pharmacol Biochem Behav 13:209–213

Majewska MD, Harrison NL, Schwartz RD, Barker JL, Paul SM 1986 Steroid hormone metabolites are barbiturate-like modulators of the GABA receptor. Science (Wash DC) 232:1004–1007

Morse D 1989 Neuroendocrine responses to nicotine and stress: enhancement of peripheral stress responses by the administration of nicotine. Psychopharmacology 98:539–543

Rubin RP, Warner W 1975 Nicotine induced stimulation of steroidogenesis in adreno-cortical cells in the cat. Br J Pharmacol 53:357–362

Schachter S, Silverstein B, Kozlowski LT, Perlick D, Herman CP, Liebling B 1977 Studies of the interaction of psychological and pharmacological determinants of smoking. J Exp Psychol (Gen) 106:3–40

Final discussion

Withdrawal syndrome

Collins: The scientific community has developed a considerable data base regarding the acute effects of nicotine as well as development of tolerance. But most people who have dealt with the dependence issue would argue that dependence involves more than a changed sensitivity to nicotine. In particular, for many drugs there's the issue of withdrawal syndrome. The animal studies of nicotine action have provided little evidence for nicotine withdrawal symptoms. This is reminiscent of the situation in humans 10 or 12 years ago, when there was a great deal of debate as to whether or not tobacco was addictive; it wasn't well established whether there was a withdrawal syndrome.

We have some preliminary data which indicate that we can demonstrate a withdrawal syndrome for nicotine in laboratory animals. We have been using minimitters (developed by Minimitters Inc in Oregon in the United States). The minimitter is a small radiotransmitter which sends out pulses that are directly proportional to the animal's temperature. It can also be used to measure EEG or heart rate .or locomotor activity. You put the minimitter in animals in individual cages. The radiotransmitter has receivers that track the movements of the animal. You can also get lick counters to look at drug self-administration by oral intake.

In one strain of mouse, we assessed the effects of chronic nicotine infusion on body temperature and mean activity during the day. The animals were infused for seven days with saline, then with 2 mg/kg per hour nicotine. The body temperature went down over a couple of days, then the animals developed tolerance to this effect. We increased the dose to 4 mg/kg per hour and the body temperature went down and once again the animals developed tolerance. After withdrawal of the nicotine, there was short-term hypothermia followed by a hyperthermia that lasted about four days. Locomotor activity in the home cage was depressed during nicotine infusion. We recorded activity continuously for 12 days after the infusion was stopped. After withdrawal there was an initial depression of activity but about a week later there was an explosive increase in locomotor activity. These animals are hyperactive and very aggressive.

We also looked at oral intake of nicotine. We presented the animals with a choice between a solution containing 1% saccharin or one containing nicotine plus saccharin. We then infused with 4 mg/kg per hour nicotine for seven days, took them off the infusion and continued to look at nicotine intake. After cessation of nicotine infusion, the animals showed a profound increase in oral

240

intake of nicotine. I don't know if I believe our own data—there were 12 animals—but it looks like we get a withdrawal syndrome. Furthermore, if we chronically treat the animals with the drug we can get them to increase their oral intake of nicotine.

West: There are two important points to make in relation to tobacco withdrawal syndrome. It is clearly established that there is such a syndrome in human beings and it is related to nicotine. The other point is that there is a great deal of doubt about the extent to which the withdrawal syndrome itself is the factor which mediates dependence. A number of people have tried prospectively to look at the association between the severity of the withdrawal during the acute abstinence phase and the extent to which they subsequently stay off cigarettes. It has been very difficult to show a relationship. We have found a very weak relationship, and it relates specifically to an increase in depression and to craving (West et al 1990). For other withdrawal symptoms, e.g. instability, we were unable to show any relationship at all. So the significance of withdrawal syndrome for dependence in its broader sense I think is questionable.

Gray: What are the key symptoms of the human withdrawal syndrome?

West: Irritability, restlessness, difficulty concentrating, hunger; I also include craving because I believe, and there is evidence to support the view, that craving is not simply a desire for something in the same way that you desire chocolate or television; there is evidence that it is specifically linked to loss of nicotine.

Collins: In our animal model, the animals have a 50% increase in their food intake.

Gray: But your withdrawal syndrome is over in a couple of weeks; what's the human time span?

West: Similar, except for hunger, which persists.

Grunberg: In the biology of nicotine dependence, it is critical to understand the withdrawal phenomenon. 10 years ago we began studying the effects of nicotine cessation and smoking cessation. We found parallel results in humans and animals (Grunberg 1986a,b). We went on to look at various biochemical changes. We found an inverse dose–response relationship between chronic nicotine administration in animals using a minipump and plasma levels of insulin (Grunberg et al 1988).

In that same study, we looked at catecholamines, corticosteroids and glucose, building on the work of Dr Fuxe and Dr Svensson. In our chronic continuous infusion model, nicotine increased the levels of these biochemicals, but these effects adapted over a few days. In contrast, and this surprised us, the decrease in plasma insulin caused by nicotine became more pronounced with time, becoming highly significant and most marked after two weeks of chronic administration. After cessation of nicotine, we saw increases in body weight and in specific food consumption. However, there are a few caveats. We have followed this for several months after cessation. In those models we are getting several effects consistent with Allan Collins' and some additional ones. In rats, chronic nicotine administration for two weeks enhances physical activity. This is using doses relevant to the human smoker. There is a sex difference: we get an increase in males but not in females. After cessation of nicotine there are significant decreases in locomotor activity in males but not in females.

In terms of eating behaviour, we get decreased body weight during nicotine administration, increased body weight after. There is a decrease during nicotine administration in intake of sweet tasting and high carbohydrate foods and an increase after. In the males it is only the sweets and carbohydrates. In females there is increased intake of all foods after nicotine cessation. With insulin we are seeing the decrease during and an increase after cessation of nicotine. The time course is interesting, it takes a few days to develop.

We have extended these studies to the brain. Preliminary results indicate that the effect of nicotine on hypothalamic insulin is the opposite of its effect on plasma insulin.

Balfour: Some years ago we showed that the chronic administration of nicotine to rats evoked regionally selective reductions in the concentration and bio-synthesis of serotonin in the hippocampus (Benwell & Balfour 1979a, 1982). More recently we have investigated the changes in brain serotonin levels in tissue, taken at post-mortem, from subjects who were tobacco smokers and whose smoking habits could be clearly established from their clinical notes. None of the subjects selected had shown any signs of neurological or psychiatric disease. We compared the 5-hydroxytryptamine (5HT) levels in these subjects with those measured in tissue taken from a group of age and sex-matched non-smokers. The results showed that smoking was associated with reductions in 5HT and 5-hydroxyindoleacetic acid (5HIAA) in two areas of the hippocampus, the hippocampal neocortex and the hippocampal formation. No significant changes were observed in the gyrus rectus, cerebellum or medulla oblongata. In the median raphe nuclei, however, an area of the brain which provides a significant serotonergic innervation to the hippocampus, a small, but significant, reduction in the concentration of 5HIAA was observed.

In addition to the reductions in 5HT and 5HIAA, the density of $5HT_{IA}$ receptors in the hippocampus was found to be increased in the tissue taken from the subjects who had smoked. No changes in the density of these receptors was observed in the other brain areas studied. We believe that the regionally selective changes in the concentrations of 5HT and 5HIAA and in the density of the $5HT_{IA}$ receptors in the hippocampus are consistent with the hypothesis that tobacco smoking reduces 5HT secretion in this area of the brain. We were able to establish that all the subjects who had been tobacco smokers had smoked regularly up to within 48 hours of death. Nevertheless, a majority of these subjects had not smoked for some hours prior to death and, therefore, it could be argued that the measurements were made in nicotine-withdrawn subjects. However, in the studies with rats (Benwell & Balfour 1979a, 1982), reduced levels of 5HT and 5HIAA were found in both nicotine-treated and nicotine-withdrawn animals, which suggests that the reductions in the levels and biosynthesis of 5HT are evoked by exposure to nicotine and that they persist for many hours following withdrawal of the drug. In addition, since the results suggest that the regionally selective changes in 5HT which we found in the hippocampus of rats given daily injections of nicotine also occur in the brains of humans who habitually smoke tobacco, they provide some support for the hypothesis that the effects of the drug on this system may be relevant to its role in the tobacco smoking habit.

Professor Gray has already told us that nicotine does not appear to exert any direct effects on 5HT secretion in the hippocampus. We have also failed to find any direct effects of nicotine on 5HT secretion in this area of the brain. We currently believe that the effects of nicotine on this system are probably indirect and reflect an adaptation to its effects on other systems rather than a direct action on the serotonergic neurons which innervate the hippocampus.

In this context it is interesting that corticosterone can also evoke regionally selective changes in hippocampal 5HT. In rats, if the plasma corticosterone concentration is reduced by pretreatment with betamethasone, reductions in hippocampal 5HT and 5HIAA, similar to those found in animals given chronic nicotine, are seen (Benwell & Balfour 1979b). Thus, nicotine appears to alter the concentration of 5HT in the hippocampus in a way which is equivalent to removing the corticosterone from the plasma and, presumably, the brain. The psychopharmacological consequences of this effect remain to be established, although 5HT probably exerts a tonic influence on the responsiveness of hippocampal cells to other neurotransmitters and this aspect of hippocampal function is altered by chronic exposure to nicotine.

Grunberg: With regard to nicotine, and probably other drugs, there appears to be a qualitative difference between a short-term withdrawal and a more protracted withdrawal. That is interesting, because, as Dr West said, irritability and other withdrawal symptoms are relatively short-term, lasting days or weeks. But the altered eating behaviour, the body weight changes, and perhaps sleep disturbance, may last longer after nicotine cessation.

This is an interesting puzzle in terms of pharmacokinetics. The pharmacokinetics may help explain the short-term withdrawal, but a simple presence or absence of nicotine does not explain the protracted withdrawal symptoms. We are therefore interested in whether or not there is a permanent change, or at least a very long-term change, in some aspects of neuronal non-responsivity and receptors, with respect to nicotine and perhaps other drugs. If there is, that may be relevant for prevention or treatment. There may be permanent brain changes in receptors, as Dr Heinemann suggested.

Heinemann: I am suggesting that drug addiction could involve long-term changes in the efficiency of synapses, brought about by exposure to the drug. These drug-induced changes might involve the same mechanisms that occur during the phenomenon of long-term potentiation, which is thought to play a role in the early events of memory acquisition. These changes can be very long lasting, perhaps even permanent.

Collins: I can comment on the relationship between behaviour and the return to control levels of brain nicotinic receptors, as measured by [^{3}H]nicotine and bungarotoxin binding. There is no relationship for bungarotoxin binding, but the depressed behaviour, the return to baseline by 8–10 days after withdrawal of nicotine, pretty much parallels what we saw in terms of the rate of return of [^{3}H]nicotine binding to control (Marks et al 1985). The hyperactivity that we see after that time can't be readily explained by alterations in the number or affinity of receptors. If it has anything to do with nicotinic receptors at all, it might be the sort of thing that Steve Heinemann was talking about—an altered functional status of the receptors.

Heinemann: This has been studied most in the glutamate system in terms of long-term potentiation. There were some reports that it was due to a change in the number of receptors on the basis of binding studies. These initial conclusions are now thought to be incorrect. One has to be very careful with binding studies; we need much more specific probes.

Henningfield: It seems that there is a risk in attempting to develop a sophisticated neuropharmacological explanation of behavioural consequences of nicotine administration and withdrawal. The risk is that the behavioural phenomena themselves are often poorly documented. For example, elaborate explanations for nicotine's anxiolytic and cognitive enhancing effects may be based on the assumption that nicotine is more effective in these areas than has been demonstrated.

Collins: That was my point: we have to do more behavioural work in animals before we start trying to equate withdrawal symptoms in animals with the human withdrawal phenomena.

Possible pharmacological therapies for nicotine dependence

Iversen: The discovery that the nicotinic receptors in the brain are radically different in their pharmacology from those in the periphery seems to me a major advance in this field. However, it is not clear which centrally acting nicotinic antagonist is most suitable for use in animal studies. Should mecamylamine continue to be used?

Kellar: Dihydro-β-erythroidine is another nicotinic antagonist that has been used a little. It may have more competitive properties than mecamylamine. The problem is one of availability; it is supplied by Merck, but at the moment there is not great demand for it and it is scarce.

Clarke: I think it may be useful, but I am not sure how well it penetrates the brain if given systemically. It is competitive in that it inhibits [^{3}H]nicotine binding. Interestingly, in the literature on electrophysiology, whereas mecamyl-amine has been shown to block the effects of iontophoresed excitatory amino acids, in addition to the effects of nicotine, dihydro-β-erythroidine, at least in a couple of studies where this has been tested, has not blocked the excitatory amino acid response. That may suggest that it acts at the agonist binding site, and so it may be more selective for the nicotine response.

Schwartz: Did they do dose–response curves?

Clarke: No.

Gray: If it doesn't cross the blood:brain barrier, it is going to be hard to use in behavioural studies.

Stolerman: I think dihydro-β-erythroidine may be interesting for a different reason. We injected it into the lateral ventricles of rats and tested responses to nicotine in the drug discrimination procedure. We failed to get any blocking effect, however high we pushed the dose of dihydro-β- erythroidine. We went up to the threshold dose for convulsions and then we stopped. This compound does not block all central effects of nicotine.

Changeux: Catherine Vidal in my laboratory has shown that dihydro-β-erythroidine blocks the response to nicotine in slices of rat prefrontal cortex. Christopher Mulle has shown a similar effect in the response to nicotine of neurons isolated from the medial habenula.

Kellar: Is it a channel blocker or a competitive blocker?

Heinemann: Dihydro-β-erythroidine blocks all the subtypes of the nicotinic receptor that have been tested, α2β2, a3β2, a4β2 (Luetje & Patrick 1989).

Colquhoun: Very few of these agents have been characterized in detail, even on neuromuscular junctions. If you look carefully at the action of tubocurarine on the neuromuscular junction, it's a much better channel blocker than it is a competitive blocker, if you are talking about equilibrium constants of the open channel and of the agonist binding site. Under physiological conditions ACh is present for such a short time that little channel block can develop.

Clarke: You referred to mecamylamine as an NMDA receptor antagonist. It may be possible to find a dose of mecamylamine that blocks central nicotinic receptors but does not block central NMDA receptors.

Gray: Where is this NMDA antagonism reported?

Clarke: The best evidence is from Snell & Johnson (1989). There are 2–3 papers from an older literature showing that mecamylamine can inhibit responses to excitatory amino acids; admittedly, in these earlier papers, the excitatory amino acids were delivered iontophoretically, so you don't know what the local concentration was.

Gray: But is there no study in which it's been shown that systemic injection of mecamylamine blocks a glutamatergic response? We use mecamylamine systemically to check that we can block the central effects of nicotine, and we ally it to systemic hexamethonium to check that blockade of the peripheral effects of nicotine is ineffective. I have heard at this meeting that neither of these is reliable and now I am very worried. Is there any evidence that the results obtained in the iontophoretic experiments can be generalized to the systemic injection of the whole animal?

Clarke: Not that I know of.

Colquhoun: There's a tradition in pharmacology of quantitative use of drug antagonists to classify receptors by determining their equilibrium constants for binding to different receptor types. That worked well up to a point, as long as proper equilibrium constants were measured, for example by the Schilde method. In real pharmacology the idea that you could learn anything reliable by putting in 1 µM of a antagonist and seeing if the response went away was abandoned 30 years ago. But people continue to do this in these studies; they haven't any option of course because in most cases you can't do things properly. But to ask whether mecamylamine at a certain concentration specifically blocks certain receptors is pointless; if it is a channel blocker the answer will depend on properties such as the membrane potential and how much agonist is present.

Heinemann: I would like to reiterate what I said before. We have tested mecamylamine on cloned nicotinic receptor subtypes under controlled conditions. I don't think you can control the concentration of a drug in different parts of the brain.

Colquhoun: And even if somebody measures the channel blocking characteristics precisely, that won't help in a whole brain experiment because there are too many unknowns in the brain, for example, the time course of membrane potential.

Heinemann: Because whether a channel blocker works depends on the situation. We need competitive blockers that bind to the ligand binding site and not channel blockers. We know that the ligand-gated channels all have a similar structure, they are evolutionarily related, so it will be hard to find channel blockers that are specific.

Steinbach: Neosuragotoxin appears to be quite selective, but it is almost totally unavailable.

Even competitive blockers may not be easily found, for example d-tubocurarine has a higher affinity for $5HT_3$ receptor recognition sites than it does for nicotinic receptor recognition sites. If these ligand-gated channels are encoded by an extended gene family, some of the protein structure around the recognition site may be shared, and these regions may be recognized by antagonists. There is a lot of pharmacology to do before we come up with a really selective blocker.

Colquhoun: Competitive antagonists have the advantage that they are likely to be less sensitive to things like membrane potential and local agonist concentration.

Gray: What about the other half of the problem? I have heard conflicting stories here: one statement was that hexamethonium doesn't do anything peripherally, and another statement was that it does.

Clarke: In the cat it is well established that hexamethonium and mecamylamine are equipotent. In the rat there are very few data on this; the only systematic study is by Romano (1981). He looked at the effects of nicotine in the rat colon. He found a potency ratio of 25:1 in favour of mecamylamine. If one extrapolates from that, it suggests that hexamethonium given at a dose of 5 mg/kg systemically will not block peripheral responses to nicotine.

Coloquhoun: I think that such potency ratios are not well defined, for the reasons that we have already discussed. The actions of hexamethonium on rat ganglia are quite complex (e.g. Gurney & Rang 1984).

Clarke: I don't know whether that work is applicable to the whole animal where hexamethonium is given systemically.

Colquhoun: Why should it not be? It is well established that hexamethonium affects humans when given systemically. Gurney & Rang showed that it was an almost irreversible blocker, unless you opened the channel with agonist to let the stuff out—it was trapped inside the closed ion channel.

Balfour: One of the problems is that it's rapidly excreted from the rat. Therefore in behavioural tests, which may last an hour, after about half an hour you have overcome the hexamethonium blockade because the drug simply isn't there.

Gray: Is there an alternative compound?

Stolerman: Chlorisondamine is an alternative. The doses needed to produce peripheral nicotinic blockade in the rat *in vivo* were determined by Morrison et al (1969) to be less than 0.01 mg/kg. However, in order to demonstrate convincingly that a behavioural effect is of central origin, it may be necessary to compare the effects of systemic and central injections of chlorisondamine. As Dr Clarke noted earlier, very small doses of chlorisondamine injected by the intracerebroventricular route have blocked behavioural effects of nicotine.

Steinbach: Chlorisondamine has been characterized as a good channel blocker for invertebrate glutamate receptors (Lingle et al 1980).

Changeux: It is clear that the number of brain nicotinic receptor agonists/ antagonists available is very small. On the other hand, there is the interesting finding that the sensitivity of neuronal nicotinic receptors to neuronal bungaro-toxin varies with different combinations of subunits. It is a challenge to the pharmacologist to develop compounds that are specific for different categories of neuronal receptors.

Gray: Paul Clarke said that chlorisondamine given intracerebroventricularly had an effect for five weeks. What happens if you inject it peripherally?

Clarke: In the human literature it is always described as a long acting ganglion blocking drug when given systemically. It does seem to wear off, although that needs to be looked at again.

Iversen: Are some of the peripheral effects of nicotine, particularly those on heart rate, really peripherally mediated or do they represent a central effect on sympathetic output?

Collins: In the mouse we showed that nicotine effects on heart rate give only a decrease—it is difficult to take a heart rate of 780 beats per minute and make it go up. You see a nicotine-induced decrease in heart rate; mecamylamine will block it, hexamethonium has very little effect. However, as David Balfour mentioned, there might not have been any hexamethonium in the animal at the time of the challenge. We waited about 10–15 minutes, but David is absolutely right, hexamethonium is very rapidly metabolized. I gave you the data, I also give you my doubt.

Benowitz: There are major differences in the heart rate response to nicotine between animals and humans; in most animals nicotine decreases the heart rate; in humans, where nicotine is usually given at lower doses, it accelerates the heart rate. Nicotine appears to produce general sympathetic neural activation in people; plasma noradrenaline levels rise at the same time as the heart rate rises, adrenaline rises more slowly (Cryer et al 1976). It is argued that the neural effects, reflected in the changes in noradrenaline levels, occur very quickly, while stimulation of the adrenal medulla, reflected in increases in adrenaline, occurs later. At the lowest concentrations of nicotine, cardiovascular effects seem to be mediated by actions on aortic and carotid chemoreceptors, while effects on the adrenal gland and on autonomic ganglia occur at higher concentrations.

Iversen: This seems to me to be a key issue. If you are thinking about agents that might replace nicotine, we have to say what's wrong with nicotine itself as a drug. In humans the cardiovascular risk is significant. One would like to eliminate that and retain the psychostimulant properties.

Benowitz: The impact of nicotine on heart rate in people is an average increase of seven beats per minute over the whole day, which is overwhelmed by any form of exercise. And the effect of nicotine on blood pressure is nil.

Iversen: So where does the extra cardiovascular risk come from?

Benowitz: It is not clear whether it is caused by nicotine or by other components of cigarette smoke. The adverse effect of smoking on acute coronary events is probably the hypercoagulable state, the thrombotic propensity, which may be due to some component of tobacco smoke other than nicotine.

Clarke: You were recommending selective peripheral nicotinic antagonists so that people could continue to smoke while avoiding the peripheral effects of nicotine. I would like to turn that round and say what we want is selective *central antagonists* of nicotine, because I personally feel that the way ahead for the second generation of pharmacotherapy for smoking is, rather than replacing nicotine with an agonist, to have people smoking cigarettes with their nicotinic receptors blocked in the central nervous system. Then each time they smoke they unlearn the operant reinforcement link, that is, the link between each puff and each delivery of nicotine. If you can re-programme the brain so that there is no longer an expectation from smoking, you psychologically extinguish your cigarette.

Rose: That's why it is so important to clarify the situation with performance enhancement or stress reduction by nicotine. Your treatment may alleviate the addiction, but if people feel a lack of something that smoking gives them, the long-term prognosis for abstinence from smoking is not very good.

Henningfield: The model for treatment of drug dependence with an antagonist is based on observations on opiate use. But certain facts have been overlooked. First, whereas relatively pure antagonists are available for mu receptors, e.g. morphine, the only available nicotine blockers have extensive side effects. Secondly, even in opioid dependence, where there is a selective and long-acting antagonist, i.e. naltrexone, therapy is successful for only 5–10% of addicts, namely those who are highly motivated, well adjusted and employed. These characteristics may be more prevalent among tobacco users than among opioid addicts, but the potential of treating nicotine dependence with antagonists should not be overstated.

Clarke: I can perhaps suggest here the use of chlorisondamine. It blocks nicotine in the rat for a very long time when given intraventrically. It doesn't easily pass the blood:brain barrier, but if you give very large systemic doses, it does enter the central nervous system, and has the same long-term blocking effect (Clarke 1984). If compliance is the problem, I recommend chlorisondamine. Give it once in a large supraganglion-blocking dose and the patient no longer needs to take the medication!

Collins: I am very concerned about giving nicotinic antagonists that affect the peripheral autonomic ganglia. I don't think we have good patient compliance with one dose.

Clarke: Let's not forget that we are trying to treat a potentially life-threatening condition. Let us assume that chlorisondamine, given on one occasion, doesn't block nicotinic receptors in the periphery for ever. To treat cigarette smokers, you give chlorisondamine in a big peripheral dose. It gets into the brain and it blocks nicotine's actions in the brain for a very long time but it will be washed out of the periphery—so after three days of bed rest . . . !

Gray: You are confusing two different issues. You are talking about extinguishing the behavioural routine that leads to the stimulation of nicotine receptors in brain and which is all part of smoking. There is already a pharmacological strategy for that—a cigarette from which the nicotine has been removed.

Cue exposure methods are already being tried in the treatment of other conditions, e.g. alcoholism and opiate addiction (Powell et al 1990). These techniques haven't worked very well yet but they do look quite promising. In applying those techniques you don't need a pharmacological blockade. You need a pharmacological blockade so that you don't get re-acquisition of the drug-taking habit if there is a lapse *after* you have treated the subject.

Clarke: I think you are right!

Fuxe: I believe that dopamine is important for the euphoric action of nicotine in smoking, especially dopamine in the nucleus accumbens. Perhaps one could use a patch with a dopamine agonist, to provide a treatment like methadone for heroin addicts. If the dopamine receptors are already activated, the smoker will get a reduced euphoric response from nicotine and the craving for nicotine will be reduced. It would be interesting to test whether or not D1 or D2 receptors are involved in smoking behaviour.

One important avenue of research for the benefit of new treatments will be to understand the action of nicotine on the afferents, the interneurons, and the efferents of the subcortical forebrain and their transmitters, including the frontal and hippocampal afferents.

Gray: But if you treat with a dopamine agonist, there's a high risk that the patient will become psychotic. If you treat with a dopamine antagonist, it will be extremely unacceptable and have some unpleasant side effects.

Fuxe: I am not speaking of dopamine antagonists, but of dopamine agonists. Dopamine agonists are used to treat Parkinson's disease, together with L-dopa. A small number of patients are predisposed to develop psychotic episodes, but these are always reversible and disappear when the treatment is stopped.

Henningfield: Concerning medication development, a wide range of effects of nicotine and nicotine withdrawal may be important in motivating smoking and precipitating relapse. Even the route or vehicle of administration may be significant. This has important implications for the development of medications to help people quit smoking. It seems unlikely that a single medication will be or could be all things to all people. Therefore, we should be looking for more selective medications. We could develop some that mimic specific desirable effects of nicotine, perhaps involving dopaminergic agonists, while also looking for medications that alleviate specific adverse effects of quitting smoking.

Changeux: For we molecular biologists to work efficiently in this field, it is important to have more information about the neural networks involved. Looking at nicotine effects in humans and animals, it would be useful to know exactly which cells or centres in the brain are involved in these phenomena. Then one could approach these mechanisms at the molecular level in a more pertinent manner.

Use of transdermal nicotine patches to help people give up smoking

Howald: At the moment we have only one approach to prevent withdrawal symptoms on cessation of smoking, this is nicotine replacement, which has been accepted for quite a long time with nicotine-containing gum. Several companies are developing a nicotine transdermal therapeutic system. At CIBA-GEIGY we have used our experience with other transdermal systems, like scopolamine or nitroglycerine, to develop a nicotine skin patch. We showed that there is a dose-relationship between the amount of nicotine in the patch and plasma concentrations of nicotine. A patch delivering 7, 14 or 21 mg of nicotine is worn for 24 hours. The maximum concentration of nicotine in plasma is reached about eight hours after application of the patch. This falls during the night, but there is still a significant concentration the next morning. Repeated administration doesn't lead to accumulation. Measuring the nicotine plasma concentration of smokers before smoking a cigarette and then immediately after, and that of people wearing a nicotine patch shows that in the latter we reached the so-called 'footpoint' plasma concentrations found in smokers.

Is this effective in helping people to give up smoking? We have done two large studies with placebo-controlled administration of the transdermal nicotine system. One lasted for three months: during the first month the subjects wore a 30 cm^2 patch, which administers 21 mg/day of nicotine. There were two weaning phases of four weeks using patches of 20 and 10 cm^2 that delivered 14 and 7 mg/day, respectively. This study was done in 199 patients of general practitioners in Switzerland.

The second study, which lasted nine weeks, was on university students, and the two weaning phases were of three weeks. We have the follow-up results for abstinence at three, six and nine months after stopping this programme.

In terms of abstinence rate, there was a significant difference between subjects wearing the nicotine patch and the placebo group in both studies. Abstinence rates collapsed after cessation of the treatment phase but even after one year there was still a difference in favour of those who had been treated with the patch.

We asked the participants to rate six different withdrawal symptoms. The average of these scores was always less (i.e. less severe withdrawal symptoms) in the actively treated group. In individual symptoms, such as difficulty of concentration, at least in students we often found a significant effect of the nicotine transdermal treatment.

So we are quite confident that one can improve the rate of abstinence from smoking by using this nicotine patch, even in a situation of almost no psychological support. Most smoking cessation programmes include strong psychological support, and we are aware that this is preferable, especially after treatment, to prevent relapse.

The major adverse affect of the patch is skin irritation. A marked reaction occurs in about 5% of the users—quite severe reddening, even some oedema, itching, and some subjects had to stop the treatment because of these problems. However, there is no obvious risk of allergy; some of the subjects who gave up the treatment because of skin irritation tried again later and experienced no more skin reactions.

Rose: We recently completed a clinical trial using the American version of the CIBA-GEIGY nicotine patch, which had technical problems of greater irritation to the skin. Concerning skin irritation, it might be interesting to look at hexamethonium or some blocker in that context. It has been shown in some animal models that nicotine irritation could be blocked with peripheral nicotine antagonists (Jancso et al 1961). So one might retain a central effect of nicotine and block the irritation by including a peripheral nicotinic antagonist in the patch. There are other solutions, such as reducing flux rate through the skin.

There has been quite a controversy about whether craving is affected by nicotine in the same way as other withdrawal symptoms. We did a separate analysis of different withdrawal symptoms over a three week duration (Rose et al 1990). Transdermal nicotine relieved difficulty in concentration, and relieved irritability but did not significantly relieve craving. Abelin et al (1989), using a much larger sample, also essentially got no effect on craving in the first three weeks when craving was high. With many repeated t tests there were some significant points later on when craving was not as high.

While there is clearly a therapeutic potential for nicotine patches and transdermal nicotine is a great way of giving nicotine while eliminating bad taste and compliance problems of nicotine gum, as well as the oral and habit factors that are still present with nicotine gum, the lack of these behavioural factors may limit their therapeutic efficacy. Ultimately, we will probably need a combination treatment of some sort, such as a nicotine patch used in combination with a cigarette substitute that provides some of the inhalational cues of smoking.

Initially in smoking cessation the biggest problem for many smokers is to alleviate withdrawal symptoms, but later there are problems with re-addiction liability. So maybe early in smoking cessation treatment nicotine replacement is most useful, but centrally acting nicotine blockers will have a role to combat subsequent re-addiction.

Gray: What stops the transdermal patch delivering nicotine at levels closer to the peak levels that occur during smoking? Is it the way you design the patch or can it not deliver that much?

Howald: The major problem is the concentration of nicotine on the patch itself. When it is too high, there is too much skin irritation.

Russell: You could just increase the surface area of the patches, or even apply two patches at a time, to increase the plasma nicotine concentration without increasing the amount of nicotine going through a given area of skin.

Howald: The other thing is that not all the nicotine from the patch is delivered to the blood, about half remains in the patch, because a gradient is needed for penetration into the skin. The data I presented were from prototypes. We are also studying 40 cm^2 patches, which will deliver 28 mg/day of nicotine, because we felt that heavy smokers might have been underdosed with our 30 cm^2 patch.

Iversen: In a survey done last year in Sweden, 2000 people representing the Swedish adult population—men and women, smokers and non-smokers, town dwellers and country dwellers—were asked to rate a number of items of modern life on two arbitrary scales: the degree of risk that they perceived to be associated with these items, and the degree of benefit that was likely to be obtained from them. Some were very obvious—having your appendix out had a certain degree of perceived risk but also a high degree of perceived benefit. Food additives were regarded as having almost no benefit and having definite risk. Drugs for treating AIDS were perceived to have a high risk but also a high benefit. Cigarette smoking lay at the extreme of this particular analysis, in having a high perceived risk and very low perceived degree of benefit. That seems to help define it as a drug dependence problem.

References

Abelin T, Buehler A, Muller P, Imhof PR 1989 Controlled trial of transdermal nicotine patch in tobacco withdrawal. Lancet i:7–10

Benwell MEM, Balfour DJK 1979a Effects of nicotine administration and its withdrawal on plasma corticosterone and brain 5-hydroxyindoles. Psychopharmacology 63:7–11

Benwell MEM, Balfour DJK 1979b Betamethasone-induced pituitary-adrenocortical suppression and brain 5-hydroxytryptamine in the rat. Psychoneuroendocrinology 4:83–86

Benwell MEM, Balfour DJK 1982 The effects of nicotine administration on 5-HT uptake and biosynthesis in rat brain. Eur J Pharmacol 84:71–77

Clarke PBS 1984 Chronic central nicotinic blockade after a single injection of the bisquarternary ganglion blocking drug chlorisondamine. Br J Pharmacol 83:527–535

Cryer PE, Haymond MW, Santiago JU, Shah SD 1976 Norepinephrine and epinephrine release and adrenergic mediation of smoking-associated hemodynamic and metabolic events. N Engl J Med 295:573–577

Grunberg NE 1986a Nicotine as a psychoactive drug: appetite regulation. Psychopharm Bull 22:875–881

Grunberg NE 1986b Behavioral and biological factors in the relationship between tobacco use and body weight. In: Katkin ES, Manuck SB (eds) Advances in behavioral medicine. Vol 2. JAI Press, Greenwich, Connecticut, p 97–129

Grunberg NE, Popp KA, Bowen DJ, Nespor SM, Winders SE, Eury SE 1988 Effects of chronic nicotine administration on insulin, glucose, epinephrine, and norepinephrine. Life Sci 42:161–170

Gurney AM, Rang HP 1984 The channel-blocking action of methonium compounds on rat submandibular ganglion cells. Br J Pharmacol 82:623–642

Jancso N, Jancso-Gabor A, Takats J 1961 Pain and inflammation induced by nicotine, acetylcholine and structurally related compounds and their prevention by desensitizing agents. Acta Physiol Hung 9:113–132

Lingle C, Eisen JS, Marder E 1980 Block of glutamatergic excitatory synaptic channels by chlorisondamine. Mol Pharmacol 19:349–353

Luetje CW, Patrick JW 1989 Soc Neurosci Abstr p677

Marks MJ, Stitzel JA, Collins AC 1985 Time course study of the effects of chronic nicotine infusion on drug response and brain receptors. J Pharmacol Exp Ther 235:619–628

Morrison CF, Goodyear JM, Sellers CM 1969 Antagonism by antimuscarinic and ganglion-blocking drugs of some of the behavioural effects of nicotine. Psychopharmacologia 15:341–350

Powell J, Gray JA, Bradley BP, Kasvikis Y, Barratt L, Marks I 1990 The effects of exposure to drug-related cues in detoxified opiate addicts: a theoretical review and some new data. Addict Behav, in press

Romano C 1981 Nicotine action on rat colon. J Pharmacol Exp Ther 217:828–833

Rose JE, Levin ED, Behm F, Adivi C, Schur C 1990 Transdermal nicotine facilitates smoking cessation. Clin Pharmacol Ther 47:323–330

Snell LD, Johnson KM 1989 Effects of nicotinic agonists and antagonists on N-methyl-D-asparate-induced ^{3}H-(1-[1-(2-Thienyl)cyclohexyl]-piperidine) binding in rat hippocampus. Synapse 3:129–135

West RJ, Hajek P, Belcher M 1990 Severity of withdrawal symptoms as a predictor of outcome of an attempt to quit smoking. Psychol Med 19:971–980

Index of contributors

Non-participating co-authors are indicated by asterisks. Entries in bold type indicate papers; other entries refer to discussion contributions.

Indexes compiled by Liza Weinkove

Subject index